Rapid Diagnosis of Mycoplasmas

FEDERATION OF EUROPEAN MICROBIOLOGICAL SOCIETIES SYMPOSIUM SERIES

Recent FEMS Symposium volumes published by Plenum Press

1991 • MICROBIAL SURFACE COMPONENTS AND TOXINS IN RELATION TO PATHOGENESIS
Edited by Eliora Z. Ron and Shlomo Rottem
(FEMS Symposium No. 51)

1991 • GENETICS AND PRODUCT FORMATION IN STREPTOMYCES
Edited by Simon Baumberg, Hans Krügel, and Dieter Noack
(FEMS Symposium No. 55)

1991 • THE BIOLOGY OF *ACINETOBACTER*: Taxonomy, Clinical Importance, Molecular Biology, Physiology, Industrial Relevance
Edited by K. J. Towner, E. Bergogne-Bérézin, and C. A. Fewson
(FEMS Symposium No. 57)

1991 • MOLECULAR PATHOGENESIS OF GASTROINTESTINAL INFECTIONS
Edited by T. Wadström, P. H. Mäkelä, A.-M. Svennerholm, and H. Wolf-Watz
(FEMS Symposium No. 58)

1992 • MOLECULAR RECOGNITION IN HOST-PARASITE INTERACTIONS
Edited by Timo K. Korhonen, Tapani Hovi, and P. Helena Mäkelä
(FEMS Symposium No. 61)

1992 • THE RELEASE OF GENETICALLY MODIFIED MICROORGANISMS—REGEM 2
Edited by Duncan E. S. Stewart-Tull and Max Sussman
(FEMS Symposium No. 63)

1993 • RAPID DIAGNOSIS OF MYCOPLASMAS
Edited by Itzhak Kahane and Amiram Adoni
(FEMS Symposium No. 62)

1993 • BACTERIAL GROWTH AND LYSIS: Metabolism and Structure of the Bacterial Sacculus
Edited by M. A. de Pedro, J.-V. Höltje, and W. Löffelhardt
(FEMS Symposium No. 65)

A Continuation Order Plan is available for this series. A continuation order will bring delivery of each new volume immediately upon publication. Volumes are billed only upon actual shipment. For further information please contact the publisher.

Rapid Diagnosis of Mycoplasmas

Edited by

Itzhak Kahane

The Hebrew University–Hadassah Medical School
Jerusalem, Israel

and

Amiram Adoni

Hadassah University Hospital, Mount Scopus
Jerusalem, Israel

PLENUM PRESS • NEW YORK AND LONDON

Library of Congress Cataloging-in-Publication Data

Rapid diagnosis of mycoplasmas / edited by Itzhak Kahane and Amiram
Adoni.
        p.   cm. -- (FEMS symposium ; no. 62)
    "Proceedings of a symposium held under the auspices of the
Federation of European Microbiological Societies, held August 11-23,
1991, in Jerusalem, Israel"--T.p. verso.
    Includes bibliographical references and index.
    ISBN 0-306-44621-9
    1. Mycoplasma diseases--Diagnosis--Congresses.   I. Kahane,
Itzhak. II. Adoni, Amiram. III. Series.
QR201.M97R37 1993
616'.014--dc20   93-41675
                                                           CIP

Proceedings of a symposium held under the auspices of the Federation of European
Microbiological Societies, August 11-23, 1991, in Jerusalem, Israel

ISBN 0-306-44621-9

©1993 Plenum Press, New York
A Division of Plenum Publishing Corporation
233 Spring Street, New York, N.Y. 10013

Printed in the United States of America

PREFACE

This compendium is the result of the FEMS Workshop on "Rapid Diagnosis of Mycoplasmas" which I organized and which took place in Jerusalem, Israel, August 11-23, 1991.

The first week's sessions were held at a resort on the outskirts of Jerusalem and consisted of lectures and discussions. This part was modelled along the lines of the Gordon Conference in the USA, i.e., in an intimate atmosphere in which everyone could mix and exchange ideas, and was very beneficial. About 100 scientists from around the world attended the first week. During the first week, the biology, molecular biology and pathophysiology of mycoplasmas, as well as all the main diagnostic methods were covered, including both conventional and the newer technologies. The session on mycoplasmas in the human urogenital tracts was held in conjunction with the Israel Society for the Study and Prevention of Sexually Transmitted Disease.

The second week was a laboratory session and was held at the Hebrew University-Hadassah Medical School campus in Ein Karem, Jerusalem. All experiments were conducted by eminent specialists in their field. The lab session had 36 participants from 19 countries who used the most modern techniques for the diagnosis of mycoplasmas in medicine, veterinary medicine and agriculture. The efficacy of several commercial kits were also tested at this time.

I want to again thank everyone who helped and supported this workshop, as well as the authors of the various chapters.

Itzhak Kahane
Jerusalem

CONTENTS

INTRODUCTION

Itzhak Kahane

Department of Membrane and Ultrastructure Research
The Hebrew University-Hadassah Medical School
POB 1172, Jerusalem 91010, Israel

The class *Mollicutes*, whose members are commonly known as myco-plasmas, now include more than 120 species, most of which are parasites and many are pathogens of a vast variety of hosts. Until recently, the detection of mycoplasmas was slow and proven only within days or even weeks. This would not be so problematic if the mycoplasmas would cause only mild and chronic disease. However, in recent years, data are accumulating that in sever-al instances, mycoplasmas cause diseases which are acute and may be fatal. This was dramatically illustrated very recently when a 20-year old patient died from *Mycoplasma pneumoniae* infection, as reported in the case records of Massachusetts General Hospital published in the New England Journal of Medicine, (Case 5, 1992). It should be noted that this pathogen is the cause of pneumonia in about 30% of the children hospitalized with all kinds of pneu-monia in developed countries. Another mycoplasma which is documented as causing fatal disease is *Ureaplasma urealyticum* which causes respiratory dis-tress syndrome and which is life threatening to infants of low birth weight (Cassell *et al.*, 1988; Quinn, P.A., 1988). The final example is linked to infection with *Mycoplasma fermentans*, incognitus strain. This organism is highly path-ogenic and was reported to cause severe systemic disease that is potentially fatal. In addition, it was also incriminated in setting the stage for HIV infect-ion and AIDS (Lo *et al.*, 1989). These aspects illuminate the great need for methods for rapid detection of mycoplasmas in order to allow the early diag-nosis of infection and prevent the severe consequences which are even more threatening if the link of HIV activation to mycoplasma infection is true.

Needless to say, similar aspects of importance in rapid detection are in-volved in mycoplasma diseases in veterinary medicine. Here, the commer-cial aspects are an important factor as well. Finally, the need for rapid detect-ion is also of major importance in all areas where cells in culture are used, since mycoplasmas can be considered pests of these cells. With the aforemen-

Rapid Diagnosis of Mycoplasmas, Edited by I. Kahane
and A. Adoni, Plenum Press, New York, 1993

tioned threats that mycoplasma may cause, there is no wonder that health authorities demand that all products from cell cultures be from mycoplasma-free sources.

With all of this in mind, and with the approaches and methods for rapid detection of mycoplasmas that started to imerge and that were discussed in the workshop, I felt that it would be important for many more mycoplas-mologists to have this basic information and the detailed approaches and methods included in this book, believing that in this way, more laboratories around the world will have the skills and will be able to detect the mycoplas-mas and, hopefully be able to design new methods or improve the current ones for rapid detection and fast diagnosis of mycoplasma infections.

REFERENCES

Case 5-1992: Presentation of a Case. 1992. New England J. Med. 326: 324-336

Cassell, G. H., Crouse, D. T., Canupp, K C., Waites, K. B., Rudd, P. T., Stagnos, S. and Cutter, G. R. 1988. Association of *Ureaplasma urealyticum* infection of the lower respiratory tract with chronic lung disease and death in very low- birth- weight infants. Lancet 2:240-244.

Lo, S.-C., Dawson, G., Wong, D. M.,Newton III, P. B., Sonoda, M. A., Engler, W. F., Wang, R. Y.-H. Shih, J. W.-K., Alter, H. J. and Wear, D. J.1989. Identification of *Mycoplasma incognitus* infection in patients with AIDS: an immunohistochemical, *in situ* hybridization and ultra-structural study. Am. J. Trop. Med. Hyg. 41:601.

Quinn, P. A. 1988. Mycoplasma infection in fetus and newborn in: "Trans-placental Effects on Fetal Health" (D. G. Scarpelli and G. Migaki, Eds.) Alan R. Liss, New York, pp. 107-151.

BIOLOGY OF MOLLICUTES

Joseph G. Tully

Mycoplasma Section, National Institute of Allergy and Infectious Diseases, National Institutes of Health Frederick, MD, USA

INTRODUCTION

Mollicutes are bacteria that lack a cell wall, one of the principal cellular and morphological structures of most prokaryotes. These wall-less organisms, earlier called either "pleuropneumonia-like organisms" or "mycoplasmas", are also the smallest free-living, self-replicating forms currently known in biology. They share a small size and filterability with a number of viruses, which helps explain why many mollicutes were earlier mistaken for viruses. On the other hand, mollicutes are structurally different from viruses and are capable of sustained growth on cell-free media of varying complexity. Within the past twenty-five years, an enormous increase in our knowledge and understanding of mollicutes has taken place. These microbial forms are now known to occur in most vertebrates, in numerous insect and other arthropods, and within and on the surfaces of many plants. While it is also obvious now that many of these organisms can be considered part of the normal commensal flora of the host, other mollicutes have become well established pathogens of man, animals, plants, and arthropods.

The discussion to follow will focus on some recent developments affecting our current thinking about several specific areas in the biology of mollicutes, rather than attempt to provide a comprehensive coverage of the topic. For a more adequate background on the biology of mollicutes, particularly with regard to members belonging to the various genera within the class *Mollicutes* and to the unclassified mycoplasma-like organisms of plants, one should consult a number of recent reviews (Kirkpatrick, 1991; Razin, 1991; Tully and Whitcomb, 1991; Whitcomb and Tully, 1989) or other contributions to this volume.

Rapid Diagnosis of Mycoplasmas, Edited by I. Kahane
and A. Adoni, Plenum Press, New York, 1993

Table 1. Taxonomy of Mollicutes.

Division *TENERICUTES* - Class *MOLLICUTES*

Order I	*Mycoplasmatales*
Family I	*Mycoplasmataceae*
Genus I	*Mycoplasma*

-92 species described
-Genome size ranges 450-900 MDa
-DNA G + C base composition 23-41 mol %
-Requires cholesterol for growth
-Glucose and/or arginine pathways in most
-Animal, plant, and insect habitat.

Genus II	*Ureaplasma*

-5 species described
-Genome size ranges 470-740 MDa
-DNA G + C base composition 25-31 mol %
-Requires cholesterol for growth
-Hydrolyzes urea
-Animal habitat

Family II	*Spiroplasmataceae*
Genus I	*Spiroplasma*

-11 species described
-Genome size averages 1000 MDa
-DNA G + C base composition 25-31 mol %
-Requires cholesterol for growth
-Glucose and arginine pathway in most
-Insect and plant habitat

Order II	*Acholeplasmatales*
Family I	*Acholeplasmataceae*
Genus I	*Acholeplasma*

-12 species described
-Genome size averages 1000 MDa
-DNA G + C base composition 27-36 mol %
-No cholesterol requirement
-Most glucose fermenters
-Animal, insect, and plant habitat

Order III	*Anaeroplasmatales*
Family I	*Anaeroplasmataceae*
Genus I	*Anaeroplasma*

-4 species described
-Genome size averages 1000 MDa
-DNA G + C base composition 29-33 mol %
-Cholesterol requirement for growth
-Strict anaerobe
-Bovine/ovine rumen habitat

Genus II	*Asteroleplasma*

-1 species described
-Genome size 1000 MDa
-DNA G + C base composition 40 mol %
-Strict anaerobe
-Bovine/ovine rumen habitat

CURRENT CLASSIFICATION AND TAXONOMY OF MOLLICUTES

Bacterial taxonomists and phylogenists presently hold different opinions as to the proper classification of bacteria at higher taxa (Domain, Kingdom, etc.). However, there seems to be some consensus now that most wall-less organisms should be assigned to a separate Division (*Tenericutes*) and Class (*Mollicutes*). Table 1 presents a summary of the current taxonomic scheme for the class *Mollicutes*, including the number of species presently recognized in each genus and some brief information on nutritional and habitat markers.

GENOME SIZE AS A TAXONOMIC MARKER IN MOLLICUTES

The genome of mollicutes is the smallest among any known self-replicating organism, and is about one-half to one-fifth that of most other bacteria. In early studies on the DNA of mollicutes, using renaturation kinetics (RK), it was found that most species fell into two clusters. Sterol-requiring species had a genome of about 500 MDa (or near 750 kb), and the genome of non-sterol species averaged about 1000 MDa (or near 1500 kb) (Bak *et al.*, 1969). These genomic differences were confirmed in a number of later studies (Askaa *et al.*, 1973), and genome size eventually came to represent an important criterion for taxonomic assignment of mollicutes at the Family level. Mycoplasmas and ureaplasmas have genomes of about 500 MDa, while acholeplasmas, spiroplasmas, and the anaeroplasmas have a genome of about 1000 MDa.

However, Finch and co-workers in 1988 (Pyle *et al.*, 1988) suggested that the genome size of some *Mycoplasma* and *Ureaplasma* species was considerably larger than the reported range. Using pulse-field gel electrophoresis (PFGE) to measure the size of fragments obtained from digestion of genomic DNA, they found that the genomes of some species examined were as large as 900 to 1300 kb. Further evidence of size variation in genome measurements made by PFGE and RK, within some mollicute species, has now been confirmed in a number of other laboratories.

As noted by Neimark and Lange (1990), size estimates of the mollicute genome obtained by PFGE and RK agree well in mollicutes with the largest and smallest chromosomes. In the intermediate range, however, RK consistently provides lower values than PFGE (see Table 2). The evidence now available would suggest that the *Mycoplasma* and *Ureaplasma* chromosomes span a continual range of sizes between about 600 kb and 1300 kb (400 MDa and 800 MDa). These new findings clearly indicate that genome size is an inappropriate taxonomic indicator and that current taxonomic descriptions for species within the Family *Mycoplasmataceae* should be revised.

NEW STEROL-NONREQUIRING MOLLICUTES OF PLANTS AND INSECTS. ARE THEY MEMBERS OF THE GENUS ACHOLEPLASMA?

Sterol-nonrequiring mollicutes now assigned to the genus *Acholeplasma* were first isolated from soil and sewage more than fifty years ago. Later, these organisms and other acholeplasmas were found to occur in a wide variety of animal hosts (for early history see Tully, 1979). Sterol-nonrequiring mol-

Table 2. Comparison of mollicute genome sizes as measured by two methods.

Species	PFGE[a]	RK[b]	Ref.
M. genitalium	600[c]	ND[d]	5
M. arginini	735	606	4, 13
U. urealyticum biotype 1	760	645	3, 14
M. pneumoniae	840	727	4, 12
U. urealyticum biotype 2	890	666-712	1, 3, 12
MLO (Oenothera)	1050	ND	8
M. gallisepticum	1070	780	1, 12
M. bovis	1080	666	4, 13
M. capricolum	1120	ND	4
U. urealyticum biotype 2	1140	675	3, 14
M. fermentans	1160	720	4, 12
U. felinum	1170	ND	9
MLO (Aster yellows)	1185	ND	6
M. iowae 695	1315	1607	1, 10
M. iowae PPAV	1300	1571	10
M. mycoides	1240-1330	760-860	1, 3, 13
S. mirum	1310	ND	11
S. apis	1350	1644	2, 11
Acheloplasma hippikon	1540	ND	4
Acheloplasma laidlawii	1600	1660	3, 4, 7, 12
S. citri	1780	1365	2, 11

[a]Pulse-field gel electrophoresis
[b]Renaturation kinetics
[c]Kilobase pair
[d]ND = not done

References: (1) Pyle et al., 1988; (2) Bové et al., 1989; (3) Robertson et al., 1990; (4) Neimark and Lange, 1990; (5) Su and Baseman, 1990; (6) Neimark and Kirkpatrick, 1990; (7) Whitley and Finch, 1990; (8) Lim and Sears, 1991; (9) Kakulphimp et al., 1991; (10) Grau et al., 1991; (11) P. Carle and J. M. Bové, personal communication; (12) Bak et al., 1969; (13) Askaa et al., 1973; (14) Black et al., 1972.

licutes were first established as plant inhabitants in 1979 (Eden-Green and Tully), and further isolations reported shortly thereafter (McCoy et al., 1979; Somerson et al., 1982; Whitcomb et al., 1982). Similar mollicutes were also identified from insects in 1986 (Clark et al.).

In early investigations on animal acholeplasmas, it was observed that strains of one species (A. axanthum), contrary to other acholeplasmas, grew very poorly in medium without serum or cholesterol. However, supplements of small amounts (0.01%) of a fatty acid mixture (Tween 80) to serum-free medium provided enhanced growth (Table 3) (Tully and Razin, 1969, 1970). These observations indicated the likelihood that other acholeplasmas might not have a specific need for cholesterol, but possess unique fatty acid requirements for growth. These impressions were soon confirmed when several strains of the first putative plant acholeplasma were characterized. However, the three serologically identical strains isolated by McCoy et al. (1979) from plant surfaces failed to show sustained growth in the usual amounts (0.01%) of Tween 80. Further studies found that slight additions (0.04%) of this fatty acid supplement would provide the necessary requirements for sustained growth (Table 3), and the organism was eventually described as A. florum (McCoy et al., 1984).

Since that time, numerous other plant and insect isolates with similar growth requirements for the Tween 80 fatty acid mixture have been made by our collaborative group (Tully et al., 1989, 1990b). Several of these serologically distinct sterol-nonrequiring mollicutes were eventually characterized and given taxonomic designations of Acholeplasma entomophilum (Tully et al., 1988) and Acholeplasma seiffertii (Bonnet et al., 1991). Although these new species do differ in some important biologic properties from animal-derived acholeplasmas, their lack of a sterol requirement for growth is certainly similar to other mollicutes within this taxonomic entity. Our collaborative group in Bordeaux, Beltsville, and Frederick (Tully et al., 1990b) has recently focused efforts on investigating whether these insect-plant isolates really belong to the genus Acholeplasma.

The results of a recent phylogenetic study of over 40 mollicutes by Weisburg et al., (1989) provided important information on this point. Using sequence analysis of 16S rRNA, they divided the mollicutes into five phylogenetic units, acholeplasma-anaeroplasma, asteroleplasma, spiroplasma-mycoides, hominis, and pneumoniae. The so-called classic acholeplasmas, as represented by A. laidlawii and A. modicum, were placed in the acholeplasma-anaeroplasma branch. The analysis suggested that this branch had split at some early evolutionary time from the main spiroplasma-mycoides line, the ancestoral origin of most sterol-requiring mollicutes.

In contrast to classic acholeplasmas, the sterol nonrequiring, insect-plant isolates (represented by A. florum and A. entomophilum) were phylogenetically related to the spiroplasma-mycoides group, and more specifically, clustered within a group of sterol-requiring Mycoplasma species of both animal (M. mycoides, M. putrefaciens, etc.) or insect-plant (M. ellychniae, etc.) origin. Although this placement mixed sterol-requiring and sterol-nonrequiring mollicutes in a close phylogenetic relationship, other biologic characteristics established for the insect-plant isolates suggested the validity of the placement.

Table 3. Modified test for measuring sterol growth requirements of mollicutes

Medium composition	Acholeplasma axanthum	Acholeplasma florum & A. entomophilum	Mycoplasma lactucae
Serum Fraction Broth (Control)	9.38[a]	3.12	6.50
Serum-Free base	2.51	<0.02	<0.02
Base medium with:			
- albumin/palmitate supplements[b]	4.95	<0.02	<0.02
- supplements + Tween 80 (0.01%)	10.43	<0.02	<0.02
- supplements + Tween 80 (0.04%)	ND[c]	2.45	<0.02
Base medium with supplements and added cholesterol of:			
-1 μg/ml	10.45	2.55	2.50
-5 μg/ml	10.45	2.25	6.00
-10 μg/ml	10.45	2.75	8.20
-20 μg/ml	11.43	2.55	6.80

[a]Milligrams of cell protein from 100 ml of culture when organism grown in particular medium.
[b]Supplements included 0.5% albumin and 10 μg/ml of palmitic acid.
[c]Not done.

Recent genome size measurement on a number of established species or strains within this group, especially those performed using PFGE (P. Carle and J. M. Bové, unpublished data), would suggest a genome much smaller than that recorded for classic acholeplasmas (Table 4). Interestingly, the genome size range (540-900 MDa) is also compatible with recent measurements reported on sterol-requiring *Mycoplasma* species of both animal and plant-insect origin in this phylogenetic grouping (Tully *et al.*, 1989, 1990a; Rose *et al.*, 1990; Williamson *et al.*, 1990) (see also Table 2).

Thus, we now believe there is fairly strong evidence that the new sterol-nonrequiring mollicutes from insects and plants are genetically and phylogenetically distinct from some and, perhaps all, classic acholeplasmas from animals. The position of *Acholeplasma axanthum* is still somewhat uncertain, since this organism was not examined in the 16S rRNA analysis, and the genome size has yet to be determined by PFGE. This organism has been isolated from several animal hosts (see review of Tully, 1979), frequently from

Table 4 Comparison of biological characteristics of classic *Acholeplasma* and new sterol nonrequiring, insect and plant mollicutes.

I.   **Classic *Acholeplasma* species**
-Phylogeny established through 16S rRNA sequence analysis
         (*A. laidlawii, A. modicum*).
-Most isolates from variety of animal hosts, with only few found on plant surfaces or in insects.
-No cholesterol requirements for growth
-Tween 80 supplements (0.04%) not required for growth.
-Genome size averages 1000 MDa.

A. laidlawii	1012-1064 MDa	
A. granularum	-950	
A. hippikon	-1026	
A. modicum	-906	

II.   **Insect-Plant Mollicutes**
-Phylogenically distinct from classic acholeplasmas, with evolutionary relationships to spiroplasma/mycoides branch (florum and entomophilum)
-All current isolates from insects or flowers.
-No cholesterol requirements for growth.
-Tween 80 supplements (0.04%) necessary for growth in serum-free medium.
-Genome size ranges from 540 to 900 MDa.

A. florum	- 540-596 MDa
A. entomophilum	- 616
A. seiffertii	- 886-897 (renaturation)
Strain YJS	- 573
Strain CHPA-2	- 589
Strain ELCA-2	- 589

some plants, but never from insect hosts (Tully *et al.*, 1990b), so it has a habitat range shared by both the groups in question. Further efforts are underway to establish other phenotypic and genotypic markers that will help to differentiate *A. axanthum, A. florum, A. entomophilum, A. seiffertii,* and at least seven other serologically distinct insect isolates with similar characteristics from classic animal acholeplasmas. We believe these markers will then be sufficient to establish a new taxonomic entity, perhaps within the Family *Mycoplasmataceae,* for a group of sterol-nonrequiring mollicutes. This reclassification would be in line with recent efforts to make taxonomy compatible with phylogenetic properties whenever possible.

COMMENTS ON THE CURRENT MOLLICUTE FLORA OF HUMANS

Several developments in our understanding of the mollicute flora of man has occurred over the past few years, including characterization of a number of new species. In addition, suggestions have been made that other species heretofore regarded as not playing a role in human disease might be pathogens. The comments to follow will briefly outline some general impressions that relate only to these two points and will omit most discussion on infect-

Table 5. Properties of mycoplasmas that infect man.

Species	Primary Site of Colonization		Principal Metabolic Marker	Comment
	Respiratory	Genito-urinary		
M. salivarium	+	-	A	Common
M. orale	+	-	A	Common
M. buccale	+	-	A	Rare
M. faucium	+	-	A	Rare
M. lipophilum	+	-	A	Rare
M. pneumoniae	+	-	G	Pathogen
M. hominis	+	+	A	Common
M. genitalium	+	+	G	Common?
M. fermentans	+	+	G + A	Common?
M. primatum	-	+	A	Rare
M. spermatophilum	-	+	A	Rare
M. pirum	?	?	G + A	Rare
U. urealyticum	+	+	U	Common
A. laidlawii	+	-	G	Rare

A = arginine hydrolysis; G = glucose fermentation
U = urea hydrolysis.

ions with *M. pneumoniae* and *U. urealyticum*, since these topics will be covered elsewhere in this volume.

Fourteen species of mollicutes are now recognized as infecting man (Table 5). About half of this number is now considered to be part of the normal human flora. This includes the first five arginine-hydrolyzing mollicutes in the list that colonize the human oropharynx. *M. salivarium* has been isolated on a few occasions from the arthritic joints of immunocompromised patients, as has other mollicutes found in the respiratory or urogenital tracts.

M. hominis is a common inhabitant of the lower genital tract of both women and men. Isolation rates from normal women generally average 40-50%, with rates increasing to 90-100% in women attending sexually transmitted disease (STD) clinics, while rates in men vary from about 5% under normal conditions to 40% in men attending STD clinics. However, *M. hominis* is an important pathogen and has been repeatedly documented in post-partum or post-abortal infections, arthritis in immunocompromised hosts, and in a variety of septicemias from traumatic wounds, or from prosthetic, transplant and surgical infections. Invasion of the brain and central nervous system in neonates has also recently been described.

M. genitalium is still an enigma. Aside from the two initial isolates from the human urogenital tract, no other strains have been isolated. Whether this is related to the fastidious growth requirements of the organism or to its absence at this site is uncertain. Some studies with molecular probes for the organism suggest its presence in the urogenital tract. The organism has been established as occurring in the human respiratory tract, and on one occasion in arthritic joints, so far always in conjuction with *M. pneumoniae*. It is uncertain at present whether the organism plays any role in respiratory disease. Current serologic assays for *M. pneumoniae* infections do not differentiate between this organism and *M. genitalium* (Tully and Baseman, 1991). Specific molecular probes have been developed for both organisms and their application to clinical infections should resolve the role of each mollicute in human disease.

M. fermentans occurs infrequently in the lower genital tract of men and women. However, the organism has recently been isolated from the normal respiratory tract and from post-mortem lung tissues of respiratory disease patients (R. Dular, personal communication). Further details of these infections and confirmation of the identification will be published elsewhere. In other recent studies, the organism has been identified in various post-mortem tissues of patients with and without acquired immunodeficiency disease (AIDS) (Lo *et al.*, 1989a, b) and from the blood of AIDS patients (Montagnier *et al.*, 1990). The availability of genetic probes and gene amplification techniques (PCR) (Wang *et al.*, 1992) for the organism should help delineate its occurrence in health and disease.

M. pirum was first isolated from eukaryotic cell culture infections in 1968 and defined as a new species in 1985 (DelGiudice *et al.*). However, since its original isolation, the organism has never been identified with any particular animal host, including bovine serum or other animal-derived material used in cell culture supplements. Numerous isolations of the organism have been made from early passage of primary human tumor cells and human lymphocyte (or other blood cell) lines. These isolations have never been docmented in the primary tissues or blood cells, although the general impression persisted that *M. pirum* was probably coming from the primary human specimens. Several isolations of the organism have been reported from laboratory cultivation of lymphocytes from AIDS patients (Montagnier *et al.*, 1990). Additional confirmation of these findings will help to establish this organism as part of the human flora. Likewise, the presence of *M. pirum* in blood of AIDS patients would also suggest that the organism might be part of the urogenital tract flora of AIDS patients and occurs, perhaps, in the absence of disease.

At present, the three remaining organisms, *M. primatum*, *M. spermatophilum*, and *A. laidlawii* appear to be infrequent inhabitants and, for now, apparently play no role in human disease. Less than six total isolates of both *M. primatum* and *M. spermatophilum* have been reported from humans, all from the urogenital tract. *A. laidlawii* has been isolated on occasion from the oropharynx and from skin surfaces of humans.

At this point, one might ask whether we now are close to knowing the definitive mollicute flora of man or are other new species yet to be identified? The unequivocal answer from past experiences is that other new mollicutes will be found in man. As new culture medium is developed and other technical advances are made in the detection and isolation of mollicutes, and these procedures applied to a variety of patient populations, new mollicutes will continue to be encountered and isolated.

REFERENCES

Askaa, G, Christiansen, C. and Ernø, H. (1973) Bovine mycoplasmas: genome size and base composition of DNA. J. Gen. Microbiol. 75:283-286.

Bak, A. L., Black, F. T., Christiansen, C. and Freundt, E. A. (1969) Genome size of mycoplasmal DNA. Nature 244:1209-1210

Black, F. T., Christiansen, C. and Askaa, G. (1972) Genome size and base composition of deoxyribonucleic acid from eight human T-mycoplasmas. Int. J. Syst. Bacteriol. 22:241-242.

Bonnet, F., Saillard, C., Vignault, J. C., Garnier, M., Carle, P., Bové, J. M., Rose, D. L., Tully, J. G. and Whitcomb, R.F. (1991) *Acholeplasma seiffertii* sp. nov., a mollicute from plant surfaces. Int. J. Syst. Bacteriol. 41:45-49.

Bové, J. M., Carle, P., Garnier, M., Laigret, F., Renaudin, J. and Saillard, C. (1989) Molecular and cellular biology of spiroplasmas, in: "The Mycoplasmas" (Whitcomb, R. F., and Tully, J. G., Eds.). Vol. V, pp. 243-364.

Clark, T. B., Tully, J. G., Rose, D. L., Henegar, R. and Whitcomb, R. F. (1986) Acholeplasmas and similar non-sterol-requiring mollicutes from insects: missing link in microbial ecology. Curr. Microbiol. 13:11-16.

DelGiudice, R. A., Tully, J. G., Rose, D. L. and Cole, R. M. (1985) *Mycoplasma pirum* sp. nov., a terminal structured mollicute from cell cultures. Int. J. Syst. Bacteriol. 35:285-291.

Eden-Green, S. and Tully, J. G. (1979) Isolation of *Acholeplasma* spp. from coconut palms affected by lethal yellowing disease in Jamaica. Curr. Microbiol. 1:311-316.

Grau, O., Laigret, F., Carle, P., Tully, J. G., Rose, D. L. and Bové, J. M. (1991) Identification of a plant-derived mollicute as a strain of an avian pathogen, *Mycoplasma iowae*, and its implications for mollicute taxonomy. Int. J. Syst. Bacteriol. 41:473-478.

Kakulphimp, J., Finch, L. R., and Robertson, J. A. (1991) Genome sizes of mammalian and avian ureaplasmas. Int. J. Syst. Bacteriol. 41:326-327.

Kirkpatrick, B. C. (1991) Mycoplasma-like organisms-plant and invertebrate pathogens, in: "The Prokaryotes" (Balows, A., Truper, H. G., Dworkin, M., Harder, W. and Schleifer, K.-H., Eds.), 2nd Ed., Vol. IV, pp. 4050-4067. Springer-Verlag, New York.

Lim, P.-O., and Sears, B. B. (1991) The genome size of a plant pathogenic mycoplasma-like organism resembles those of animal mycoplasmas. J. Bacteriol. 173: 2128-2130.

Lo, S.-C., Dawson, M. S., Newton, P. B., III, Sonoda, M. A., Shih, J. W.-K., Engler, W. F., Wang, R. Y.-H., and Wear, D. J. (1989a) Association of the virus-like infectious agent originally reported in patients with AIDS with acute fatal disease in previously healthy non-AIDS patients. Amer. J. Trop. Med. Hyg. 41:364-376.

Lo, S.-C., Dawson, M. S., Wong, D. M., Newton, P. B., III , Sonoda, M.A., Engler, W. F., Wang, R. Y.-H., Shih, J. W. K., Alter, H. J. and Wear, D. J. (1989b) Identification of *Mycoplasma incognitus* infection in patients with AIDS. Amer. J. Trop. Med. Hyg. 41:601-616.

McCoy, R. E., Williams, D. S., and Thomas, D. L. (1979) Isolation of mycoplasmas from flowers, in: "Proceedings of the Republic of China - U.S. Cooperative Science Seminar" (McCoy, R. E., and Su, H., Eds.), pp. 75-80. National Science Council, Taipai, Taiwan.

McCoy, R. E., Basham, H. G., Tully, J. G., Rose, D. L., Carle, P. and Bové, J. M. (1984) *Acholeplasma florum,* a new species isolated from plants. Int. J. Syst. Bacteriol. 34:11-15.

Montagnier, L., Berneman, D., Guetard, D., Blanchard, A., Chamaret, S., Rame, V., Van Rietschoten, J., Mabrouk, K. and Bahraoui, E. (1990) Inhibition of HIV prototype strain infectivity by antibodies directed against a peptide sequence of mycoplasma. Compte Rendu Acad. Sci. (Paris) 311:425-430.

Neimark, H. C. and Lange, C. S. (1990) Pulse-field electrophoresis indicates full-length mycoplasma chromosomes range widely in size. Nucleic Acids Res. 18:5443-5448.

Pyle, L. E., Corcoran, L. N., Cocks, B. G., Bergemann, A. D., Whitley, J.C. and Finch, L. R. (1988). Pulsed-field electrophoresis indicates larger-than-expected sizes for mycoplasma genomes. Nucleic Acids Res. 16:6015-6025.

Razin, S. (1991) The Genera *Mycoplasma, Ureaplasma, Acholeplasma, Anaeroplasma,* and *Asteroleplasma,* in: "The Prokaryotes" (Balows, A., Truper, H. G., Dworkin, M., Harder, W. and Schleifer, K.-H., Eds.), 2nd Ed., Vol. II, pp. 1937-1959. Springer Verlag, New York.

Robertson, J. A., Pyle, L. E., Stemke, G. W., and Finch, L. R. (1990) Human ureaplasmas show diverse genome sizes by pulsed-field electrophoresis. Nucleic Acids Res. 18:1451-1456.

Rose, D. L., Kocka, J. P., Somerson, N. L., Tully, J. G., Whitcomb, R. F., Carle, P., Bové J. M., Colflesh, D. E. and Williamson, D. L. (1990) *Mycoplasma lactucae* sp. nov., a sterol-nonrequiring mollicute from a plant surface. Int. J. Syst. Bacteriol. 40:138-142.

Somerson, N. L., Kocka, J. P., DelGiudice, R. A. and Rose, D. L. (1982) Isolation of acholeplasmas and a mycoplasma from vegetables. Appl. Environ. Microbiol. 43:412-417.

Su, C. J., and Baseman, J. B. (1990) Genome size of *Mycoplasma genitalium.* J. Bacteriol. 172:4705-4707.

Tully, J. G. (1979) Special features of the acholeplasmas, in: "The Mycoplasmas" (Barile, M. F. and Razin, S., Eds.), Vol. I, pp. 431-449. Academic Press, New York.

Tully, J. G., and Baseman, J. B. (1991) Mycoplasma. Lancet 337, 1296.

Tully, J. G., and Razin, S. (1969) Characteristics of a new sterol-nonrequiring *Mycoplasma.* J. Bacteriol. 98:970-978.

Tully, J. G. and Razin, S. (1970) *Acholeplasma axanthum,* sp.n.: a new sterol non-requiring member of the *Mycoplasmatales.* J. Bacteriol. 103:751-754.

Tully, J. G. and Whitcomb, R. F. (1991) The Genus *Spiroplasma,* in: "The Prokaryotes" (Balows, A., Truper, H. G., Dworkin, M., Harder, W. and Schleifer, K.-H., Eds.), 2nd Ed., Vol. II, pp. 1960-1980. Springer-Verlag, New York.

Tully, J. G., Rose, D. L., Whitcomb, R. F., Hackett, K. J., Clark, T. B., Henegar, R. B., Clark, E., Carle, P. and Bové, J. M. (1987) Characterization of some new insect-derived acholeplasmas. Israel J. Med. Sci. 23:699-703.

Tully, J. G., Rose, D. L., Carle, P., Bové, J. M., Hackett, K. J. and Whitcomb, R. F. (1988) *Acholeplasma entomophilum* sp. nov. from gut contents of a wide range of host insects. Int. J. Syst. Bacteriol. 38:164-167.

Tully, J. G., Rose, D. L., Hackett, K. J., Whitcomb, R. F., Carle, P., Bové, J. M., Colflesh, D. E. and Williamson, D. L. (1989) *Mycoplasma ellychniae* sp. nov., a sterol-nonrequiring mollicute from the firefly beetle *Ellychnia corrusca.* Int. J. Syst. Bacteriol. 39, 284-289.

Tully, J. G., Rose, D. L., McCoy, R. E., Carle, P., Bové, J. M., Whitcomb, R. F. and Weisburg, W. G. (1990a) *Mycoplasma melaleucae* sp. nov., a sterol-non-requiring mollicute from flowers of several tropical plants. Int. J. Syst. Bacteriol. 40:143-147.

Tully, J. G., Whitcomb, R. F., Rose, D. L., Hackett, K. J., Clark, E., Henegar, R.B., Carle, P. and Bové, J. M.   (1990b) Current insight into the host diversity of acholeplasmas. Zbl. Hyg. suppl. 20, 461-467.

Wang, R. Y·-H, Hu, W. S., Dawson, M. S., Shih, J. W.-K., and Lo, S.-C. (1992) Selective detection of *Mycoplasma fermentans* by polymerase chain reaction and by using a nucleotide sequence within the insertion sequence- like element. J. Clin. Microbiol. 30:245-248.

Weisburg, W. G., Tully, J. G., Rose, D. L., Petzel, J. P., Oyaizu, H., Yang, D., Mandelco, L., Sechrest, J., Lawrence, T. G., Van Etten, J., Maniloff, J. and Woese, C.R. (1989) A phylogenetic analysis of the mycoplasmas: basis for their classification. J. Bacteriol. 171:6455-6467.

Whitcomb, R. F. and Tully, J. G. (Eds.) (1989) *Spiroplasmas, Acholeplasmas, and Mycoplasmas* of Plants and Arthropods, in: "The Mycoplasmas", Vol. V. Academic Press, New York.

Whitcomb, R. F., Tully, J. G., Rose, D. L., Stephens, E. B., Smith, A., McCoy, R. E. and Barile, M. F. (1982) Wall-less prokaryotes from fall flowers in central United States and Maryland. Curr. Microbiol. 7:285-290.

Whitley, J. C. and Finch, L. R. (1990) Ligated mycoplasma genomes as DNA size markers for PFGE. Nucleic Acids Res. 18:6167-6168.

Williamson, D. L., Tully, J. G., Rose, D. L., Hackett, K. J., Henegar, R., Carle, P., Bové, J. M., Colflesh, D. E., and Whitcomb, R. F. (1990) *Mycoplasma somnilux* sp. nov.,*Mycoplasma luminosum* sp. nov. and *Mycoplasma lucivorax* sp. nov., new sterol-requiring mollicutes from firefly beetles (*Coleoptera: Lampyridae*). Int. J. Syst. 40:160-164.

MOLECULAR BIOLOGY OF *SPIROPLASMAS* : 1991

Joseph M. Bové

Laboratoire de Biologie Cellulaire et Moléculaire
INRA et Universite de Bordeaux II
Domaine de la Grande Ferrade - B.P. 81
33883 Villenave D'Ornon Cedex, France

An extensive review of the molecular and cellular biology of spiroplasmas has been published in 1989 (Bové *et al.*, 1989). The purpose of the present chapter is to update the 1989 review.

Indeed, major developments have occurred since. Introduction of pulse field gel electrophoresis (PFGE) has prompted a re-evaluation of the genome sizes of mollicutes and has been used to determine a restriction map of the *Spiroplasma citri* genome, as well as the location of several genes on these genomes. Ribosomal RNA genes and their promoters have been cloned, sequenced and analyzed.

Two tryptophan transfer RNAs have been identified and sequenced, one recognizing the universal tryptophan codon UGG, and the other reading not only UGG, but also UGA. Codon UGA is one of the three stop codons in the universal genetic code, but codes for tryptophan in *Spiroplasma* (Renaudin *et al.*, 1986) as well as *Mycoplasma* (Yamao *et al.*, 1985). Therefore, *Spiroplasma* and *Mycoplasma* genes cannot be fully translated in bacterial clones, where UGA on the messenger RNA (mRNA) means: stop translation. This difficulty can be overcome by using a UGA suppressor clone, but more directly by using spiroplasmas as expression hosts. This goal has now been achieved by using the replicative form of spiroplasma virus SpV1 as a vector to introduce foreign genes into *S. citri* by electroporation. Transformation of *S. citri* to tetracycline resistance by plasmid pAM120 carrying transposon Tn 916 was also achieved by electroporation.

Rapid Diagnosis of Mycoplasmas, Edited by I. Kahane
and A. Adoni, Plenum Press, New York, 1993

Several *S. citri* genes have been cloned, sequenced and located on the spiroplasma genome, while other *S. citri* genes have been identified and located on the genome by use of various gene probes. The presence of SpV1 viral DNA sequences in the *S. citri* genome has been further documented. DNA sequences of virus SpV1-R8A2 B are present throughout the genome, except for one region extending over about 20% of the genome. A second SpV1 virus has been discovered in strain S102 of *S. citri* . DNA of this virus, SpV1- S102, is present in only 2 small regions of the genome.

Finally, transcription promoters and terminators of the eubacterial type initially identified on the basis of their sequences have now been shown to be functional by primer extension and S1 nuclease mapping.

GENOME SIZE

By renaturation kinetics, the genome of *S. citri* and other spiroplasmas was found to be in the range of 10 megadaltons (mDa) or 1500 kbp (Bové *et al.*, 1989). By pulsefield gel electrophoresis (PFGE), with non-restricted *S. citri* genomic DNA, a single band was obtained and estimated to be 1700 kbp by comparison with yeast chromosomal DNAs (P. Carle and J. M. Bové, unpublished). When the DNA was restricted with *Apa*I, *Bss*HII, or *Sal*I, enzymes that recognize respectively GGGCCC, GCGCGC or GTCGAC sites, the C-G poor (26%) *S. citri* DNA was cut into 9, 9 or 8 fragments; the sum of the fragments from a given enzyme yielded 1780 kbp (O. Grau, F. Laigret and J. M. Bové, unpublished). The genome size of other spiroplasmas was in the range of 1350 kbp, a value smaller than that for *S. citri* . The presence of large amounts of SpV1 viral DNA sequences in the *S. citri* genome could explain, at least partly, the larger size of this genome.

RESTRICTION MAP OF *S. CITRI* R8A2 HP GENOME

Figure 1 shows the restriction map of the spiroplasmal genome when analyzed by endonucleases *Apa*I, *Bss*HII, *Not*I, and *Sal*I (F. C. Yee, F. Laigret and J. M. Bové, unpublished). These enzymes have been chosen because their recognition sequences are 6 to 8 base pairs long and contain only C and G, with the exception of the *Sal*I site which contains one A and one T (see above). The spiroplasmal genome containing only 26% G+C, the number of sites where these enzymes cut is small, 9 for *Apa*I and only 1 for *Not*I, the recognition site of this endonuclease being GCGGCCGC. As shown on Figure 1, most of the sites recognized by these enzymes cluster in two regions of the genome, suggesting that these regions are richer in G and C than the others.

POSITIONING VARIOUS GENES ON THE *S. CITRI* GENOME

*Apa*I, *Bss*HII and *Sal*I were used singly or in combination to generate restriction fragments. These fragments were separated by PFGE and blot-transferred to nylon membranes for hybridization according to Southern with ^{32}p-labelled DNA probes of various homologous genes, *i.e.*, *S. citri* genes or heterologous genes (*i.e.*, genes from other mollicutes) (Table I). This identifies the

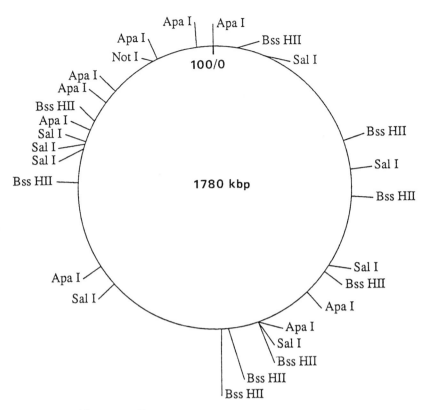

Figure 1. Restriction map of the genome of
Spiroplasma citri R8A2 HP

restriction fragments hybridizing with the probes and thus containing the relevant genes. The position of the hybridizing fragment on the restriction map (Fig. 1) gives the position of the gene on the map (Fig. 2). (The circular map is divided into 100 units and begins arbitrarily with zero at the "left"*Apa*I restriction fragment). In this way, the following genes have been located on the *S. citri* genomic map starting from zero and going clockwise (Fig. 2): fib (Fibrillar protein); the spiralin gene cluster with 2 divergent promoters rpsB (ribosomal protein S2) being transcribed in one direction, while the following genes are transcribed in the opposite direction; tsf (polypeptide chain elongation factor EF-Ts), X (unknown protein), spi (spiraline), pfk (6-phosphofructo-kinase), pyk (pyruvate kinase); genes for tRNAs Ile and Ala; gyrA (A subunit of DNA gyrase), gyrB (β-subunit); *rpo*B (β-subunit of RNA polymerase), rpoC (β' subunit), GlyA (serine-hydroxymethyl transferase), atp (membrane bound ATP synthetase); pyrG (CTP synthetase), purA (adenylosuccinate synthetase), purB (adenylosuccinate lyase); gene cluster of ribosomal proteins (similar to the "a" cluster of *B. subtilis*); *rpo*D (σ subunit of RNA polymerase); rrn (rRNA operon); tRNA gene cluster for tRNAs Val-Thr-Gln-Lys-Leu; gene for 4.5 S RNA (F. C. Ye, F. Laigret and J. M. Bové, unpublished).

Regarding the genes surrounding the spiralin gene, it is noteworthy that in *S. citri* the genes for two key enzymes of glycolysis, 6-phosphofructokinase (pfk) and pyruvate kinase (pyk) are part of the same transcription unit; in *E. coli*, these genes occur on different regions of the genome. In *S. citri* , the genes

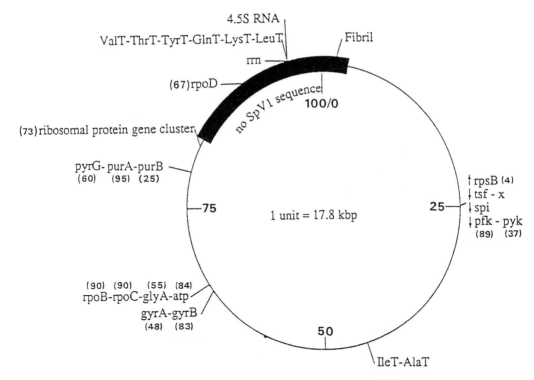

Figure 2. Gene location on the *Spiroplasma citri* genome

The numbers associated with certain genes refer to the position of these genes on the *E. coli* map subdivided in 100 units (100/0).

for ribosomal protein S2, (rpsB) and EF-Ts (tsf) are divergent; in *E. coli* they are transcribed in the same direction and belong to a single transcription unit.

The genes (gyrA and gyrB) for the two subunits of DNA gyrase are linked in *S. citri* as well as in *B. subtilis*; they are far apart on the *E. coli* genome.

In both *S. citri* and *E. coli*, the genes (rpoB and rpoC) for the β and β' subunits of RNA polymerase are adjacent and part of the same transcription unit. In the bacterium, the so-called β operon additionally encodes two ribosomal proteins (L10 and L7/L12), the genes (rplJ and rplL) which are upstream of rpoB and rpoC, i.e., 5' rplJ, rplL, rpoB, rpoC. In the spiroplasma, the rpoB and rpoC genes are followed by glyA (serinehydroxymethyltransferase) and atp (ATP synthetase). In *E. coli*, glyA, atp and the β operon are in different regions of the chromosome. Similarly, in both *E. coli* and *Bacillus subtilis*, purG, purA, and purB, three genes involved in nucleotide synthesis, are in separated regions; in *S. citri*, these three genes are part of the same transcription unit.

18

RIBOSOMAL RNA GENES

By the use of various ribosomal rDNA probes and different restriction enzymes, it was shown by Southern blot hybridzation that *S. citri*, as well as 13 other spiroplasma species tested, contain only one rDNA operon, while *S. apis* and *S. sp* MQ4 have two. The gene order is 5'-rrs-rrl-rrf-3', coding respectivel for 16 S RNA, 23 S RNA and 5S RNA. In *E. coli* and *B. subtilis*, there are respectively 7 and 10 rDNA operons and they contain transfer RNA genes between rrs and rrl and/or after rrf. No tRNAs occur in the rrn operon of *S. citri*. In several plant MLOs, a tRNA gene is present between rrs and rrl. In *M. capricolum*, 2 tRNAs precede rrs.

The mollicutes are seen as having evolved from ancestors of *Clostridia* (Weisburg *et al.*, 1989). The bacteria that are phylogenetically closest to the mollicutes are *Clostridium innocuum* and *C. ramosum*. Interestingly, the first has 5 rDNA operons and the second 4, thus fewer than *B. subtilis* with 10, but more than the mollicutes with only 1 or 2. *Mycoplasma lactucae* 831-C4T is, so far, the only mollicute tested with 3 rDNA operons.

The 16 S rDNA of *S. citri* was sequenced as part of a 4.2 kbp *Hind*III restriction fragment cloned in plasmid pBR322 (Laigret *et al.*, 1990; Grau *et al.*, 1990, unpublished). The upstream (5') and downstream (3') regions were also sequenced. The total region sequenced extends from nucleotide -320 (*Alu*1 site) to 1899 (*Hind*III site), +1 being the 5' end of the 16 S RNA as determined by Woese *et al.* (1980). The 5' end of the primary transcription product has been determined by S1 mapping. In fact, two primary transcription products have been detected, one starting at nucleotide -272, the other at nucleotide -196. This result indicates that there are two tandem promoters, P1 and P2; P1 for the transcript starting at -272, and P2 for that starting at -196. The -10 and -35 regions of P1 are, respectively, 5' -288TACTAA 3' and 5' -310TTGTAA3'; those of P2 are, respectively, 5' -210 CATAAT3' and 5' -233TTGGGA3'. These regions, experimentally determined by S1 mapping, are different from those proposed earlier on the basis of sequence analysis only (Bové *et al.*, 1989).

The 3'OH end of the 16 S RNA has also been determined by S1 mapping; it occurs at adenine 1529. When the conserved 3'OH terminal sequences of the 16 S RNAs of *S. citri*, *B. subtilis* and *E. coli* are aligned, it appears that the 3'OH end of *S. citri* 16 S RNA has, respectively, 4 and 7 terminal nucleotides more than *B. subtilis* and *E. coli* 16 S RNA:

S. citri	3'OH AGG<u>UAUCUUUCCUCCACUAGGU</u>...5'
B. subtilis	AUCUUUCCACCACUAGGU...5'
E. coli	AUUCCACCACUAGGU...5'

M. capricolum and *Mycoplasma sp.* PG50, resemble *S. citri* as they also have the 3' OH terminal AGGU sequence; they belong to the same phylogenetic group as *S. citri*.

The prokaryotic messenger RNA (mRNA) has a ribosome binding site, 5 to 10 nucleotides upstream of the initiation codon AUG. This so-called Shine-Dalgarno sequence is complementary to the 3'OH end of the 16S RNA.

In the initiation step of protein synthesis, the 30 S ribosomal subunit containing the 16 S RNA is able to bind to the mRNA by hydrogen bonding between the Shine-Dalgarno sequence and the 3'OH end of the 16 S RNA. We have examined the Shine-Dalgarno regions of the 12 open reading frames (ORFs) of spiroplasma virus SpV1, the 9 ORFs of SpV4, and those of the following protein genes: fib, rspB, tsf, X, spi, pfk, pyk, pyrG, purA and purB. It turns out that the Shine-Dalgarno regions, when hydrogen-bonded to the 3'OH end of S. citri of 16 S RNA, involve several of the 17 nucleotides underlined above. In the case of gram negative bacteria, the number of nucleotides involved in ribosome binding on the mRNA is much smaller.

Ribosomal RNAs are obtained by maturation of the primary transcription product. 16 S RNA and 23 S RNA occur on the primary transcripts as giant loops carried by double stranded stems. These stems carry recognition sites for RNase III cleavage; in the case of B. subtilis, the recognition site is 12 nucleotides long (boxed sequence):

```
5' ... A|T C T T T|G A A A A C T|A A A ......   .   .
        .     .   .           .      . . .
        .|.   .   .|.   .   .   .|. . .         16 S RNA
3' ... T|A G A G A|C T T T T G A|T T T ......
                                              .   .
```

Identical or very similar sequences occur also in mollicutes including S. citri , but not in E. coli, where the recognition signal is different.

TRANSFER RNA GENES

A tRNA gene cluster for 10 tRNAs (Cys, Arg, Pro, Ala, Met, Ile, Ser, fMet, Asp, Phe) has been identified in S. melliferum (see Bové et al., 1989). We have recently cloned and sequenced a tRNA gene cluster from S. citri for the tRNAs of 5' Val, Thr, Tyr, Gln, Lys, Leu 3' and two tRNA gene clusters for Ile and Ala tRNAs (C. Citti, C. Saillard and J. M. Bové, unpublished). However, the most relevant results regarding S. citri tRNAs concern tryptophan tRNAs. As indicated above, in spiroplasmas UGA is not a stop codon but codes for tryptophan (trp). There are, thus, two trp codons in spiroplasmas: UGA and the universal trp codon UGG. Are there also two trp tRNAs, one with anticodon 3' ACC 5' recognizing UGG, the other with anticodon 3' ACU 5' recognizing UGA? A priori, the tRNA with anticodon 3' ACU 5' is sufficient, since this anticodon, because of wobble, could recognize not only UGA but also UGG. We have, therefore, looked for trp tRNAs in S. citri (C. Citti, L. Marechal Drouard, C. Saillard, J. Weil and J. M. Bové, unpublished). We were able to isolate and purify two tRNAs that could be charged in vitro with tryptophan. When enzymes from S. citri were used for tryptophanyl synthesis, both tRNAs could be charged, but with enzymes from E. coli, only one tRNA could be aminoacylated with tryptophan. The two tRNAs have been sequenced directly by the method of Stanley and Vassilenko (1978). One is the universal trp with anticodon 3' ACC 5' and is aminoacylated with the enzymes from both S. citri and E. coli, while the second has the anti-codon 3' ACU 5' and can only be used by S. citri enzymes.

On the basis of the sequences of the two trp tRNAs, an oligonucleotide probe has been chemically synthesized and has been used to locate the genes for the two trp tRNAs on the *S. citri* map.

In *M. capricolum* and *M. gallisepticum*, there are also two trp tRNAs, one for UGG and one for UGA. In *M. pneumoniae* as in *M. genitalium*, only one trp tRNA is present. This trp tRNA possesses the 3' ACU 5' anticodon which can read both UGA and UGG.

GENES FOR PROTEINS

Spiralin Gene and Adjacent Genes

The gene for spiralin is of particular interest. Spiralin is the major membrane protein of *Spiroplasma citri*. It is apparently a transmembrane amphiphilic protein and it is acylated (see Bové *et al.*, 1989). Acylation seems to be a characteristic of several membrane proteins of mollicutes. The role of spiralin is not known. However, it must be a key protein of the spiroplasmal membrane, since spiralin-like proteins occur in *Spiroplasma* species other than *S. citri* and probably in all spiroplasmas (see below). Sequence determination of the spiralin gene was made possible by the fact that we have previously cloned the gene. A library of cloned genomic sequences of *S. citri* R8A2 was constructed by incorporation of *Hind*III restriction fragments into plasmid pBR328 and cloning in *Escherichia coli*. The bacterial clone harboring recombinant plasmid pES1 was selected by its ability to express spiralin. Spiralin was indeed expressed in *E. coli* and was the first mollicute gene product to be fully expressed in a bacterium.

Recombinant plasmid pES1 was subcloned into plasmid pES3'. The 5-kilobase-pair (kbp) spiroplasmal insert of pES3' has been entirely sequenced. Sequence analysis of the 5-kbp spiroplasmal insert of pES3' made it possible to identify the spiralin gene and five additional open reading frames (ORFs) (Chevalier *et al.*, 1990a). The translational products of four of these ORFs were identified by their amino acid sequence homologies with known proteins: ribosomal protein S2, elongation factor Ts, phosphofructokinase, and pyruvate kinase, respectively, encoded by the genes rpsB, tsf, pfk, and pyk. The product of the fifth ORF remains to be identified and was named protein X (X gene). The order of the above genes was tsf-X-spi-pfk-pyk. These genes were transcribed in one direction, while the gene for ribosomal protein S2 (rpsB) was transcribed in the opposite direction; rpsB and tsf are thus divergent genes with overlapping promoters. This is the first description of divergent genes in mollicutes. The region between the promoter of rpsB and the ATG initiation codon contains an inverted repeat, 28 bp upstream of the ATG codon. This sequence is such that a protein dimer with dyad symmetry would be able to bind to the same side of the DNA helix, one monomer in contact with the direct sequence, the other with the inverted sequence. Hence, the inverted repeat would represent a region where a polypeptide with regulatory functions could bind to control transcription in both directions. It would be interesting to investigate whether protein X may function as a regulatory protein that acts at the inverted repeat (within the divergent transcription unit) to control transcription of the nonregulatory S2 protein.

In *E. coli*, the genes for S2 (rpsB) and EF-Ts (tsf) are not divergent as they are in *S. citri*. They belong to a single transcription unit, with rspB being promoter proximal, and are transcribed in the same direction.

A protein similar to spiralin occurs in the membrane of *Spiroplasma melliferum*, an organism related to *S. citri*. A restriction fragment of the spiralin gene has been used as a probe to detect the gene encoding *S. melliferum* spiralin. A 4.6 -kilobase-pair ClaI DNA fragment from *S. melliferum* strongly hybridized with the probe. This fragment was inserted in pBR322 and cloned in *Escherichia coli*.. It was further subcloned in the replicative forms of M13mp18 and M13mp19 and its nucleotide sequence was determined (GenBank accession number M33991). An open reading frame showing 88.6% base sequence homology with the *S. citri* spiralin gene could be identified and was assumed to be the gene encoding *S. melliferum* spiralin. The deduced amino acid sequence of the protein has 75% homology with the *S. citri* spiralin sequence. In particular, the two proteins possess a well conserved sequence of 20 amino acids which can form an α-helix with the size required for membrane spanning (Chevalier *et al.*, 1990b).

Axial projection of this α-helix shows that the distribution of the amino acid residues determines a hydrophobic face and a hydrophilic face, involving one-third and two-thirds of the α-helix surface, respectively. The amphiphilic nature of the α-helix suggests that several spiralin molecules assemble in the membrane to form a homooligomer in such a way that the hydrophobic faces of their α-helices are on the outside of the oligomer, turned towards the lipid bilayer, while the hydrophilic domains are turned towards the inside of the oligomer, away from the hydrophobic environment of the lipid bilayer. This interpretation agrees with biochemical data on spiralin. Indeed, spiralin seems to occur as dimers, tetramers, and large oligomers in the spiroplasmal membranes.

Spiralin gene sequences can be amplified by polymerase chain reaction (PCR). PCR has been used on several *S. citri* strains to demonstrate spiralin gene polymorphism as well as the presence of a spiralin gene in all the spiroplasmas of group I (X. Foissac, C. Saillard and J. M. Bové, unpublished).

Fibrillar Protein Gene

We have now cloned and sequenced the fibrillar protein in the following way (Williamson *et al.*, 1991). The protein was purified by polyacrylamide gel electrophoresis (PAGE). Two peptides generated by V8 protease were sequenced at their N- terminal. The sequences were used to construct oligonucleotides, based on the codon usage of spiroplasmas. Oligonucleotide 23C was used as a probe to screen a phage λ library. Clone B selected in this way contained an 11.3 kbp spiroplasmal insert, of which a 3.3 kbp EcoRI fragment strongly hybridized with probe 23C. The sequence of the 3.3 kbp fragment showed it to contain two open reading frames (ORFs). Comparison of the N terminal amino sequences of the V8 protease peptides to the amino acid sequences of the translation products of the two ORFs showed ORF 1 to be the fibrillar protein gene. The gene contains 1548 nucleotide residues. The amino acid sequence of the protein comprises 515 amino acids, including 4 cysteine residues and 7 tryptophan residues. Six of the 7 tryptophan residues are encoded by triplet TGA and 1 by TGG. By Northern blot hybridization with a fibrillar protein specific probe, one single mRNA transcript of 1.7 kb was detected. Primer extension was used to determine the 5' end of the mRNA, as well as the transcription promoter. The 3'OH end of the mRNA terminates with a row of Us following a terminator structure of the rho independent type. The 5' and 3' ends determined experimentally in this way lead to a transcript of precisely 1.7 kbp.

This fibrillar protein possesses four α-helices. Axial projection of the three most prominent ones shows that the hydrophobic and hydrophilic amino acids are distributed to opposite sides of the helices. This arrangement may offer a mechanism for the attachment of the fibrillar protein to the plasma membrane, with the hydrophobic side associated with the membrane and the hydrophilic side facing the cytoplasm. An actin-like protein found in spiroplasmas may be linked to the fibrils and be involved in motility, but there is presently no evidence of their association.

Pyr G, Pur A and Pur B

In *M. capricolum*, UGA is read as a tryptophan codon (Yamao *et al.*, 1985). The tRNA recognizing UGA has been sequenced. We have used the sequence of the 3' end of this tRNA to synthetize a 24 mer oligonucleotide and use it as a probe to identify the tryptophan tRNA gene in *S. citri*. A strong hybridization signal was obtained with *Eco*RI restricted *M. capricolum* DNA, a weak but clear-cut signal with *S. citri* DNA and no signal with *Acholeplasma laidlawii* DNA. The hybridization of *S. citri* DNA fragment was cloned and sequenced. To our surprise, no tRNA gene was detected, but two complete and two partial open reading frames (ORFs) were identified! (C. Citti, C. Saillard and J. M. Bové, unpublished). They were positioned as follows: 5'-(3' end of ORF I), (ORF II), (ORF III), (5' end of ORF IV)-3'. ORF II, ORF III and ORF IV were identified by protein sequence comparisons as pyr G, pur A and pur B. These genes code for enzymes involved in pyrimidine and purine nucleotide metabolism. Pyr G is the gene for CTP synthetase which converts UTP to CTP; the reaction is an amination of UTP at the expense of ATP; glutamine is the preferred nitrogen donor in the presence of GTP as a positive effector. PurA codes for adenylosuccinate synthetase which converts IMP to succinyl AMP in the presence of aspartate and GTP; succinyl AMP is cleaved to AMP and fumarate by adenylosuccinate lyase, the gene product of pur B. In the condensation of aspartate with IMP, cleavage of GTP to GDP and phosphate provides energy to drive the reaction.

IDENTIFICATION OF *S. CITRI* GENES BY HETEROLOGOUS PROBES

Table I indicates genes or gene clusters from four mycoplasma species that have been analyzed by various authors. These DNAs have been kindly made available to us and we have used them to search for similar genes in

Table 1. Heterologous probes

Genes Obtained from	Product	Source	
gyrA	DNA gyrase subunit A	*M. pneumoniae*	Hu, P. C.
gyrB	DNA gyrase subunit B		(1)
rpoB	RNA polymerase β subunit	*Mycoplasma* PG50	
rpoC	RNA polymerase β' subunit		
glyA	Serine hydroxymethyltransferase		Christiansen, C.
atp	Membrane bound ATP synthase		(2)
sRNA	Small 4, 5S RNA	*M. mycoides*	Samuelsson, T. (3)
rplP	50S ribosomal protein L16	*M. capricolum*	
rpmC	50S ribosomal protein L29		
rpsQ	30S ribosomal protein L14		
rplN	50S ribosomal protein L17		
rplX	50S ribosomal protein L24		
rplE	50S ribosomal protein L5		
rpsN	30S ribosomal protein S14		Muto, A
rpsH	30S ribosomal protein S8		(4)
rplF	50S ribosomal protein L6		
rplR	50S ribosomal protein L18		
rpsE	30S ribosomal protein S5		
rplO	50S ribosomal protein L15		
secY	protein export (prlA)		

---

(1)   Coleman, S. D., Hu, P.-C and Bott, K. F. (1990) *Mycoplasma pneumoniae* DNA gyrase genes. Mol. Microbiol. 4:1129-1134.

(2)   Rasmussen, O. F. and Christiansen, C. (1990) A 23 kb region of the *Mycoplasma* PG50 genome with three identified genetic structures, Zbl. Bakt. Suppl. 20:315-324.

(3)   Samuelsson, T. and Guindy, Y. (1990) Nucleotide sequence of a *Mycoplasma mycoides* RNA which is homologous to *E. coli* 4.5S RNA. Nucleic Acids Res. 18:4938.

(4)   Ohkubo, S., Muto, A., Kawauchi, Y., Yamao, F. and Osawa, S. (1987) The ribosomal protein gene cluster of *Mycoplasma capricolum*. Mol. Gen. Genet. 210:314-322.

S. citri by Southern hybridization. Hybridization signals have indeed been obtained for all these genes; Figure 2 indicates their position on the *S. citri* map (F. C. Ye, F. Laigret and J. M. Bové, unpublished).

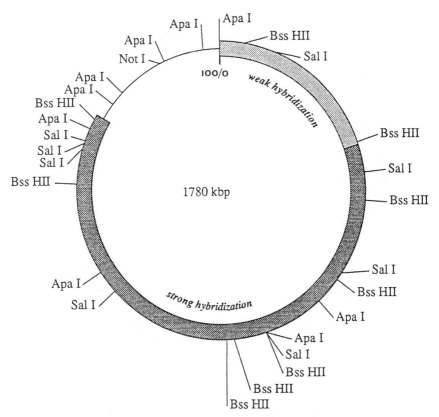

Figure 3. Hybridization map of *S. citri* genome
with SpV1-R8A2B viral DNA

PRESENCE OF SpV1 VIRAL DNA SEQUENCES IN THE *S. CITRI* GENOME

We have reported earlier on the presence of SpV1 viral DNA sequences in the *S. citri* genome (see Bové *et al.*, 1989). The spiroplasma strain used in this work is *S. citri* strain R8A2 HP. This high passage strain produces no SpV1 virus spontaneously and contains no extra-chromosomal DNA. However, this strain can be experimentally infected with SpV1-type viruses. The SpV1 virus strains used are SpV1-R8A2 B, from the low passage *S. citri* strain R8A2 B, SpV1-78 from a low passage culture of a Turkish isolate of *S. citri*, and SpV1-S102 from a low passage culture of a Syrian isolate of *S. citri*.

When Southern hybridization is carried out between restricted *S. citri* -R8A2 HP DNA and the DNA of virus SpV1-R8A2B or SpV1-78 as the probe, many chromosomal DNA bands are found to hybridize, suggesting that viral sequences are probably present at several sites in the spiroplasma chromosome (Renaudin *et al.*, 1990 b). This has recently been confirmed by showing that SpV1-R8A2 B viral DNA used as a probe hybridized with the majority of the PFGE- separated fragments generated by rare cutting enzymes (*Apa*I, BssHII,

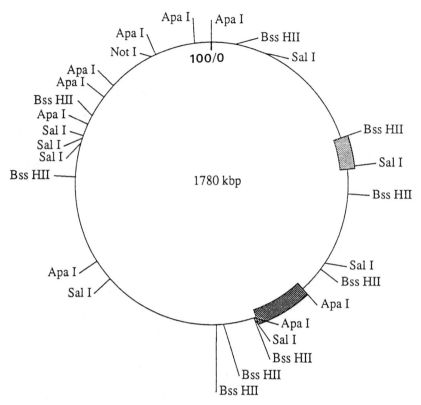

Figure 4. Hybridization map of *S. citri* genome with SpV1-S102 viral DNA

*Sal*I) acting on *S. citri* -R8A2 HPDNA embedded in agarose blocks (F. C. Ye, F. Laigret, J. Renaudin and J. M. Bové, unpublished). As shown in Figure 3, more than 3/4 of the *S. citri* R8A2 HP genome contained SpV1-R8A2 B DNA sequences. Only one region, about 20% of the genome, contained no viral DNA sequences (Fig. 3). Similar results were obtained with several *S. citri* pV1 viruses, including SpV1 R8A2 B and SpV1-78. These viral strains show strong cross hybridization among themselves. Recently however, virus strain SpV1- S102 was selected because its DNA had a size of 7.0 kb, a value smaller than the 8.3 kb of SpV1-R8A2 B DNA. To our surprise, there was practically no cross-hybridization between the DNAs of viral strains R8A2 B and S102 and, furthermore, only one small region of the *S. citri* R8A2 HHP genome gave a strong hybridization signal with SpV1-S102 DNA as a probe; an even shorter region gave only a faint hybridization signal (Fig. 4). These results suggest that the problem of SpV1 viral DNA sequences in the *S. citri* genome is even more complex than was thought.

The DNA of SpV1-R8A2 B has been fully sequenced and contains 8,273 nucleotide residues (Renaudin *et al.*, 1990a). The sequence of this virion DNA has been compared with the viral sequences present in the spiroplasmal chromosome (Renaudin *et al.*, 1990b; P. Aullo, J. Renaudin and J. M.Bové, unpub-

lished). To that purpose, a genomic DNA library of *S. citri* R8A2 HP DNA has
been established in a phage λ derived vector. Several recombinant λ clones hybridizing with SpV1-R8A2 HP DNA have been detected. One clone (L10) has
been further analyzed. The DNA of clone L10 was shown to contain a full-
length SpV1 genome; the junctions between viral DNA and spiroplasmal chromosomal DNA have been sequenced, thus identifying the side where the
circular viral RF DNA has to be cut (linearization) for insertion as a linear
viral DNA into the *S. citri* chromosome. The mechanism by which this insertion process occurs is unknown. It is, however, interesting to note that one
of the SpV1 ORFs codes for a protein that shows partial homology with the
integrase of phage P22.

The full viral genome of clone L10 shows more than 95% homology
with the virion DNA of SpV1-R8A2 B. Alignment of the two sequences reveals that the L10 viral DNA contains point mutations, insertions and delet-
ions without effects on the reading frames. There is, however, the insertion of
one base at the beginning of viral ORF 1 (the longest ORF) which interrupts
the reading frame. This one insertion would probably be enough to explain
why *S. citri* strain R8A2 HP produces no virus in spite of the presence of full
length viral DNA.

TOWARDS A VIRUS-DERIVED VECTOR FOR GENE CLONING AND
EXPRESSION IN SPIROPLASMA

We have recently shown that the replicative form (RF) of *S. citri* virus
SpV1- R8A2 B can be used as a vector to insert and amplify genes into cells of
S. citri strain R8A2 HB (Stamburski *et al.*, 1991).   The gene for chloramphenicol acetyl transferase (CAT) and responsible for resistance to chloramphenicol was used as the model gene. Indeed, it was possible to insert the CAT
gene into the intergenic region I3 at the single *Mbo*I site of the viral RF, trans-
fect the spiroplasma cells by electroporation with the recombinant RF, get transcription and translation of the CAT gene in the spiroplasmal host, and recover SpV1 viruses containing the CAT sequences as an insert (SpV1-CAT).
Expression of the CAT gene in the transfected *S. citri* cells was demonstrated
by the presence of strong CAT activity in cell-free extracts from SpV1-CAT
infected cells, but not in cells infected with "CAT"-free SpV1.

The CAT gene, being of bacterial origin, does not contain TGA tryptophan codons. To show that the presence of such codons in a gene does not
block translation of the gene in the *S. citri* host we have introduced a TGA
codon in the CAT gene by changing the first tryptophan TGG codon into TGA
by uracil-DNA mediated site-directed mutagenesis in *E. coli* (Kunkel *et al.*,
1987). In this technique, the CAT gene was inserted in the RF of phage M13.
The recombinant phage was called M13-CATTGG before mutation, and M13-
CATTGA upon mutation. That fact that TGG was indeed mutated into TGA
was verified by sequencing. As expected, the *E. coli* cells (DH5aF') infected by
mutated phage M13-CATTGA did not express CAT activity, as compared to *E.
coli* cells infected with non-mutated phage M13-CATTGG. In contrast to the
situation in *E. coli,* the *S. citri* R8A2 HP cells expressed CAT activity equally
well whether they were infected by the SpV1 virus containing mutated CAT

gene (SpV1-CA TGA) or by the SpV1 virus containing non-mutated CAT gene (SpV1CAT TGG) (C. Stamburski, J. Renaudin and J. M. Bové, unpublished). From these experiments, we conclude that SpV1-RF can be used as a gene vector to transform *S. citri* cells, and these cells are able to express a foreign gene in which TGA codes for tryptophan.

TRANSFORMATION OF *S. CITRI* BY TRANSPOSITION

Transformation of *Acholeplasma laidlawii* and *M. pulmonis* to tetracycline resistance by plasmid pAM120 was achieved in 1987 (Dybvig and Cassell, 1987). In this plasmid, the determinant for tetracycline resistance, tetM, is contained within transposon Tn916. In the transformed tetracycline resistant mollicutes, transposons Tn916 with the enclosed tetM was found to be inserted in the cell chromosome indicating that both the tetM determinant and the Tn916 genes required for transposition were expressed in the mollicutes.

Similar results have now also been obtained with *S. citri*, but only when electroporation was used as the technique to introduce DNA in the cells. Under these conditions, plasmid pAM120 was able to transform *S. citri* cells to tetracycline resistance. Nine tetracycline resistant clones have been obtained in which transposon Tn916 with the enclosed tetM was inserted in the spiroplasma genome. The site of insertion differed from one clone to the other (C. Stamburski, J. Renaudin and J. M. Bové, unpublished).

CONCLUSION

Molecular biology of spiroplasmas has advanced rapidly over the last five years and has essentially confirmed the eubacterial nature of these organisms. We now know that many aspects of the molecular biology of the spiroplasmas are similar to those of other eubacteria, even though the spiroplasmas use UGA in addition to UGG as tryptophan codons. Among the questions that remain unanswered are those, for instance, that concern gene regulation, but also those that refer to properties that are specific of the spiroplasmas, which make these organisms unique within the eubacterial world. Why are spiroplasmas helical and motile? What are the functions of spiralin and the fibrillar protein? Why do all *S. citri* strains contain vast amounts of viral SpV1 DNA in their genome? What is the mechanism of phytopathogenicity of the sieve-tube restricted spiroplasmas? Why are certain *S. citri* strains transmissible by leafhopper vectors while others are not? These problems and others probably require new approaches. Spiroplasma mutants for genetic work are urgently required. Complementation of such mutants by transposition or transfection is now possible.

ACKNOWLEDGEMENTS

The author is indebted to his colleagues F. Laigret, J. Renaudin and Colette Saillard for unpublished material and helpful discussions.

REFERENCES

Bové, J. M., Carle, P., Garnier, M., Laigret, F., Renaudin, J. and Saillard, C. (1989) Molecular and cellular biology of spiroplasmas In: "The Myco-plasmas", Vol. V (Whitcomb, R. F. and Tully, J. G., Eds.), pp. 244-364. Academic Press, New York.

Chevalier, C., Saillard, C. and Bové, J. M. (1990 a) Organization and nucleotide sequences of the *Spiroplasma citri* genes for ribosomal protein S2, elong-ation factor Ts, spiralin, phosphofructokinase, pyruvate kinase, and an unidentified protein. J. Bacteriol. 172:2693-2703.

Chevalier, S., Saillard, C. and Bové, J. M. (1990 b) Spiralins of *Spiroplasma citri* and *Spiroplasma melliferum*: amino acid sequences and putative organization in the cell membrane. J. Bacteriol. 172, (10): 6069-6097.

Coleman, S. D., Hu, P.-C and Bott, K. F. (1990) *Mycoplasma pneumoniae* DNA gyrase genes. Mol. Microbiol. 4:1129-1134.

Dybvig, K. and Cassell, G. H. (1987) Transposition of gram positive transposon Tn196 in *Acholeplasma laidlawii* and *Mycoplasma pulmonis*. Science 235: 1392-1394.

Grau, O., Laigret, F. and Bové, Staneke, J. M. (1990) Analysis of ribosomal RNA genes in two spiroplasmas, one acholeplasma and one unclassified mollicute, In: "Recent Advances in Mycoplasmology" (Stanek, G., Cassell, G. H., Tully, J. G. and Whitcomb, R. F., Eds.) Zbl. Bakteriol. Suppl. 20. pp. 895-897. Gustav Fischer Verlag, Stuttgart, New York.

Kunkel, T. A. (1985) Rapid and efficient site-specific mutagenesis without phenotypic selection. Proc. Natl. Acad. Sci. USA 82:488-492.

Laigret, F., Grau, O. and Bové, J. M. (1990) Comparison of 16S rDNA sequences of various mollicutes In: "Recent Advances in Mycoplasmology" (Stanek, G., Cassell, G. H., Tully, J. G. and Whitcomb, R. G., Eds.) Zbl. Bakteriol. Suppl. 20, pp. 435-440. Gustav Fischer Verlag, Stuttgart, New York.

Ohkubo, S., Muto, A., Kawauchi, Y., Yamao, F. and Osawa, S. (1987) The ribosomal protein gene cluster of *Mycoplasma capricolum*. Mol. Gen. Genet. 210:314-322.

Rasmussen, O. F. and Christiansen, C. (1990) A 23 kb region of the *Myco-plasma* PG50 genome with three identified genetic structures, Zbl. Bakt. Suppl. 20:315-324.

Renaudin, J., Pascarel, M. C., Saillard, C., Chevalier, C. and Bové, J. M. (1986) Chez les spiroplasmes le codon UGA n'est pas non sens et semble coder pour le tryptophane. C.R. Acad. Sc. Paris 303, série III, no 13:539-540.

Renaudin, J., Aullo, P., Vignault, J. C. and Bové, J. M. (1990a) Complete nucleotide sequence of the genome of *Spiroplasma citri* virus SpV1-R8A2 B. Nucleic Acid Res. 18:1293-1294.

Renaudin, J., Bodin-Ramiro, C., Vignault, J. C. and Bové, J. M. (1990 b) Spiro-plasma virus 1: presence of viral DNA sequences in the spiroplasma genome In: "Recent Advances in Mycoplasmology" (Stanek, G., Cassell, G. H., Tully, J. G. and Whitcomb, R. F., Eds.) Zbl. Bakteriol. Suppl. 20, pp. 125-130. Gustav Fischer Verlag, Stuttgart, New York.

Samuelsson, T. and Guindy, Y. (1990) Nucleotide sequence of a *Mycoplasma mycoides* RNA which is homologous to *E. coli* 4.55 RNA. Nucleic Acids Res. 18:4938.

Stanley, J. and Vassilenko, S. (1978) A different approach to RNA sequencing. Nature 274:87-89.

Weisburg, W. G., Tully, J. G., Rose, D. L., Petzel, J. P., Oyaizu, H., Yang, D., Mandelco, L., Sechrest, J., Lawrence, T. G., Van Etten, J., Maniloff, J. and Woese, C. R. (1989) A phylogenetic analysis of the mycoplasmas: basis for their classification. J. Bacteriol. 171:6455-6467.

Williamson, D. L., Renaudin, J. and Bové, J. M. (1991) Nucleotide sequence of the *Spiroplasma citri* fibril protein gene. J. Bacteriol. 174 (14)4353-4362.

Woese, C. R., Maniloff, J. and Zablen, L. B. (1980) Phylogenetic analysis of the mycoplasmas. Proc. Natl. Acad. Sci. USA 77:494-498.

Yamao, F., Muto, A. Kawauchi, Y., Iwami, M., Iwagami, S., Zumi, Y. and Osawa, S. (1985) UGA is read as tryptophan in *Mycoplasma capricolum*. Proc. Natl. Acad. Sci. USA 82:2306-2309.

Note added in proof. The following relevant articles have now appeared:

Stamburski, C., Renaudin, J. and Bové, J. M. (1991) First step toward a virus-derived vector for gene cloning and expression in spiroplasmas, organisms which read UGA as a tryptophan codon: synthesis of chloramphenicol acetyltransferase in *Spiroplasma citri*. J. Bacteriol. 173:2225-2230.

Citti, C., Maréchal-Drouard, L., Saillard, C., Weil, J. H. and Bové, J. M. (1992) *Spiroplasma citri* UGG and UGA tryptophan codons: sequence of the two tryptophanyl-tRAs and organization of the corresponding genes. J. Bacteriol. 174:6471-6478.

Stamburski, C., Renaudin, J. and Bové, J. M. (1992) Mutagenesis of a tryptophan codon from TGG to TGA in the *cat* gene does not prevent its expression in the helical mollicute *Spiroplasma citri*. Gene 110:133-134.

Ye, F., Laigret, F., Whitley J. C., Citti, C., Finch, L. R., Carle, P., Renaudin, J. and Bové, J. M. (1992) A physical and genetic map of the *Spiroplasma citri* genome. Nucleic Acids Res. 20:1559-1565.

Marais, A., Bové, J. M., Dallo, S. F., Baseman, J. B. and Renaudin, J. (1993) Expression in *Spiroplasma citri* of an epitope carried on the G fragment of cytadhesin P1 gene from *Mycoplasma pneumoniae*. J. Bacteriol. 175:2783-2787.

MYCOPLASMAS IN THE HUMAN UROGENITAL TRACT

David Taylor-Robinson

Division of Sexually Transmitted Diseases, Clinical
Research Centre, Harrow, Middlesex and Jefferiss Wing
St. Mary's Hospital, Paddington, London W1 1NY, U.K.

MYCOPLASMAS OF HUMAN ORIGIN

Twelve species in the genus *Mycoplasma*, two in the genus *Acholeplasma*, and one in the genus *Ureaplasma* have been isolated from humans, mostly from the oropharynx. Eight *Mycoplasma* species (*M. fermentans*, *M. genitalium*, *M. hominis*, *M. penetrans*, *M. pneumoniae*, *M. primatum*, *M. salivarium*, *M. spermatophilum*) and *U. urealyticum* have been isolated from the urogenital tract, *M. hominis* and ureaplasmas most frequently. Their role in disease is mentioned briefly.

NON-GONOCOCCAL URETHRITIS (NGU) AND ITS SEQUELAE

M. fermentans, *M. pneumoniae*, *M. primatum* and *M. salivarium* have been isolated so rarely from the genital tract as to make their significance in NGU improbable, although for some it is not known whether their rarity is a reflection of inadequate culture media or a truly rare existence. For *M. penetrans* and *M. spermatophilum*, the information is, as yet, insufficient to draw conclusions. In the case of *M. hominis*, isolation may be achieved from about one-fifth of patients with NGU, but there are insufficient data to incriminate it as a cause (Taylor-Robinson, 1985). On the other hand, there is evidence to implicate ureaplasmas as one of the causes of non-chlamydial NGU (Taylor-Robinson, 1985). This comes mainly from animal (chimpanzee) and human volunteer inoculation studies in which urethritis has been produced, and observations on immunocompromised patients (see below), together with information from serological and controlled antibiotic studies. The proportion of cases for which ureaplasmas are responsible remains unclear, but their occurrence in the urethra of about 20% of asymptomatic men suggests that only

Rapid Diagnosis of Mycoplasmas, Edited by I. Kahane
and A. Adoni, Plenum Press, New York, 1993

certain serotypes are pathogenic or that predisposing factors, such as impaired mucosal immunity or a particular HLA type, exist in those who develop disease. The role of *M. genitalium* in NGU is gradually being resolved. This mycoplasma may be detected by use of the polymerase chain reaction (PCR) (Palmer *et al.*, 1991a) and has been found in 23% of men with acute NGU, but in only 6% of matched controls (p<0.006) (Horner *et al.*, 1993) and in about 20% of patients with recurrent or persistent NGU, many of whom respond to a prolonged course of erythromycin (P. E. Hay, C. B. Gilroy and D. Taylor-Robinson, unpublished data). Tetracycline-resistant ureaplasmas have also been associated with persistent NGU (Stimson *et al.*, 1981). So far as other sequelae of NGU are concerned, there is no evidence that any of the *Mycoplasma* species or the ureaplasmas are a cause of chronic abacterial prostatitis, biopsy specimens taken transperineally to avoid the urethra not yielding the organisms (Doble *et al.*, 1989). On the other hand, the isolation of ureaplasmas from an epididymal aspirate of a patient suffering from non-chlamydial, non-gonococcal acute epididymitis, together with a rise in the titre of antibody and response to tetracycline therapy (Jalil *et al.*, 1988) seem sufficient to incriminate the organisms and suggest that they may cause this disease occasionally. Although ureaplasmas have been associated with altered sperm motility, specimens from fertile and infertile subjects contain the organisms with similar frequency and the results of antibiotic trials are not in favour of ureaplasmas alone causing male infertility (Taylor-Robinson, 1986). In view of the role of ureaplasmas in NGU, it would not be surprising to find that they were involved in sexually acquired reactive arthritis (SARA). Stimulation of synovial mononuclear cells from some SARA patients by ureaplasmal antigens (Ford *et al.*, 1980; Ford, 1986) is consistent with such involvement, but the notion needs stronger support.

URINARY INFECTION AND CALCULI

M. hominis, frequent in the lower urogenital tract, has been isolated from the upper urinary tract only of patients with symptoms of acute pyelonephritis, often accompanied by an antibody response (Thomsen, 1978a, b). This has not been accomplished recently but, nevertheless, *M. hominis* is thought to cause probably about 5% of such cases, obstruction or instrumentation of the urinary tract being predisposing factors. No evidence has accrued to suggest that ureaplasmas are involved in the same way. However, the fact that they produce urease, induce crystallization of struvite and calcium phosphates in urine when introduced experimentally (Grenabo *et al.*, 1988) and stimulate the formation of calculi in animal models (Texier-Maugein *et al.*, 1987) raises the question of whether they cause calculi in the human urinary tract. In this regard, the occurrence of ureaplasmas more often in the urine and calculi of patients with infection stones than in those with metabolic stones (Grenabo *et al.*,1988) suggests that they may have a causal role, but the question is not settled.

REPRODUCTIVE TRACT DISEASE AND SEQUELAE IN WOMEN

M. hominis organisms and, to a lesser extent, ureaplasmas are found in much larger numbers in the vagina of women who have bacterial vaginosis than in healthy women (Taylor-Robinson and Munday, 1988). The significance of such increased numbers is hard to assess in view of the profusion of various bacteria, but they may contribute to the pathogenesis of the condition. Likewise, it is not inconceivable that ureaplasmas contribute to the development of the urethral syndrome, but evidence that they do so is weak (Schiefer and Weidner, 1990).

M. hominis is a likely cause of pelvic inflammatory disease (PID), although the proportion of cases attributable to it is probably small. It has been isolated from the endometrium, and from the Fallopian tubes of about 10% of Swedish women with acute salpingitis diagnosed by laparoscopy (Mardh and Westrom, 1970), some of whom had significant specific antibody responses. Comparable observations have been made in the United Kingdom (Munday et al., 1987; Stacey et al., 1992). Ureaplasmas have also been isolated directly from affected Fallopian tubes, but the absence of antibody responses and failure to produce salpingitis in subhuman primates makes them a much less likely cause of disease (Taylor-Robinson and Munday, 1988; Stacey et al., 1992). M. genitalium has been shown to occur, by use of the PCR, in the lower genital tract of women attending a sexually transmitted disease clinic (Palmer et al., 1991b). Thus, the possibility exists that this mycoplasma could cause PID. However, such a role for M. genitalium suggested by some serological data (Moller et al., 1984) needs a great deal more support. The minor part that M. hominis plays in PID makes its role, if any, in infertility inevitably small and somewhat speculative. The notion that ureaplasmas, by themselves, may be a cause of involuntary infertility was first raised more than 20 years ago, but none of the observations made subsequently (Taylor-Robinson, 1986) has helped to consolidate the idea and convince the sceptics.

DISEASES ASSOCIATED WITH PREGNANCY AND THE NEWBORN

M. hominis and ureaplasmas have been isolated in large numbers, mainly as part of the flora of bacterial vaginosis, from the lower genital tract of women. This occurs significantly more often in women who experience preterm labour than in those who have normal births (Lamont et al., 1987) and bacterial vaginosis in early pregnancy has been shown to be a marker for preterm labour (Hay et al., 1993). Thus, a bacterial, including mycoplasmal, cause for the phenomenon is postulated. Further support comes from the isolation of M. hominis and ureaplasmas from the amniotic fluids of women with severe chorioamnionitis who had preterm labour (Cassell et al., 1983). In addition, ureaplasmas have been isolated from spontaneously aborted foetuses and stillborn or premature infants more frequently than from induced abortions or normal full-term infants. The ability to isolate ureaplasmas from the internal organs of aborted foetuses, together with some serological responses and an apparent diminished occurrence following antibiotic therapy, have supported a role for these organisms in abortion (Taylor-Robinson and Munday, 1988). Nevertheless, whether ureaplasmas are pathogenic on their own and whether abortion occurs because ureaplasmas invade the foetus to cause its death, or whether the foetus dies for some other reason and is then invaded are questions that remain unanswered. So, too, is the question of whether genital mycoplasmas, particularly ureaplasmas, cause low birth weight in otherwise normal infants. The association of ureaplasmas with low birth weight, seen by some (Kass et al., 1986), is supported by serological data and by a study in which women given erythromycin in the third trimester delivered larger babies than those given a placebo (McCormack *et al.*, 1987). However, it has not been excluded that women who are predisposed to smaller babies for some reason are selectively colonised, and the possibility that ureaplasmas do not act alone but do so in conjunction with other microorganisms, perhaps as part of bacterial vaginosis, needs to be explored more fully. Although there is uncertainty surrounding this problem, ureaplasmas, in particular, appear to be involved in respiratory disease of very low birth-weight infants (Cassell *et al.*, 1988), and premature infants in some population groups are prone to invasion of the cerebrospinal fluid by both *M. hominis* and ureaplasmas within the first few days of life (Waites *et al.*, 1988). Meningitis may occur without sequelae or with damage leading to permanent handicaps.

Fever that occurs after an abortion or normal delivery appears to be caused by *M. hominis* occasionally (Taylor-Robinson and Munday, 1988). Thus, it has been isolated from the blood of about 10% of the aborting febrile women, half of them exhibiting an antibody response, but not from aborting afebrile women, nor from normal pregnant women. In addition, *M. hominis* has been recovered from the blood of about 5-10% of women experiencing fever after a normal birth, but seldom from the blood of afebrile women. Similar observations have been made for ureaplasmas (Eschenbach, 1986) and it seems that both microorganisms induce fever by causing endometritis although, again, disentangling what can be attributed to mycoplasmas alone from a plethora of bacteria is not straight-forward.

INFECTIONS IN IMMUNOCOMPROMISED PATIENTS

A small proportion of hypogammaglobulinaemic patients develop suppurative arthritis for which mycoplasmas, particularly those in the urogenital tract, are responsible, having been isolated repeatedly from the joints (Taylor-Robinson *et al.*, 1986). In some of the cases involving ureaplasmas, the arthritis has been associated with subcutaneous abscesses, persistent urethritis, and chronic urethrocystitis/cystitis. Although responding usually to tetracyclines, it has been known for the organisms and disease to persist for months or years despite treatment with various antibiotics, success being achieved only by coupling antibiotic therapy with the administration of ureaplasmal antibody of high titre. Septicaemia due to *M. hominis* has occurred after trauma and genitourinary manipulations and the mycoplasma has been found in brain abscesses and osteomyelitis, but haematogenous spread leading to septic arthritis, surgical wound infections and peritonitis seems to occur more often after organ transplantation and in other patients on immunosuppressive therapy (Madoff and Hooper, 1990). Particularly common are sternal wound infections caused by *M. hominis* in heart/lung transplant patients (Steffenson *et al.*, 1987). Furthermore, polyarthritis with recovery of both *M. hominis* and ureaplasmas has been seen in a kidney allograft patient on an immunosuppressive regime (Taylor-Robinson *et al.*, 1986). Evidence that strains of *M. fermentans* exist in the blood and internal organs of some patients suffering from the acquired immunodeficiency syndrome (AIDS) (Lo *et al.*, 1989; Montagnier *et al.*, 1990) has been confirmed (Katseni *et al.*, 1993). However, whether this mycoplasma or others have a role in the development of AIDS will be established only through continued careful investigation.

TREATMENT OF UROGENITAL MYCOPLASMAL INFECTIONS

Chlamydiae, even more than ureaplasmas and *M. genitalium*, are a cause of NGU, so that patients should receive a tetracycline which will inhibit all these microorganisms. However, at least 10% of the ureaplasmas are resistant to tetracyclines (Taylor-Robinson and Furr, 1986) so that patients who fail to respond to such therapy should then be treated with a six-week course of erythromycin to which most tetracycline-resistant ureaplasmas are sensitive and to which *M. genitalium*-positive patients with chronic disease are likely to respond. A tetracycline should also be included for the treatment of PID so that chlamydiae and *M. hominis* are covered. However, since an increasing proportion (≥20%) of *M. hominis* strains are resistant to tetracycline (Koutsky *et al.*, 1983), other antibiotics, such as lincomycin or clindamycin, may need to be considered. Fever following abortion or childbirth often settles within a few days, but if it does not do so, tetracycline therapy should be started, while, at the same time, keeping tetracycline resistance in mind. It is premature to think of antibiotic therapy for AIDS patients until the role of putative mycoplasmal infections has been properly defined.

REFERENCES

Cassell, G. H., Davis, R. O., Waites, K. B., Brown, M.B., Mariott, P. A., Stagno, S. and Davis, J. K. (1983) Isolation of *Mycoplasma hominis* and *Ureaplasma urealyticum* from amniotic fluid at 16-20 weeks of gestation: potential effect on outcome of pregnancy. Sex. Transm. Dis. Suppl. 10:294-302.

Cassell, G. H., Waites, K. B., Crouse, D. T., Rudd, P. T., Canupp, K. C., Stagno, S. and Cutter, G. R. (1988) Association of *Ureaplasma urealyticum* infection of the lower respiratory tract with chronic lung disease and death in very low-birth-weight infants. Lancet ii, 240-245.

Doble, A., Thomas, B. J., Furr, P. M., Walker, M. M., Harris, J. R. W., Witherow, R. O'N. and Taylor-Robinson, D. (1989) A search for infectious agents in chronic abacterial prostatitis using ultrasound guided biopsy. Brit. J. Urol. 64:297-301.

Eschenbach, D. A. (1986) *Ureaplasma urealyticum* as a cause of postpartum fever. Pediatr. Infect. Dis. Suppl. 5:258-261.

Ford, D. K. (1986) Synovial lymphocyte responses show that ureaplasmas cause sexually transmitted reactive arthritis. Pediatr. Infect. Dis. Suppl. 5:353.

Ford, D.K., da Roza D. M., Shah, P. and Wenman, W. M. (1980) Cell-mediated immunoresponses of synovial mononuclear cells in Reiter's syndrome against ureaplasmal and chlamydial antigens. J. Rheumotol. 7:751-755.

Grenabo, L., Hedelin, H. and Pettersson, S. (1988) Urinary infection stones caused by *Ureaplasma urealyticum*: a review. Scand. J. Infect. Dis. Suppl. 53:46-49.

Hay, P. E., Lamont, R. F., Taylor-Robinson, D., Morgan, D. J., Ison, C. and Pearson, J. (1993) Abnormal bacterial colonisation of the genital tract as a marker for subsequent preterm delivery and late miscarriage. Brit. Med. J. (In press).

Horner, P. J. , Gilroy, C. B. Thomas, B. J., Naidoo, O. and Taylor Robinson, D. (1993) The association of Mycoplasma genitalium with acute non-gonococcal urethritis. Lancet. (In press).

Jalil, N., Doble, A., Gilchrist, C. and Taylor-Robinson, D. (1988) Infection of the epididymis by *Ureaplasma urealyticum*. Genitourin. Med. 64:367-368.

Kass, E. H., Lin, J.-S. and McCormack, W. M. (1986) Low birth weight and maternal colonization with genital mycoplasmas. Pediatr. Infect. Dis. Suppl. 5:279-281.

Katseni, V. L., Gilroy, C. B., Ryait, B.K., Ariyoshi, K., Bieniasz, P.D., Weber, J. N. and Taylor-Robinson, D. (1993) *Mycoplasma fermentans* in individuals seropositive and seronegative for HIV-1. Lancet 341:271-273.

Koutsky, L. A., Stamm, W. E., Brunham, R. C., Stevens, C. E., Cole, B., Hale, J., Davick, P. and Holmes, K. K. (1983) Persistence of *Mycoplasma hominis* after therapy: importance of tetracycline resistance and of coexisting vaginal flora. Sex. Transm. Dis. Suppl. 10:374-381.

Lamont, R. F., Taylor-Robinson, D., Wigglesworth, J. S., Furr, P. M., Evans, R. T. and Elder. M. G. (1987) The role of mycoplasmas, ureaplasmas and chlamydiae in the genital tract of women presenting in spontaneous early preterm labour. J. Med. Microbiol. 24:253-257.

Lo, S.-C., Dawson, M. S., Wong, D. M., Newton, P. B. III, Sonoda, M. A., Engler, W. F., Wang, R. Y.-H., Shih, J. W. K., Alter, H. J. and Wear, D. (1989) Identification of *Mycoplasma incognitus* infection in patients with AIDS: an immuno-histochemical, *in situ* hybridization and ultrastructural study. Amer. J. Trop. Med., Hyg. 41:601-616.

Madoff, S. and Hooper, D. C. (1990) Nongenitourinary tract infections in adults caused by *Mycoplasma hominis*: a review in: "Recent Advances in Mycoplasmology" (Stanek, G., Cassell, G. H., Tully, J. G. and Whitcomb, R. F., Eds.), pp. 373-378. Gustav Fischer Verlag, Stuttgart.

Mardh, P.-A. and Westrom, L. (1970) Tubal and cervical cultures in acute salpingitis with special reference to *Mycoplasma hominis* and T-strain mycoplasmas. Brit. J. Vener. Dis. 46:179-186.

McCormack, W. M., Rosner, B., Lee, Y.-H., Munoz, A., Charles, D. and Kass, E. H. (1987) Effect on birth weight of erythromycin treatment of pregnant women. Obstet. Gynecol. 69:202-207.

Moller, B. R., Taylor-Robinson, D. and Furr, P. M. (1984) Serological evidence implicating *Mycoplasma genitalium* in pelvic inflammatory disease. Lancet i, 1102-1103.

Montagnier, L., Berneman, D., Guetard, D., Blanchard, A., Chamaret, S., Rame, V., van Tietschoten, J., Mabrouk, K. and Bahraoui, E. (1990) Inhibition de l'infectiosite de souches prototypes due VIH par des anticorps diriges contre une sequence peptidique de mycoplasme. C.R. Acad. Sci., Paris, 311:425-430.

Munday, P. E., Stacey, C. M., Ison, C. A., Thomas, B. J. and Taylor-Robinson, D. (1987) Clinical and microbiological investigation of women with acute salpingitis and their consorts. Brit. J. Obstet. Gynaecol. 94:281-282.

Palmer, H. M., Gilroy, C. B., Furr, P. M. and Taylor-Robinson, D. (1991a) Development and evaluation of the polymerase chain reaction to detect *Mycoplasma genitalium*. FEMS Microbiol. Lett. 77:199-204.

Palmer, H. M., Gilroy, C. B., Claydon, E. J. and Taylor-Robinson, D. (1991b) Detection of *Mycoplasma genitalium* in the genitourinary tract of women by the polymerase chain reaction. Int. J. STD and AIDS 2:261-263.

Schiefer, H. G. and Weidner, W. (1990) Urethral syndrome in women: aetiologic and cytologic studies, in: "Recent Advances in Mycoplasmology" (Stanek, G., Cassell, G. H., Tully, J. G. and Whitcomb, R. F., Eds.), pp. 756-757, Gustav Fischer Verlag, Stuttgart

Stacey, C. M., Munday, P. E., Taylor-Robinson, D., Thomas, B. J., Gilchrist, C., Ruck, F., Isoon, C. A. and Beard, R. W. (1992). A longitudinal study of pelvic inflammatory disease. Brit. J. Obstet. Gynaecol. 99:994-999.

Steffensen, D. O., Dummar, J. S., Granick, M. S., Pasculle, A. W., Griffith, B. P. and Cassell, G H. (1987) Sternotomy infections with *Mycoplasma hominis.* Ann. Intern. Med. 106:204-208.

Stimson, J. B., Hale, J., Bowie, W. R. and Holmes, K. K. (1981) Tetracycline resistant *Ureaplasma urealyticum*: a cause of persistent nongonococcal urethritis. Ann. Intern. Med. 94:192-194.

Taylor-Robinson, D. (1985) Mycoplasmal and mixed infections of the human male urogenital tract and their possible complications, in: "The Mycoplasma", Vol. 4 (Razin, S. and Barile, M. F., Eds.) pp. 27-63. Academic Press, New York.

Taylor-Robinson, D. (1986) Evaluation of the role of *Ureaplasma urealyticum* in infertility. Pediatr. Infect. Dis. Suppl. 5:262-265.

Taylor-Robinson, D. and Furr, P. M. (1986) Clinical antibiotic resistance of *Ureaplasma urealyticum.* Pediatr. Infect. Dis. Suppl. 5:335-337.

Taylor-Robinson, D. and Munday, P. E. (1988) Mycoplasmal infection of the female genital tract and its complications, in:" Genital Tract Infection in Women" (Hare, M. J., Ed.), pp. 228-247. Churchill Livingstone, Edinburgh.

Taylor-Robinson, D., Furr, P. M. and Webster, A. D. B. (1986) *Ureaplasma urealyticum* in the immunocompromised host. Pediatr. Infect. Dis. Suppl. 5:236-238.

Texier-Maugein, J., Clerc, M., Vekris, A. and Bébéar, C. (1987) *Ureaplasma urealyticum*-induced bladder stones in rats and their prevention by flurofamide and doxycycline. Isr. J. Med. Sci. 23:565-567.

Thomsen, A. C. (1978a) Occurrence of mycoplasmas in urinary tracts of patients with acute pyelonephritis. J. Clin. Microbiol. 8: 84-88.

Thomsen, A. D. (1978b) Mycoplasmas in human pyelonephritis: demonstration of antibodies in serum and urine. J. Clin. Microbiol. 8:197-202.

Waites, K. B., Rudd, P. T., Crouse, D. T., Canupp, K. C., Nelson, K.G., Ramsey, C. and Cassell, G. H. (1988) Chronic *Ureaplasma urealyticum* and *Mycoplasma hominis* infections of central nervous system in preterm infants. Lancet ii, 17-21,

MYCOPLASMA INFECTIONS OF MAN:
RESPIRATORY AND MALE GENITAL TRACT DISEASES

Helmut Brunner

Institut für Chemotherapie, Bayer AG
Wuppertal, Germany

INTRODUCTION

Mycoplasmas are of major importance in many diseases of animals. In addition, *Mycoplasma pneumoniae* is a frequent cause of respiratory tract infections of man. *Mycoplasma hominis* and *Ureaplasma urealyticum* are involved in infections of the urogenital tract and *M. fermentans* appears to cause disease as a facultative pathogenic organism in patients with the Acquired Immuno-Deficiency Syndrome (AIDS).

MYCOPLASMA PNEUMONIAE

The illness. The disease, caused by *M. pneumoniae* in the respiratory tract, has been extensively studied and described (Denny *et al.*, 1971; Murphy *et al.*, 1981; Putman *et al.*, 1975)). Most persons are infected several times with *Mycoplasma pneumoniae* during the 70 to 80 years of their average lifetime. The majority of infected individuals does not suffer from any symptoms. Sometimes a mild, self-limiting disease of the upper respiratory tract is apparent. Approximately, one tenth of the infected persons present the clinical syndrome of primary atypical pneumonia to the physician.

The pneumonia caused by *M. pneumoniae* has been designated "primary atypical" to distinguish it from the "typical" pneumonia, caused by *Streptococcus pneumoniae*, the pneumococcus. The difference is obvious during the clinical course, which is more acute and severe in pneumococcal pneumonia, compared to the mild onset and benign nature of *M. pneumoniae* disease.

This is also reflected on X-ray films. A confluent dense shadow is usually seen in pneumococcal infections, whereas patchy infiltrates occur in *M. pneumoniae* lung involvement. Sometimes *M. pneumoniae* disease appears

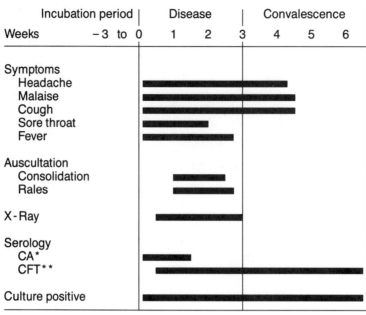

	Incubation period	Disease	Convalescence
Weeks	− 3 to 0	1 2 3	4 5 6

*CA : Coldagglutinins   **CFT : Complement fixation test

Figure 1. Natural course of mycoplasmal pneumonia

as a bronchitis only but, in many cases, a surprising discrepancy exists between the mildness of the clinical symptoms and the rather extended, yet scattered, infiltrates seen on chest X-rays of persons with *M. pneumoniae* disease. In the military community, where *M. pneumoniae*-induced inflammation of the lung can occur frequently, the term "walking pneumonia" has been used.

After an incubation period of approximately two to three weeks, similar to virus-infections, and unlike pneumococcal pneumonia, the disease starts with uncharacteristic symptoms (Fig.1). The illness might last for several weeks. It is usually mild, but can require bed rest. This means a loss of working days and, thus, suffering of the patient and a financial burden for society.

Complications. In addition, complications from other organs have been reported (Table 1). The etiology of these complications remains largely unsolved. Autoimmune reactions have been discussed but, in most cases, the connection with *M. pneumoniae* infections is unclear (Assaad *et al.*, 1980; Biberfeld, 1979; Pönkä, 1980)

Epidemiology. A detailed definition of the epidemiology of *M. pneumoniae* disease has emerged (Chanock et al., 1967; Foy, et al., 1979; Lind and Bentzon, 1976). The organisms account for 15 to 20% of the total number of pneumonias. The attack rate is low. Therefore, the disease spreads slowly in communities with close contact among their members (children at school, university students, military recruits). Transmission by droplets requires a rather high inoculum unless the host is immunocompromised.

Table 1.   Symptoms at non-respiratory organs in *M. pneumoniae* disease

Organ	Symptoms
Ear	Myringitis
CNS	Guillain-Barre-Syndrome Polyradiculitis Encephalitis Meningitis
Heart	Pericarditis
Intestinal tract	Pancreatitis
Skin	Stevens-Johnson-Syndrome
Blood	Haemolytic anaemia (Cold agglutinins)

The disease occurs worldwide with a higher incidence every four years (Lind and Bentzon, 1976; Noah, 1974; Niitu, 1985). This pattern is changing in countries with an increase in the number of children in day care centers as, *e.g.,* shown by Lind and Bentzon for Denmark (Lind and Bentzon, 1990). Under these conditions, the four year period changes into a more continuous occurrence of the disease over the years.

The age distribution of *M. pneumoniae* disease also follows a certain pattern with the highest frequency in school age and in young adults (5-20 years).

This has been explained by the fact that the first contact with *M. pneumoniae* usually occurs when children enter school. This high rate of occurrence continues during a time when susceptible persons are together during school and at the university. It ends when a sufficiently powerful immune response has developed which protects the majority of adults. During later years, reinfections booster the immune system and the disease becomes apparent, usually with mild symptoms only.

An interesting finding is in disagreement with these rather logical conclusions. *M. pneumoniae* has been isolated from healthy children less than five years of age with similar frequency as from children with respiratory tract symptoms. In a study performed from 1965 to 1968 in the Washington (DC) area, *M. pneumoniae* was recovered from 3% of 1,149 children less than five years of age who were free of respiratory tract disease (J. Canchola, H. W. Kim, C. D. Brandt, R. H. Parrott, and R. M. Chanock, unpublished observations). The frequency of recovery of *M. pneumoniae* from infants and preschool children with respiratory tract disease was 3.1%, *i.e.,* almost identical to that in the group free of respiratory tract disease (3%). This means that many children less than five years of age are infected at a susceptible age, but they do not develop disease. However, the most interesting question, whether healthy

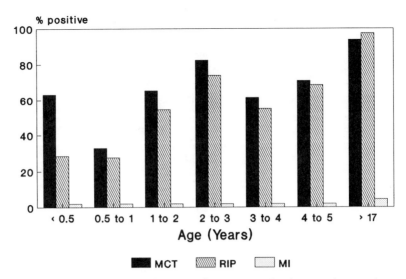

Figure 2. Age distribution of serum-antibodies as detected by various techniques (MCT: Mycoplasmacidal Test; RIP: Radioimmunoprecipitation test; MI: Metabolism inhibition test)

children possess serum antibodies to *M. pneumoniae*, remained unanswered. Complement-fixation (CF) and metabolism-inhibition (MI) tests, the conventional techniques, failed to detect antibodies in sera of children less than five years of age, but antibodies could be detected using more sensitive procedures such as the complement dependent mycoplasmacidal test (MCT) first described by Gale and Kenny (1970) and the radioimmunoprecipitation test, RIP (Brunner and Chanock, 1973a). MCT and RIP are considerably more sensitive than CF or MI for detection of antibodies to *M. pneumoniae*. Both tests use whole cells of *M. pneumoniae* as the antigen.

Antibodies, most likely of maternal origin, were detected by MCT and RIP during the first six month of life (Fig. 2). The rate of positive sera increased already during the second year. As expected, most adults possessed serum antibodies to *M. pneumoniae*. It was also of interest whether adults who are susceptible to *M. pneumoniae* possess serum antibodies. More than two thirds of individuals who later developed *M. pneumoniae* lung infiltrates had antibodies before exposure to the organisms (Fig. 2). These observations led to the hypothesis by us and Fernald *et al.*, that disease caused by *M. pneumoniae* might be, in part, immunologically determined in a host sensitized by one or more silent infections (Brunner *et al.*, 1973b; Fernald and Clyde, 1974). There was some support for this hypothesis in the volunteer study by Smith *et al.* (1967). Volunteers, who had received a killed *M. pneumoniae* vaccine and failed to develop metabolism-inhibiting (MI) antibodies in serum, exhibited a tendency towards more severe disease after challenge with the wild-type organism than did unvaccinated individuals. In recent years, animal experiments in our group and by Jacobs *et al.* (Brunner, 1980; Jacobs, 1988) have mounted further evidence in support of this hypothesis. Repeated inoculations of *M. pneumoniae* led to more extended infiltrates, which indicated a more pronounced immune response. A classical sensitization, *i.e.*, IgE-antibodies, have not as yet been demonstrated.

Clearly the findings are not conclusive to validate the sensitization-hypothesis. Antibodies to *M. pneumoniae*, measured by MCT and RIP, could be blocked not only by *M. pneumoniae* lipids, but also by lipid-extracts from vegetables (parsnip or carrots) or from *Staphylococcus aureus* and *Streptococcus pyogenes* group A (Greenberg *et al.*, 1973). It has been shown previously that the carbohydrate-chains of *M. pneumoniae* glycolipids can cross react with similar structures on other bacteria (Streptococcus MG, *Streptococcus pneumoniae*) or with those of cell surface markers such as cytolipin H or the I-antigen of human erythrocytes, but the spatial presentation, density, accessibility and binding affinities of haptenic groups may be different (Greenberg *et al.*, 1973; Marmion *et al.*, 1967; Allen and Prescott, 1978; Plackett *et al.*, 1969; Costea *et al.*, 1971).

It is possible that the antibodies detected in sera of healthy persons had been induced by related antigens, *e,g.*, cross reactive glycolipids, present in vegetables or other bacteria. The antibodies detected by sensitive methods might be meaningless as far as the hypothesis of sensitization is concerned. On the other hand, sensitization might be mediated by antibodies elicited by related, but not homologous, immunogens.

Pathogenesis. Because *M. pneumoniae* disease is rarely fatal, animal models have been developed to study the pathogenic potential of the organisms. Golden Syrian hamsters and guinea pigs have proved to be especially susceptible to *M. pneumoniae* disease (Dajani *et al.*, 1965; Brunner *et al.*, 1973c; Brunner *et al.*, 1973d). Hamsters are more suitable than guinea pigs, when the lung histopathology has to be studied because uninfected hamsters do not, like guinea pigs, exhibit lymphatic follicles in their lung tissue.

After intranasal inoculation of *M. pneumoniae*, the exudate in the bronchi of hamsters and guinea pigs contains polymorphonuclear neutrophils (PMN) and a few lymphocytes, whereas unlike in pneumococcal pneumonia, the infiltrates surrounding bronchi and blood vessels are mainly composed of lymphocytes, a few PMNs and some macrophages. Fluorescent antisera directed specifically against *M. pneumoniae* show antigenic material on the surface of the bronchial wall, but also in deeper layers of the epithelium and the submucosa of bronchi. This indicates that dead mycoplasmas are carried to the blood vessels. *M. pneumoniae* has never been cultivated from the blood stream or any organ other than the lung and the upper respiratory tract of animals. In man, such isolations have been reported in immunocompromised patients (Clyde *et al.*, 1990).

Host response. A low to moderate level of antibodies to *M. pneumoniae* detected by CF and MI in serum is not sufficient for resistance of the host against disease. Only high serum antibody titers are correlated with protection, but antibodies in local secretions of the respiratory tract have been shown to be related to resistance towards *M. pneumoniae* disease in men (Biberfeld and Sterner, 1968; Brunner *et al.*, 1973e). Serum antibody titers might merely be a concomitant reaction. At a certain time during the course of the disease, local

Table 2. Relationship of pre-existing antibodies to *M. pneumoniae* in nasal secretions and serum to resistance against subsequent disease.

Nasal IgA-antibody titer	Serum MI-antibody titer		
	<1:8	>1:8	sum
<1:3a	9/18	7/12	16/30 (53%)
>1:3	5/6	9/9	14/16 (88%)*
sum	14/24 (58%)	16/21 (76%)	

* p=0.02, Fisher's exact probability test
a) level of detectability

immunity might already be reduced, permitting recurrent illness after reinfection, while serum antibodies are still present.

Second attacks of *M. pneumoniae* lung disease occur. In studies on local immunity after infection with *M. pneumoniae*, it has been shown that 28 of 67 (42%) persons developed a threefold or greater rise in IgA-antibody-titers to the organisms in nasal secretions as measured by RIP and 49 of 67 (73%) in sputum (Brunner *et al.*, 1973e). Significant protection to subsequent disease was correlated with pre-existing local antibodies (titer greater than 1:3) but not with pre-existing serum antibodies (titer of 1:8 or greater) (Table 2).

Furthermore, autoimmune reactions due to antibodies are possible in *M. pneumoniae* infection. Cold agglutinins observed in 50% of the sera of patients with *M. pneumoniae* infections are such antibodies. They are directed against the I-antigen on erythrocytes. Cold agglutinins can be considered type II antibodies (cytotoxic antibodies) as classified by Gell and Coombs, *i.e.*, antibodies cross reactive with body tissue. It appears to be of great importance to investigate the role of "Tumor Necrosis Factor (TNF)" and other cytokines for protection against *M. pneumoniae* infection, because it has been shown that cells of the immune system respond to mycoplasmas by the release of TNF (Lin *et al.*, 1988). This cytokine may be involved in the elimination of mycoplasmas or in the induction of disease via the inflammatory response.

Diagnosis. The term "atypical" for the symptoms of disease can be replaced by the designation "nonspecific", because the clinical course cannot provide the physician with clear evidence for the etiology. Some helpful clinical information is given in Table 3. Viruses, chlamydia, common bacteria, or rickettsiae can cause chest involvement indistinguishable from mycoplasmal pneumonia. Ideally, the organism causing the infection should be identified early by the microbiological laboratory initiating specific treatment.

Conventional microbiological techniques are at present too slow and therefore unable to help the physician to clarify the etiology of atypical pneumonia in a single case and thus cannot provide the basis for proper chemo-

Table 3.   Information helpful for clinical diagnosis of *M. pneumoniae* pneumonia

> Epidemic year or season?
> Pneumonia with:
> -no apparently severe condition
> in spite of high fever and severe cough
> -no leukocytosis
> -occurrence of pneumonia in the family
> -enlargement of hilar lymph nodes
> -ear inflammation
> -no effect of β-lactam antibiotics
> -persistent cough

therapy (Table 4), but the diagnosis helps, of course, to clarify the epidemiological situation, *i.e.*, etiology for infections of contact persons of the index case and for information of the frequency of mycoplasma infections in general.

The microscopy of clinical specimens does not reveal stainable organisms with a definite structure. *M. pneumoniae* is pleomorphic and cannot be stained by standard methods. *M. pneumoniae* appears in electron microscopy as a multistructured organism which often forms filaments in fluid medium and at an early growth stadium on agar. The filaments frequently project in a special organelle, the tip, which mediates attachment of the organisms to host cells and to glass or plastic surfaces. (The molecular biology of attachment is summarized by Dr. E. Jacobs in this volume).

The pleomorphism is possible because the organisms are not surrounded by a rigid cell wall. This appearance hampers their visibility in the gram stain or other microscopic techniques, except in electron microscopy (Table 4). In fluid medium, the filamentous organisms form aggregates (clumps, spherules) which develop into colonies on agar. At an early growth phase, colonies do not show the classical fried egg appearance.

A procedure which has proved to be quite useful for rapid diagnosis of *M. pneumoniae* infection is the cover-slip chamber culture, first described by Bredt *et al.* (1975). This method is based on the filamentous appearance of *M. pneumoniae* under natural conditions together with the ability of the organisms to adhere to glass. These features permit the experienced microbiologist to identify *M. pneumoniae* with certainty. The authors were able to detected *M. pneumoniae* in the cover-slip chamber despite the presence of debris, epithelial cells and dead bacteria or bacteria inhibited by the presence of antibiotics used in the mycoplasma growth medium. Depending on the number of organisms present in the clinical specimens, a positive result could be obtained as early as 48 h after inoculation of the cover-slip chamber (E. Jacobs, Freiburg, personal communication). This is of great advantage as compared to the culture procedure, which reveals visible colonies not before 10 to 21 days after inoculation of the specimen onto agar plates. Unless modern technology, *i.e.*, gene probes, polymerase chain reaction (PCR) or immunological methods (capture-ELISA) become available, the cover-slip technique is a rather rapid, yet simple method for identification of *M. pneumoniae*.

Table 4. Validity of conventional methods for the laboratory diagnosis of *M. pneumoniae* disease

Microscopy
-Light-microscopy: not relevant
-Electron-microscopy: not feasible

Cultivation
-Growth on agar requires 2 to 3 weeks

Serology
-Cold agglutinins (not specific)
-Complement-fixation test (Requires two to three weeks for four-fold or greater titer rise)

A most peculiar and for diagnostic purposes useful feature of *M. pneumoniae* is its ability to form a confluent sheet of organisms on glass or plastic surfaces (Somerson *et al.*, 1965). This ability has considerably facilitated the purification of the organisms from media components, because the glass-adherent mycoplasmas can be washed vigorously to remove serum components of the growth medium sticking to the organisms. Tips are also exposed at the surface of a colony (Brunner *et al.*, 1979). This facilitates the identification of *M. pneumoniae*, because host cells attach to colonies on agar (Sobeslavsky *et al.*, 1968). For this purpose, red blood cells of sheep, guinea pigs, chickens or man have been employed. Since a number of other mycoplasma species can be isolated from the human respiratory tract, erythrocyte adherence is a simple way to identify *M. pneumoniae* colonies (Table 5). Colonies covered with erythrocytes can be easily visualized in the light-microscope by the classical fried egg appearance. A second possibility to identify *M. pneumoniae* colonies is epifluorescence with the use of either labelled specific antisera to the organisms or indirect fluorescence by employing labelled antiserum to the animal immuno-globulin used as the initial specific antibody to *M. pneumoniae* (DelGiudice *et al.*, 1967).

M. pneumoniae was first cultivated in 1962 by Chanock, Hayflick and Barile in a medium containing 20% horse serum and 10% fresh yeast extract (Chanock *et al.*, 1962). Even on this enriched medium, *M. pneumoniae* grows slowly. Colonies become visible microscopically two to three weeks after inoculation on agar medium. In a recent study, Kenny *et al.* showed that the sensitivity of either culture or serology was approximately 66% when the other method was set as the reference (Kenny *et al.*, 1990). Cultivation can be performed directly on agar or in a diphasic medium,*e.g.*, SP4, as recommended by Tully *et al.* (1979). Specimens should be inoculated directly in diphasic medium or on agar. For this purpose, growth medium should be freshly prepared and given directly to the physician, *e.g.*, as SP4 medium.

Agar plates can be observed once or twice weekly by using a 25 to 50-fold magnification. The plates should be viewed from the bottom through the agar without opening the lid of the plate. In diphasic medium, both a color change of the pH-indicator and spherules, *i.e.*, small colony-like aggregates can be seen. Cultures (plates or diphasic media) should not be discarded as negative before the 56th day of incubation at 37oC, especially if the plates have

Table 5.   Mycoplasmas recovered from the human respiratory tract

M. pneumoniae
M. hominis
M. salivarium
M. orale
M. buccale
M. faucium
M. genitalium
M. lipophilum
Ureaplasma urealyticum

been removed from the incubator to look for colonies at various times during incubation. This latter procedure slows down the growth.

It is critical to add 10% fresh yeast extract and 20% horse serum to the medium in order to obtain good culture results for *M. pneumoniae*.   The quality of all new media components, especially the basal medium, the horse serum and the fresh yeast extract, is strongly recommended. This should be performed by inoculating stored specimens from persons known to be positive for *M. pneumoniae* into media prepared using newly purchased media components.

Sensitive detection of *M. pneumoniae* infection in hamsters has been demonstrated by Bernet *et al.* using the polymerase chain reaction (PCR) (Bernet *et al*, 1989). The authors found: "PCR was more sensitive and more reproducible than the culture method and the PCR was completely unaffected by bacterial contamination." The detection limit of the PCR was 100 to 1,000 CFU. DNA probes were reported to detect 1,000 to 100,000 CFU. Culture can theoretically detect one organism after an incubation time of two to three weeks, whereas the PCR can provide information within two to three hours. Furthermore, direct and indirect antigen capture enzyme-immunoassays (Ag-EIA) have been developed for the detection of *M. pneumoniae* in clinical specimens by Kok (Kok, Varkanis and Marmion, 1988). Antigen was detected in some specimens which were culture negative. The Ag-EIA had a detection limit of 10,000 to 30,000 CFU/ml of sample.

All tests (PCR, DNA probes, Ag-EIA) appear to be specific. The Ag-EIA detected about 90% of specimens that were also positive by culture, but serological examination for specific IgM-antibodies was necessary in addition to the Ag-EIA in order to provide complete diagnostic coverage. Madsen *et al.* have used an immunoblot assay and a monoclonal antibody to a 43 kD membrane associated protein of *M. pneumoniae* (Madsen *et al.*, 1987). They calculated that the detection limit of their assay was 3,000 CFU.

Collier and Clyde found 100 to 1 million (geom. mean:12,600) CFU/ml in sputa of patients, naturally infected with *M. pneumoniae* (Collier and Clyde, 1974). All other methods detect dead organisms, whereas culture only detects living mycoplasmas. It is clear from the studies of Grayston *et al.* that only 50-64% of samples from the upper respiratory tract of patients with *M. pneumoniae* infection are culture positive, *i.e.*, there is a significant group with good serological evidence of current infection which is culture negative

(Kok, Varkanis and Marmion, 1988; Madsen *et al.*, 1987; Grayson, Foy and Kenny, 1969). The direct detection methods, therefore, have to be assessed against the standard of serological response as well as against culture of the organisms.

The existence of a substantial group of serologically positive, Ag-EIA negative cases means that the Ag-EIA cannot be the sole diagnostic test used for diagnosis of *M. pneumoniae* infection. A recently developed hybridization assay for a specific rRNA sequence(s) has been compared with the Ag-EIA (Harris *et al.*, 1988). Both tests proved to be highly specific. The protein and glycolipid antigens of the organism may have a better survival potential in the respiratory tract than the rRNA, once the organisms are damaged by immune reactions or antibiotics and membrane integrity is lost with access of nucleases to the rRNA target.

Therapy. Appropriate antimycoplasmal chemotherapy often results in the improvement of symptoms, but the organisms are frequently shed from the respiratory tract for months after clinical cure (Smith *et al.*, 1967; Slotkin, Clyde and Denny, 1967; Brunner and Weidner, 1981). This observation would be explainable if the levels of the antimicrobial agents at the site of the infection were below the minimal inhibitory concentration (MIC) for the organisms. Bergogne-Berezin determined the levels of antimicrobial agents in bronchial secretions (Bergogne-Berezin, 1981). The levels are well within or above the range of the MIC of the antibiotics for *M. pneumoniae*. The development of resistance of *M. pneumoniae* to erythromycin and other antibiotics has been reported (Niitu *et al.*, 1970; Niitu, Hasagawa and Kubota, 1974; Stopler, Gerichter and Branski, 1980). None of the patients treated with tetracycline developed resistance. Niitu *et al.* also reported that *M. pneumoniae* could be recovered for two to three months after clinically effective antibiotic therapy (Niitu, Hasagawa and Kubota, 1974).

Because the eradication of *M. pneumoniae* from the respiratory tract was not achieved, studies in animals had to be performed in order to elucidate the efficacy of therapy and the immune response after therapy (Brunner and Zeiler, 1985). One million CFU of the PI1428 strain of *M. pneumoniae* were inoculated intranasally. The organisms could be recovered for a long time from the upper respiratory tract and from the lungs of infected hamsters, whereas lung lesions peaked at 10 to 14 days after inoculation. Lung alterations were no longer observed three weeks after infection. The efficacy of three antimicrobial agents was studied: tetracycline-HCl, ciprofloxacin and erythromycin. The MIC for *M. pneumoniae* was determined according to Senterfit *et al.* : Tetracycline-HCl 0.5 mg/l, ciprofloxacin 0.5 mg/l, erythromycin 0.002 mg/l (Senterfit, 1983). Antimicrobial agents were administered from day one until day six after inoculation. Levels of antimicrobial agents in lung tissue of infected hamsters were above the MIC for *M. pneumoniae*. Nevertheless, organisms were still present at various time intervals after therapy using high doses of all antibiotics. Lung lesions, on the other hand, were reduced. These results are similar to those described in man (Smith *et al.*, 1967; Slotkin, Clyde and Denny, 1967).

The reasons for the persistence are unclear. As a working hypothesis we proposed that the immune response might be reduced by the chemotherapy (Brunner and Zeiler, 1990). Titers of serum antibodies were determined. Similar titers were finally reached in treated animals, but a few days later as compared to hamsters given placebo (Brunner and Zeiler, 1990). Sabato *et al.* had shown reduced lymphocyte function in children infected with *M. pneumoniae* (Sabato, Cooper and Thong, 1981). Similar findings could not be seen in hamsters during experimental *M. pneumoniae* infection (Brunner and Zeiler, 1990).

Two conclusions can be drawn from these results: First, systemic immune responses in hamsters appears not to be hampered during *M. pneumoniae* infection. Second, the hamster might not be the appropriate model to investigate immune responses to *M. pneumoniae*. Further studies on cell-mediated immune responses and chemotherapy are needed and the local immune response during and after chemotherapy of *M. pneumoniae* disease should be studied. Further reasons for the persistence must be discussed, *i.e.*, antigenic similarities between bacterium and host; adsorption of host material to the microorganisms which protect the bacterium by a coat of host proteins; and antigenic drift or shift of *M. pneumoniae* occurs which permits evasion from the host immune response.

Protection. It is known from hamster experiments that a primary infection with *M. pneumoniae* leads to rather long-lasting protection. This protection vanishes finally and reinfections connected with disease occur. Protection is correlated with a very high serum titer of metabolism-inhibiting antibodies, whereas a good correlation with protection has been shown between local antibodies in respiratory tract secretions and protection in man (Biberfeld and Sterner, 1968; Brunner *et al.*, 1973e). IgA-anti-bodies were demonstrated in secretions, but there were no IgG-antibodies.

Protection against challenge can clearly be shown in a reduction in the number of organisms in the lungs and in wash fluid of the upper respiratory tract in experimentally infected hamsters. Avirulent organisms, *e.g.*, ts-mutants, grow in the lungs but do not cause lesions (Brunner *et al.*, 1973d). Protection was achieved against virulent challenge but the mutants exhibited residual virulence (Brunner *et al.*, 1973d; Greenberg *et al.*, 1974). On the other hand, there was the finding that reinoculation in guinea pigs caused more extensive infiltrates, respectively, lesions (Brunner, 1980; Jacobs *et al.*, 1988). This could indicate a more extensive immune response in the lung, which leads to the patchy infiltrates in men seen on X-rays. These infiltrates are interpreted as lesions. Disease, on the other hand, might result from an acute inflammatory reaction. Foy *et al.* have reported the response of immuno-compromised persons to *M. pneumoniae* infection (Foy *et al.*, 1973). There was more severe disease, but minimal alterations were seen on lung X-rays.

Thus, in this rather complex and unclear situation, the question remains whether a vaccine against *M. pneumoniae* is desirable. Atypical pneumonia by *M. pneumoniae* is common in all countries. Ten percent of infected persons develop pneumonia. Very few of them exhibit autoimmune reactions, *e.g.*, hemolytic anemia, which very rarely leads to death. The disease is usually self-limiting. In a mild disease, such as *M. pneumoniae*- pneumonia, a vaccine without adverse reactions is mandatory. Certainly the vaccine should not induce any autoimmune reactions. It is doubtful that this is achievable. The availability of a rapid diagnostic method and a mycoplasma-cidal antibiotic are more pertinent goals than the development of a vaccine.

MYCOPLASMAS OF THE MALE UROGENITAL TRACT

INTRODUCTION

Mycoplasmas reside on the mucosal surface of the urogenital tract. They rarely penetrate into deeper tissue and are frequently commensals.*Ureaplasma urealyticum* is known to cause disease in males only (Shepard,1974; Bowie *et al.*, 1977; Taylor-Robinson and McCormack, 1980). Several other mycoplasma species can be isolated from the male urethra, especially *M. hominis* and, less frequently, *M. fermentans* and *M. genitalium*. This latter species has been suggested to be connected with nongonococcal urethritis (Tully *et al.*, 1981). If this holds true, the etiology of NGU has to be re-evaluated. Furthermore, *M. fermentans* has been connected with disease in patients with AIDS (Lo *et al.*, 1989a; Lo *et al.*, 1989b).

Nongonococcal urethritis (NGU)

NGU is the most frequently occurring sexually transmitted disease in industrialized countries. The etiology of NGU is rather clear. In half of the patients, the disease is caused by *Chlamydia trachomatis*. Thus, if C. *trachomatis* is isolated from urethral discharge, the etiologic diagnosis is clear and conclusions for treatment can easily be drawn. On the other hand, there is no doubt that ureaplasmas play a role in NGU. Shepard *et al.*, Bowie *et al*, and Taylor-Robinson *et al.* have demonstrated that *U. urealyticum* is involved in NGU (Shepard, 1974; Bowie *et al.*, 1977; Taylor-Robinson and McCormack, 1980), but up to 70% of healthy men harbor the organisms in their urethra. Thus, in an individual man with chlamydia-negative NGU, the search for the etiological diagnosis becomes a difficult task. In general, if these persons suffer from severe symptoms of inflammation, *i.e.*, discharge, in general, treatment is started with tetracyclines without proper diagnosis.

Colonization of the urethra with facultative pathogenic microorgan-isms is not unusual. Occasionally, these commensals cause disease. For a de-finite etiological diagnosis, three approaches have been attempted: 1) detection of antibody coated bacteria in urine or genital tract secretions; 2) quantitative determination of bacteria in urine and secretions; 3) detection of a serum anti-body response to a pathogen. The detection of a serum antibody response is usually too late even in *E. coli*-infection of the urinary tract and does not pro-vide reliable results at all in ureaplasma disease. Their size does not enable the search for antibody-coated ureaplasmas. Most reliable, useful and practical is, therefore, the quantitation of ureaplasmas.

Together with Weidner, Schiefer and Krauss in Giessen, we have quan-titated ureaplasmas and mycoplasmas in male genital tract secretions (Weid-ner *et al.*, 1982; Brunner, Weidner and Schiefer, 1983). In these studies, the pre-sence of 10,000 or more CFU/ml of urethral secretions and 1,000 or more CFU/ml of urine have been shown to be indicative of a significantly elevated number of ureaplasmas (Table 6). The study included 164 men with NGU.

Table 6.   Etiology of non-gonococcal urethritis and prostatitis

Disease	Etiologic agent	Proportion of patients*
1. Nongonococcal urethritis (NGU)	C. trachomatis U. urealyticum	ca. 50% ca. 30%
2. Acute bacterial prostatitis	E. coli other gram-negative bacteria and enterococci	ca. 80% ca. 20%
3. Chronic bacterial prostatitis (CBP)	common urinary tract pathogens as in ABP U. urealyticum	ca. 10% ca. 15%

*estimated

Approximately one-third fulfilled the quantitative criteria mentioned above. In these NGU patients, the duration of symptoms and the inflammatory response was also studied in addition to the application of quantitative culture procedures. Signs of inflammation were seen in three fourth of the patients with C. trachomatis and half of the patients with elevated numbers of U. urealyticum. All men with high numbers of U. urealyticum and those with positive culture for C. trachomatis were treated for two weeks with tetracycline. All men were cured after the end of the treatment, and the ureaplasmas had disappeared (Table 6).

Prostatitis. The localization technique, according to Meares and Stamey was used together with quantitation procedures to determine the etiology of prostatitis (Meares and Stamey, 1968). The diagnosis was rather easily obtained in patients with acute bacterial prostatitis (ABP). As can be seen in table 6, in 80% of these patients E. coli was the etiologic agent. The remaining 20% of ABP were caused by other gram-negative rods or enterococci.

The situation was entirely different in chronic bacterial prostatitis. Approximately 5-15 % of these diseases were caused by gram-negative bacteria as in ABP. The rest were uncertain. Using quantitative culture procedures, we provided evidence that in 15% of the patients with chronic prostatitis, the disease was caused by U. urealyticum (Table 6). It is therefore recommended using quantitative culture procedures for the etiological diagnosis in NGU and chronic prostatitis until less laborious, more sensitive, and/or faster procedures are available.

REFERENCES

Allen, P. Z. and Prescott, B., 1978, Immunochemical studies on a Mycoplasma pneumoniae polysaccharide fraction: cross-reactions with type 23 and 32 anti-pneumococcal rabbit sera. Infect. Immun., 20:421.

Assaad, F., Gispen, R., Kleemola, M., Syrucek, L. and Esteves, K., 1980, Neurological diseases associated with viral and *Mycoplasma pneumoniae* infections. Bull. WHO, 58: 297.

Bergogne-Berezin, E., 1981, Penetration of antibiotics into the respiratory tree. J. Antimicrob. Chemother., 8:171.

Bernet, C., Garret, M., DeBarbeyrac, B., Bébéar, C., Bonnet, J., 1989, Detection of *Mycoplasma pneumoniae* by using the polymerase chain reaction. J. Clin. Microbiol., 27:2492.

Biberfeld, G. and Sterner, G., 1968, Antibodies against *Mycoplasma pneumoniae* in bronchial secretions. Acta Pathol. Microbiol. Scand., 76:646.

Biberfeld, G., 1979, Autoimmune reactions associated with *Mycoplasma pneumoniae* infection. Zbl. Bakt. Hyg. I. Abt. Orig. A, 245:144.

Bowie, W. R., Wang, S. P., Alexander, E. R., Floyd, J., Forsyth, P. S., Pollock, H. M., Lin, J.-S. L., Buchanan, T. M., and Holmes, K. K., 1977, Etiology of nongonococcal urethritis. Evidence for *Chlamydia trachomatis* and *Ureaplasma urealyticum*. J. Clin. Invest., 59:735.

Bredt, W., Lam, W. and Berger, J., 1975, Evaluation of a microscopic method for rapid detection and identification of *Mycoplasma pneumoniae*. J. Clin. Microbiol., 2:541.

Brunner, H., Razin, S., Kalica, A. R. and Chanock, R. M., 1971, Lysis and death of *Mycoplasma pneumoniae* by antibody and complement. J. Immunol., 106:907.

Brunner, H., James, W. D., Horswood, R. L., and Chanock, R.M., 1972, Measurement of *Mycoplasma pneumoniae* mycoplasmacidal antibody in human serum. J. Immunol., 108:1491.

Brunner, H. and Chanock, R. M., 1973a, A radioimmunoprecipitation test for detection of *Mycoplasma pneumoniae* antibody. Proc. Soc. Exptl. Biol. Med., 143:97.

Brunner, H., Horswood, R. L., and Chanock, R. M., 1973b. More sensitive methods for detection of antibody to *Mycoplasma pneumoniae*. J. Infect. Dis., 127:S 52.

Brunner, H., James, W. D., Horswood, R. L. and Chanock, R. M., 1973c, Experimental *Mycoplasma pneumoniae* infection of young guinea pigs. J. Infect. Dis., 127: 315.

Brunner, H., Greenberg, H. B., James, W. D., Horswood, R. L. and Chanock, R.M., 1973d, Decreased virulence and protective effect of genetically stable temperature-sensitive mutants of *Mycoplasma pneumoniae*. Ann. N.Y. Acad. Sci., 225:436.

Brunner, H., Greenberg, H. B., James, W. D., Horswood, R. L., Couch, R. B. and Chanock, R. M., 1973e, Antibody to *Mycoplasma pneumoniae* in nasal secretions and sputa of experimentally infected human volunteers. Infect. Immun., 8:612.

Brunner, H., Prescott, B., Greenberg, H., James, W. D., Horswood, R.L. and Chanock, R. M., 1977, Unexpectedly high frequency of antibody to *Mycoplasma pneumoniae* in human sera as measured by sensitive techniques. J. Infect. Dis., 135:524.

Brunner, H., Krauss, H., Schaar, H. and Schiefer, H.-G., 1979, Electron microscopic studies on the attachment of *Mycoplasma pneumoniae* to guinea pig erythrocytes. Infect. Immun., 24:906.

Brunner, H., 1980, The role of the immune system in the lung histopathology of experimental infection with *Mycoplasma pneumoniae* (Abstr.). Fourth International Congress of Immunology, Paris.

Brunner, H. and Weidner W., 1981, Chemotherapy of human mycoplasma diseases. Isr. J. Med. Sci., 17:656.

Brunner, H., Weidner, W. and Schiefer, H. G., 1983, Studies on the role of *Ureaplasma urealyticum* and *Mycoplasma hominis* in prostatitis. J. Infect. Dis., 147:807.

Brunner, H. and Zeiler, H.-J., 1985, Efficacy of ciprofloxacin in *Mycoplasma pneumoniae* infection of hamsters. Current Clinical Practice Series, 34:77.

Brunner, H. and Zeiler, H-J., 1990, Chemotherapy of experimental *Mycoplasma pneumoniae* infection in hamsters and host response. in: "Recent Advances in Mycoplasmology" (G. Stanek, G. H. Cassell, J. G. Tully, R. F. Whitcomb, Eds.) Gustav Fischer Verlag, Stuttgart.

Chanock, R. M., Hayflick, L. and Barile, M. F., 1962, Growth on artificial medium of an agent associated with atypical pneumonia and its identification as a PPLO. Proc. Nat. Acad. Sci. U.S.A., 48:41.

Chanock, R. M., Fox, H. H., James, W. D., Gutekunst, R. R., White, R. J. and Senterfit, L. B., 1967, Epidemiology of *Mycoplasma pneumoniae* infection in military recruits. Ann. N.Y. Acad. Sci., 143:484.

Clyde, W. A., Wall, T. C., O'Connor, C. M., Kenny, R. T., Van Trigt III, P., Hill, G. B. and Corey, G. R., 1990, *Mycoplasma pneumoniae* pericarditis: two cases with isolation of the organism from pericardial fluid, in: "Recent Advances in Mycoplasmology", (G. Stanek, G. H. Cassell, J. G. Tully, R. F. Whitcomb, Eds.), Gustav Fischer Verlag, Stuttgart.

Collier, A. M. and Clyde, W. A., Jr., 1974, Appearance of *Mycoplasma pneumoniae* in lungs of experimentally infected hamsters and sputum of patients with natural disease. Am. Rev. Resp. Dis., 110:765.

Collier, A. M. and Denny, F. W., 1981, Pneumonia: an eleven-year study in a pediatric practice. Am. J. Epidemiol., 113: 12.

Costea, N., Yakulis, V. J. and Heller, P., 1971, The mechanism of induction of cold agglutinins by *Mycoplasma pneumoniae*. J. Immunol., 106:58.

Dajani, A. S., Clyde, W. A., Jr. and Denny, F.W., 1965, Experimental infection with *Mycoplasma pneumoniae* (Eaton Agent) J. Exp. Med., 121:1071.

DelGiudice, R. A., Robillard, N. F. and Carski, R. T., 1967, Immunofluorescence identification of mycoplasma on agar by use of incident illumination. J. Bacteriol., 93:1205.

Denny, F. W., Clyde, W. A., Jr. and Glezen, W. P., 1971, *Mycoplasma pneumoniae* disease: clinical spectrum, pathophysiology, epidemiology and control. J. Infect. Dis., 123: 74.

Fernald, G. W. and Clyde, W. A., Jr., 1974, Cell-mediated immunity in *Mycoplasma pneumoniae* infections. Les Colloques de l'institut National de la Sante et de la Recherche Medicale, INSERM., 33:421.

Foy, H. M., Ochs, H., Davis, S. D., Kenny, G. E. and Luce, R. R., 1973, *Mycoplasma pneumoniae* infections in patients with immunodeficiency syndromes: report of four cases. J. Infect. Dis., 127:388.

Foy, H. M., Kenny, G. E., Cooney, M. K. and Allan, I. D., 1979, Long term epidemiology of infections with *Mycoplasma pneumoniae*. J. Infect. Dis., 139: 681.

Gale, J. L. and Kenny, G. E., 1970, Complement-dependent killing of *Mycoplasma pneumoniae*, by antibody: kinetics of the reaction. J. Immunol., 104:1175.

Grayston, J. T., Foy, H. M., and Kenny, G. E., 1969, The epidemiology of mycoplasma infections of the human respiratory tract, in: "The Mycoplasmatales and L-Phase of Bacteria" (L. Hayflick, Ed.) Appleton-Century-Crofts, New York.

Greenberg, H. B., Prescott, B., Brunner, H., James, W. B. and Chanock, R. M., 1973, Sharing of glycolipid antigenic determinants by *Mycoplasma pneumoniae*, vegetables and certain bacteria. New approaches for inducing natural immunity to pyogenic organisms, in: (J. Robbins, R.E. Horton, R. M. Krause, Eds.), Bethesda.

Greenberg, H., Helms, C. M., Brunner, H. and Chanock, R. M., 1974, Asymptomatic infection of adult volunteers with a temperature sensitive mutant of *Mycoplasma pneumoniae*. Proc. Nat. Acad. Sci. 71:4015.

Harris, R., Marmion, B. P., Varkanis, G., Kok, T., Lunn, B., and Martin, J., 1988, Laboratory diagnosis of *Mycoplasma pneumoniae* infection. 2. Comparison of methods for the direct detection of specific antigen or nucleic acid sequences in respiratory exudates. Epidem. Inf., 101:685.

Jacobs, E., Stuhlert, A., Drews, M., Pumpe, K., Schaefer, H. E., Kist, M. and Bredt, W., 1988, Host reactions to *Mycoplasma pneumoniae* infections in guinea pigs preimmunized systemically with the adhesin of this pathogen. Microbial Pathogen., 5:259.

Kenny, G. E., Kaiser, G. G., Cooney, M. K., and Foy, H. M., 1990, Diagnosis of *Mycoplasma pneumoniae*: sensitivities and specificities of serology with lipid antigen and isolation of the organism on soy peptone medium for identification of infection. J. Clin. Microbiol., 28:2087.

Kok, T. W., Varkanis, G. and Marmion, B. P., 1988, Laboratory diagnosis of *Mycoplasma pneumoniae* infection. 1. Direct detection of antigen in respiratory exudates by enzyme immunoassay. Epidem. Inf., 101:669.

Lin, Y., Collins, J.L., Case, P.G. and Patek, P.Q.,1988, Effect of mycoplasmas on natural cytotoxic activity and release of tumor necrosis factor α by spleen cells. Infect. Immun., 56:3072.

Lind, K. and Bentzon, M. W., 1976, Epidemics of *Mycoplasma pneumoniae* infection in Denmark from 1958 to 1974. Int. J. Epidemiol., 5:267.

Lind, K. and Bentzon, M. W., 1990, A second change in the epidemiological pattern of *Mycoplasma pneumoniae* infection in Denmark in the 30 years period 1958-1987, in: "Recent Advances in Mycoplasmology", (G. Stanek, G. H. Cassell, J. G. Tully, R. F. Whitcomb, Eds.) Gustav Fischer Verlag, Stuttgart.

Lo, S. -C., Shih, J. W., Yang, N. Y., Ou, C. Y. and Wang, R. Y., 1989, A novel virus-like infectious agent in patients with AIDS. Am. J. Trop. Med. Hyg., 40:213.

Lo, S.- C. Wang. R. Y., Newton, P. B. , III, Yang, N. Y., Sonoda, M.A. and Shih, J. W., 1989, Fatal infection of silvered leaf monkeys with a virus-like infectious agent (VLIA) derived from a patient with AIDS. Am. J. Trop. Med. Hyg., 40:399.

Madsen, R. D., Weiner, L. B., McMillan, J. A., Saeed, F. A.,North, J. A. and Coates, S. R., 1987, Direct detection of *Mycoplasma pneumoniae* antigen in clinical specimens by a monoclonal antibody immunoblot assay. Am. J. Clin. Pathol., 89:95.

Marmion, B.P., Plackett, P. and Lemcke, R. M., 1967, Immunochemical analysis of *Mycoplasma pneumoniae*. I. Methods of extraction and reaction of fractions from *Mycoplasma pneumoniae* and from *Mycoplasma mycoides* with homologous antisera and with antisera against Streptococcus MG. Aust. J. Exp. Biol. Med. Sci., 45:163.

Murphy, T. F., Henderson, F. W., Clyde, W. A., Jr., Collier, A.M. and Denny, F.W. 1981, Pneumonia: an eleven-year study in a pediatric practice. Am. J. Epidemiol. 113:12.

Niitu, Y., Hasegawa, S., Suetake, T., Kubota, H., Komatsu, S. and Horikawa, M., 1970, Resistance of *Mycoplasma pneumoniae* to erythromycin and other antibiotics. J. Pediatr., 76:438.

Niitu, Y., Hasegawa, S., and Kubota, H., 1974, *In vitro* development of resistance to erythromycin, other macrolide antibiotics and lincomycine in *Mycoplasma pneumoniae*. Antimicrob. Agents Chemother., 5:513.

Niitu, Y., 1985, *Mycoplasma pneumoniae* infection. Acta Paediatr. Jpn., 27:73.

Noah, N. D., 1974, *Mycoplasma pneumoniae* infection in the United Kingdom 1967-1973. Br. Med. J., 2: 544.

Plackett, P., Marmion, B. P., Shaw, E. J., and Lemcke, R. M., 1969, Immunochemical analysis of *Mycoplasma pneumoniae*. 3. Separation and chemical identification of serologically active lipids. Aust. J. Exp. Biol. Med. Sci., 47:171.

Pönkä, A., 1980, Central nervous system manifestations associated with serologically verified *Mycoplasma pneumoniae* infection. Scand. J. Infect. Dis., 12:175.

Putman, C. E., Curtis, A., Simeone, J. F. and Jensen, P. , 1975, *Mycoplasma pneumoniae*. Clinical and roentgenographic patterns. Am. J. Roentgenol. Radium Ther. Nucl. Med., 124: 417.

Sabato, A. R., Cooper, D. M. and Thong, Y. H., 1981, Transitory depression on immune function following *Mycoplasma pneumoniae* infection in children. Pediatr. Res., 15:813.

Senterfit, L. B., 1983, Antibiotic sensitivity testing, in: "Methods in Mycoplasmology", Vol. II, (Tully, J. G. and Razin, S., Eds.), Academic Press, New York.

Shepard, M. C., 1974, Quantitative relationship of *Ureaplasma urealyticum* to the clinical course of nongonococcal urethritis in the human male. Les Colloques de l'institut National de la Sante et de la Recherche Medicale, INSERM, 33:375.

Slotkin, R. I., Clyde Jr., W. A. and Denny, F. W., 1967, The effect of antibiotics on *Mycoplasma pneumoniae in vitro* and *in vivo*. Am. J. Epidemiol., 86:225.

Smith, C. B., Friedewald, W. T., Alford, R. H. and Chanock, R.M., 1967, *Mycoplasma pneumoniae* infections in volunteers. Ann. N.Y. Acad. Sci., 143: 471.

Sobeslavsky, O., Prescott, B., and Chanock, R.M., 1968, Adsorption of *Mycoplasma pneumoniae* to neuraminic acid receptors of various cells and possible role in virulence. J. Bact., 96:695.

Somerson, N. L., Purcell, R. H., Taylor-Robinson, D., and Chanock, R. M., 1965, Hemolysin of *Mycoplasma pneumoniae*. J.Bact., 89:813.

Stopler, T., Gerichter, C. B. and Branski, D., 1980, Antibiotic-resistant mutants of *Mycoplasma pneumoniae*. Israel J. Med. Sci., 16:169.

Taylor-Robinson, D. and McCormack, W. M., 1980, The genital mycoplasmas. New Eng. J. Med., 302:1003.

Tully, J. G., Rose, D. L., Whitcomb, R. F. and Wenzel, R. P., 1979, Enhanced isolation of *Mycoplasma pneumoniae* from throat washings with a newly modified culture medium. J. Infect. Dis., 139:478.

Tully, J. G., Taylor-Robinson, D., Cole, R. M., and Rose, D. L., 1981, A newly discovered mycoplasma in the human urogenital tract. Lancet, 1:1288.

Tully, J. G., Taylor-Robinson, D., Cole, R. M., and Rose, D. L., 1981, A newly discovered mycoplasma in the human urogenital tract. Lancet, 1:1288.

Weidner, W., Schiefer, H. G., Krauss , H. and Engstfeld, J., 1982, Studies on the aetiology of non-gonococcal urethritis. Dtsch. med. Wschr., 107:1227.

MYCOPLASMAS AS IMMUNOMODULATORS

Yehudith Naot

Department of Immunology, Faculty of Medicine
Technion - Israel Institute of Technology
Haifa, Israel

INTRODUCTION

Following successful adherence and colonization of host tissues by invading mycoplasmas, interactions between organisms and their host immune system are initiated. Specific, protective antimycoplasmal humoral and cellular immune responses are often only partially effective, thus leading to a chronic persistent infection. In addition, mycoplasmas can induce nonspecific modulation of host immune responses thereby contributing to the immunopathological manifestations of mycoplasmal infections. Nonspecific suppression of host immune responses may affect the host's capacity to eradicate the evading mycoplasma and it also may render the host more susceptible to infections with other microorganisms. On the other hand, nonspecific-mitogenic activation of host immune mechanisms may be responsible for the massive cellular responses, lymphoid hyperplasia, cell infiltration, inflammation and chemotactic phenomena which often characterize mycoplasma infections. It is obvious that the immune mechanisms operating during any mycoplasma infection are complex and depend on both the mycoplasma species and the infected host. It is therefore crucial to clarify in each case the nature of specific as well as nonspecific interactions between the invading mycoplasma and its host immune cells. This paper will address the capacity of mycoplasmas to modulate immune responses either by suppression or by nonspecific activation.

Rapid Diagnosis of Mycoplasmas, Edited by I. Kahane
and A. Adoni, Plenum Press, New York, 1993

SUPPRESSION OF IMMUNE RESPONSES BY MYCOPLASMAS

It was first reported by Copperman and Morton (1966) that *Mycoplasma hominis* inhibits stimulation of *in vitro* cultured human leukocytes by the T-cell mitogen phytohemagglutinin (PHA). This observation was later extended by Barile and Levinthal (1968) to other non-fermentive mycoplasmas such as *M. arthritidis* and *M. orale,* and was demonstrated to be due to depletion of arginine from cell cultures.

With *M. fermentans,* which utilizes both arginine and glucose, Gabridge and Schneider (1975) showed that viable organisms, as well as high doses of mycoplasmal membranes, were toxic to mouse lymphocytes thereby suppressing the host immune potency. Following these initial reports, additional data revealed that, in fact, certain fermentive and nonfermentive mycoplasma species share a common feature of being suppressive at high doses while being mitogenic at low doses (Cole *et al.,* 1977) However, despite these observations, it is still obscure whether the same mycoplasmal cell constituents are responsible for the capacity of an organism to induce immune activation and immune suppression.

The potential to suppress and modulate immune reactions is not restricted to mycoplasmas and is also exhibited by various acholeplasma species. Extensive studies from the laboratory of Smith (1984) showed that lipoglycans isolated from *Acholeplasma axanthum, A, granularum and A. modicum* are not mitogenic, but rather exert suppressive effects on lymphocytes in cultures and their stimulation by B- and T-cell mitogens. The suppressive nature of lipoglycans isolated from acholeplasmas was also reflected by their ability to reduce immune responsiveness of mice and rabbit when injected prior to exposure of animals to antigens. However it was also observed that simultaneous administration of lipoglycans and antigens enhanced the antibody responses of animals to the specific antigens (Lynn, 1982; Smith, 1984; Al- Samarrai *et al.,* 1982).

The only mycoplasma species demonstrated to possess lipoglycans is *M. neurolyticum.* Interestingly, the lipoglycans isolated from this murine pathogen exhibited mitogenic activity toward cultured mice lymphocytes while inhibiting the responses of rabbit lymphocytes to T-cell mitogen (Sugiyama *et al.,* 1974; Smith, 1984). Considered together, the data reported so far suggest that certain arginine and glucose utilizing mycoplasmas, as well as different acholeplasma species are capable, at high doses, of suppressing *in vitro* immune responses to antigens and mitogens.

Evidence provided from *in vivo* studies indicate that these organisms are exerting immunosuppressive effects which result in host anergy to specific antigens (Kaklamanis and Pavlatos, 1972). It should be emphasized, however, that our knowledge of the mechanisms, other than depletion of arginine from culture medium, which are involved in these suppressive phenomena is still very limited. Additional studies are required to identify the mycoplasma cell constituents which induce suppression. It is also necessary to characterize the host immune cells affected by mycoplasmal and acholeplasmal suppressive constituents and to differentiate between direct cytotoxicity exerted by toxic elements and between possible activation of immune regulatory pathways which include cytotoxic and suppressor lymphocytes and activated macrophages.

At present, *M. arthritidis* is the only mycoplasma species which has been demonstrated to induce differentiation of mouse lymphocytes into cytotoxic/suppressor effector cells. The reaction was not due to direct toxic effects or to depletion of arginine from culture medium (Aldridge *et al.*, 1977a, 1977b; Cole *et al.*, 1980). More recent studies by Cole and Wells (1990) showed that lymphocytes of mice injected systemically with high doses of a mitogen derived from *Mycoplasma arthritidis* (MAM) exhibited a marked decrease in their ability to respond *in vitro* to MAM as well as other T-cell mitogens. The suppressive effect could be transferred to normal untreated lymphocytes by MAM activated T- helper lymphocyte subsets.

MITOGENIC ACTIVATION OF IMMUNE RESPONSES BY MYCOPLASMAS

It is now well recognized that mitogenic, polyclonal stimulation of immune cells is exerted by a wide range of mycoplasma, acholeplasma and spiroplasma species from human, animal and plant origin (Cole *et al.*, 1985). The first report by Ginsburg and Nicolet (1973) suggesting that *Mycoplasma pulmonis* stimulates rat lymphocytes in a non-specific, mitogenic manner was accepted with reservations. The *in vitro* proliferation of rat lymphocytes and their subsequent differentiation into blast cells may have been a result of a specific anamnestic response of presensitized lymphocytes obtained from animals previously infected with *M. pulmonis*. However, subsequent studies by Biberfeld *et al.*, (1974) and by Biberfeld and Gronowicz (1976) demonstrated that *M. pneumoniae* is mitogenic, not only for lymphocytes from healthy, seronegative individuals, but also for mouse and guinea pig lymphocytes. Cole and associates (1975) extended the results of Ginsburg and Nicolet and reported that *M. pulmonis* is mitogenic for mouse lymphocytes, whereas Kirchner *et al.* (1977) observed that *Acholeplasma laidlawii* activates human and mouse lymphocytes in a nonspecific manner. Conclusive evidence that, along with specific immune interactions between mycoplasmas and infected hosts, these organisms also possess a mitogenic potential was provided from studies by Naot *et al.* (1977) and Naot and Ginsburg (1978) which showed that lymphocytes from unprimed germ-free rats and mice were stimulated in a nonspecific manner by different mycoplasma species including *M. pulmonis* and *M. neurolyticum*.

As was thoroughly reviewed by Cole *et al.* (1985) accumulating results from different laboratories showed that the diverse group of mitogenic organisms, which includes pathogenic and nonpathogenic mycoplasmas, acholeplasmas and spiroplasmas, stimulates mitogenic responses of lymphocytes obtained from mice, rats, guinea pigs and human volunteers, even when the lymphocyte donors are not the natural hosts for these organisms. It was also revealed that certain mycoplasmas are capable of stimulating lymphocytes from several, but not all, species. For example, the human mycoplasmas, *M. fermentans* and *A. laidlawii* stimulate lymphocytes from humans and various mouse strains, but not rat lymphocytes (Cole *et al.*, 1977; Kirchner *et al.*, 1977; Naot *et al.*, 1977; Biberfeld and Nilsson, 1978).

M. pneumoniae, a well-recognized human pathogen, exerts nonspecific stimulation of lymphocytes from mice, guinea pigs and human subjects (Biberfeld and Gronowiz, 1976, Cole *et al.*, 1977; Naot *et al.*, 1977; Biberfeld, 1977; Biberfeld and Nilsson, 1978; Biberfeld *et al.*, 1974, 1983; Brunner *et al.*, 1983).

Initial attempts to characterize the mycoplasmal cell components displaying the mitogenic potential showed differences in heat resistance, sensitivity to proteolysis and to physical and chemical treatments among this diverse group of mitogenic organisms. In general, mitogenic activity is displayed by live organisms as well as by nonviable cells and crude extracts of lysed cells. Heat resistance is another common feature, with few exceptions, of mycoplasmal mitogens. As reviewed by Cole *et al.* (1985), detailed studies on the biochemical nature of mycoplasmal mitogens were performed in only few cases and were mainly focused on *M. pneumoniae*, *M. pulmonis*, *M. arthritidis* and *M. neurolyticum*, known pathogens of human and murine hosts.

M. pneumoniae mitogens are contained in crude membrane preparations, resist heating and ultrasonication and differ from the organism's antigenic glycolipids (Biberfeld *et al.*, 1974). Brunner *et al.* (1983) showed that polysaccharides and, to a lesser extent, membrane proteins from *M. pneumoniae* stimulate DNA synthesis in spleen cell from nonimmune-specific pathogen-free (SPF) mice of different strains. Extensive studies performed during the last 14 years by Cole and associates on mitogenic manifestations of *M. arthritidis* revealed that this organism produces a unique soluble T-cell mitogen which is released to culture supernatants (Cole *et al.*, 1981). This potent mitogen derived from *M. arthritidis* and termed MAM, is a small basic protein, protease-labile with a relative molecular weight of approximately 13,000-15,000 (Atkin *et al.*, 1986, Giebler *et al*, 1986) Recent studies with MAM showed that it acts as a superantigen in a manner resembling that of other microbial superantigens which are also known as potent mitogens (Tumang *et al.*, 1990; Cole *et al.*, 1990). In addition to the soluble MAM, *M. arthritidis* membranes contain a second mitogen which is heat stable and is probably activating lymphocytes (Cole *et al.*, 1982).

Our studies on the biochemical nature of *M. pulmonis* and *M. neurolyticum* mitogens demonstrated yet additional variety in mycoplasmal mitogenic moieities. *M. pulmonis* major mitogens, which are heat and protease sensitive, reside in the outer surface proteins of the mycoplasmal membranes. Membrane carbohydrates of *M. pulmonis* are also involved in mitogenic manifestations of this organism, albeit to a lesser extent than membrane proteins (Naot *et al.*, 1979a).

M. neurolyticum mitogens, which are also contained in the cell membranes are only partially sensitive to proteolytic digestion The mitogenic constituents of *M. neurolyticum*, which are not confined to a single membrane component, include lipoglycans, glycoproteins and an unidentified lipid. *M. neurolyticum* mitogens exhibit high susceptibility to oxidation with periodate and differ from the mitogens of *M. pulmonis* (Katz *et al.*, 1983).

It appears that different mycoplasmas exert their mitogenic activities via different cell components and that more than one mitogenic constituent possibly exists in certain mitogenic organisms. As might be expected, the differences observed in the biochemical nature of mycoplasmal mitogens were also reflected in studies on the lymphocyte populations activated by these organisms.

Results reported from several laboratories, reviewed by Cole *et al.* (1985), clearly demonstrated that different mitogenic mycoplasmas vary in their ability to stimulate various populations of immune cells from lymphoid and myeloid origin. These observations motivated further studies on mitogenic interactions between pathogenic organisms and their host immune system in an attempt to clarify the physiologic significance and the role of mitogenic stimulation in disease manifestations.

Cole and others studied and reported their thorough observations on *M. arthritidis* mitogenic stimulation of mouse, rat and human immune cells (Cole *et al.*, 1977, 1985, 1987, 1989, 1990; Moritz *et al.*, 1984; Kirchner *et al.*, 1984; Giebler *et al.*, 1986; Atkin *et al.*, 1986; Tumang *et al.*, 1990).

To illustrate the complex nature and multiple factors involved in mycoplasmal induced mitogenic stimulation we have chosen to describe here the data obtained with *M. pulmonis* and rat immune cells. *Mycoplasma pulmonis* is a causative agent of respiratory tract diseases and arthritis in both rats and mice (Cassell and Hill, 1979). It is important to clarify the mechanisms involved in induction of these rodent diseases, which are inflammatory in nature, not only as animal models for human diseases, but also in attempts to eradicate this common pathogen from widely used laboratory animals.

The novel suggestion by Ginsburg and Nicolet (1973) mentioned above, that *M. pulmonis* interacts with rat lymphocyte in a mitogenic manner, was based on their observations that a large proportion of cultured rat lymphocytes transformed into blast cells and were subsequently stimulated into mitosis, resembling the effects exerted by concanavalin A (ConA), a known T-cell mitogen, on cultured lymphocytes. The ability of *M. pulmonis* to induce similar responses of lymphocytes from conventional, specific pathogen-free and germ-free rats, confirmed the notion that *M. pulmonis* is mitogenic (Naot *et al.*, 1977). Further studies showed that this mycoplasma activates mainly B-lymphocytes and, to some extent, T-lymphocytes from Lewis rats (Naot *et al.*, 1979 b). Spleen cells from thymectomized, irradiated and bone-marrow reconstituted (TxBN) rats were stimulated to a similar level of proliferation as spleen cells from intact rats. Following activation of B-lymphocytes these cells differentiated into antibody producing cells-plasma cells, secreting antibodies with various specificities to nonmycoplasmal antigens. Thus, rat B-lymphocytes were triggered by *M. pulmonis* to proliferate and differentiate polyclonally into antibody producing plasma cells secreting antibodies to SRBC and TNP-SRBC. Rat T lymphocytes were also activated nonspecifically by *M. pulmonis*, but to a lesser extent than B-lymphocytes. We have first observed an increase in DNA synthesis in cultured rat thymocytes exposed to *M. pulmonis*.. Autoradiographic studies revealed that T-cells which were stimulated by ConA and Pokeweed Mitogen (PWM) and differentiated into blast cells and secondary lymphocytes responded to a certain extent when exposed to *M. pulmonis*. On the other hand, ConA and PWM stimulated only part of those lymphocytes populations which were initially activated by *M. pulmonis*.. It became evident that, while predominantly an activator of rat B-lymphocytes, *M.*

pulmonis also stimulates a portion, or possibly only certain subpopulations, of rats' T-lymphocytes. In accordance with these data, it was observed that, unlike known T-cell mitogen PHA, ConA and PWM, *M. pulmonis* is incapable of triggering the development of cytotoxic T-lymphocytes towards syngeneic or allogeneic target fibroblast monolayers (Ginsburg *et al.*, 1976). On the other hand, further studies demonstrated that *M. pulmonis* stimulates the production of interleukin-2 (IL-2) by rat lymphocytes exposed to this mitogenic mycoplasma *in vitro* (Levin *et al.*, 1985) It was also shown that depletion of macrophages from lymph node cell cultures reduced the stimulation of the remaining non-adherent cells by approximately 30% when exposed to *M. pulmonis* mitogenic activity (Katz *et al.*, 1983). A summary of the results obtained with *M. pulmonis* and Lewis rats shows that the mitogenic activity of *M. pulmonis* is predominantly exerted upon rat B-lymphocytes which proliferate and subsequently differentiate polyclonally into antibody producing cells which secret antibodies with specificities not related to mycoplasmal antigens

Only a portion of rat T-lymphocytes are activated by *M. pulmonis.*. Since differentiation of T-cells into effector cytotoxic T-lymphocytes was not observed in *in vitro* studies, whereas the T-lymphocyte population stimulated by *M. pulmonis* mitogens proliferated and produced IL-2, it was concluded that *M. pulmonis* activates T-helper cells. Macrophages or antigen presenting cells (APC) are required only to a certain degree for full expression of *M. pulmonis* mitogenicity toward rat lymphocytes. It is plausible to postulate that these accessory cells are necessary for interactions of *M. pulmonis* mitogens and the helper T-lymphocyte populations, while stimulation of B-lymphocytes by *M. pulmonis* is not affected by depletion of these accessory cells. However, at present it is not clear if the effects of *M. pulmonis* on T-helper cells is direct or if it requires the mediation of interleukin-1 by the stimulation of T-inducer cells and macrophages. Nevertheless, the biological significance of the observed production of IL-2 and other lymphokines produced by activated T-helper cells is most likely their function as amplifiers of inflammatory immune responses through augmentation of B-, T- and accessory cell reactions. It is still unknown if rat B- and T-helper lymphocytes are stimulated by different mitogenic components present in *M. pulmonis* membranes and whether *M. pulmonis*'s outer surface proteins, which are the major mitogenic constituents of this organism, stimulate B-lymphocyte while the minor mitogenic carbohydrate containing components selectively stimulate T-helper cells. To clarify this issue, we have produced a panel of rat monoclonal antibodies capable of inhibiting mitogenic stimulation of rat lymphocytes by *M. pulmonis* membranes. Preliminary data show that indeed *M. pulmonis* exhibits more than one mitogenic component and that individual monoclonal antibodies, highly potent in inhibiting *in vitro* mitogenesis, recognizes epitopes on more than one protein band in electrophoretic and immunoblotting experiments (Lapidot and Naot, 1990). The experiments described so far were performed with Lewis rats and the original mitogenic isolate of Ginsburg and Nicolet (1973). However, *M. pulmonis* mitogenic activity is not restricted to one strain of this mycoplasma species. We have demonstrated (Naot *et al.*, 1977) that the Negroni, PG34 and JB strains are also mitogenic for rat lymphocytes, although to a different extent. Studies by Davis *et al.* (1985) showed that the UAB5782 strain of *M. pulmonis* is mitogenic for rat lymphocytes; *M. pulmonis* is mitogenic for rat, mouse and human lymphocytes. However, data obtained from different laboratories indicated that different hosts and even different strains of a certain animal species responded to different levels to *M. pulmonis* mitogens. This issue of differences in lymphocyte responsiveness between rat strains was clarified in the experiments reported by Davis *et al.* (1985) and Williamson *et al.* (1986). It has been clearly demonstrated that lymphocytes obtained from Lewis rats are highly responsive to mitogenic stimulation exerted by *M. pulmonis* mitogens, PHA, PWM and *Salmonella typhimurium* mitogen (STM). Lymphocytes obtained from Fischer (F 344) rats and examined in parallel were less responsive to all these mitogens. The differences between these two rat strains were attributed to significantly higher numbers of T-helper cells found in Lewis lymphoid populations, while the number of cytotoxic suppressor T-lymphocytes were similar in Lewis and F 344 rats. In confirmation with our data (Katz *et al.*, 1983), it was observed that depletion of macrophages from spleen cell cultures decreased to a similar levels the responses of Lewis and F 344 nonadherent populations. Thus, macrophages are involved in the mitogenic activation of lymphocytes from both rat strains. *In vitro* experiments on polyclonal activation of B-lymphocytes from Lewis and F 344 rats showed that these strains also differ in spontaneous production of antibodies to staphylococcal protein A coupled to SRBC with Lewis spleen cells exhibiting higher activity than cells from F 344 cells. These *in vitro* manifestations of *M. pulmonis* mitogenic interactions with immune cells were the impetus for *in vivo* studies on the relationships between *M. pulmonis* mitogenicity and either defense or immunopathologic mechanisms. Indications for *in vivo* mitogenesis of *M. pulmonis* were obtained from studies on CBA mice intravenously injected with viable *M. pulmonis* cells (Cole *et al.*, 1975). Lymphocytes obtained from these animals, following exposure to *M. pulmonis* exhibited a significant increase in DNA synthesis in the absence of exogenous mycoplasmal antigens. During the initial phases of infection, animals exhibited marked lymphocytosis and low levels of specific antimycoplasmal antibodies. Additional support for *in vivo* mitogenic stimulation was provided by Keystone *et al.* (1982), who demonstrated that intravenous inoculation of C3H and C57BL with *M. pulmonis* stimulated nonspecific polyclonal activation of host B-lymphocytes which differentiated into plasma cells producing antibodies with different specificities, not related to *M. pulmonis* antigens, in a similar manner to the *in vitro* polyclonal activation. We have studied the role of mycoplasmal mitogens in the development of respiratory tract injuries by examining the relationship between mitogenic and pathological effects of *M. pulmonis* in Lewis rats. Mitogenic preparations of purified membranes of *M. pulmonis* induced interstitial pneumonia and tracheitis after intranasal administration to specific pathogen-free rats. The pneumonia, characterized by peribronchial, perivascular and alveolar wall infiltration by lymphocytes was indistinguishable from that produced by viable *M. pulmonis*.. Both pathologic and mitogenic effects were significantly reduced by prior treatment of membranes with heat or proteolytic enzymes, thus indicating that these activities may be related to and depend on the integrity of *M. pulmonis* membrane proteins. Intranasal administration of the T-cell mitogen, ConA, produced interstitial pneumonia, but not tracheitis, suggesting that mitogenic stimulation of Lewis T-lymphocytes is important factor in induction of pneumonic lesions (Naot *et al.*, 1981). In accordance with data on correlation between mitogenic stimulation of lymphocytes and pathologic effects exerted by *M. pulmonis* are the results reported by Davis *et al.*. (1982, 1985; Williamson *et al.* (1976) and Simecka *et al.* (1989) who demonstrated that *M. pulmonis* viable cells triggered polyclonal activation of B-lymphocytes following administration to rats, as was earlier demonstrated for mice by Keystone *et al.* (1982) and that Lewis rats, which are more responsive than Fischer rats *in vitro*, are also more severely affected by *M. pulmonis* mitogenic stimulus *in vivo*. It was also demonstrated that specific anti *M. pulmonis* antibodies produced *in vivo* in response to infection with *M. pulmonis* can not account for the differences in severity of diseases in Lewis and F 344 rats and that Lewis rats responded to specific *M. pulmonis* antigens to a similar or even greater extent than F 344 rats.

In summary, it is evident from the data presented that modulation of immune responses by either suppression or nonspecific polyclonal activation is a manifestation exhibited by many members of the *Mycoplasmatales* and is induced both *in vivo* and *in vitro*. There is accumulating evidence suggesting that, at least in certain mycoplasma host interactions, these modulatory effects on immune responses are involved not only in progression of disease and chronicity of infections, but also in the inflammatory, immunopathologic reactions of massive cell proliferation and chemotactic phenomena. Even the limited number of mycoplasma host systems studied so far, revealed the complex and multifactorial nature of these interactions between mycoplasmas and their host immune cells. To clarify the mechanisms responsible for immune modulation, further studies with purified mycoplasmal suppressive and mitogenic components should be pursued. Another area which requires additional experimentation is the role of lymphokines and cytokines in the modulating effects induced by mycoplasmas.

REFERENCES

Aldrige, K. E., Cole, B. C. and Ward, J. R. (1977a) Mycoplasma dependent activation of normal lymphocytes: Induction of a lymphocyte mediated cytotoxicity for allogeneic and syngeneic mouse target cells. Infect. Immun. 18:377-385.

Aldrige, K. E., Cole, B. C. and Ward, J. R (1977b) Mycoplasma dependent activation of normal lymphocytes: Role of arginine and non-viable mycoplasma antigen in the induction of lymphocyte mediated cytotoxicity for syngeneic mouse target cells Infect Immun 18:386-392.

Al-Samarrai, T. H., Smith, P. F. and Lynn, R. J. (1982) Isolation and characterization of the receptor on sheep erythrocytes for acholeplasmal lipoglycans Infect. Immun. 38:1078-1087.

Atkin, C. L., Cole, B. C., Sullivan, G. J , Washburn L. R. and Wiley, B. B. (1986) Stimulation of mouse lymphocytes by a mitogen derived from *Mycoplasma arthritidis* V. A small basic protein from culture supernatants is a potent T-cell mitogen. J. Immunol. 137:1581-1589.

Barile, M. F. and Leventhal, B. G. (1968) Possible mechanism for mycoplasma inhibition of lymphocyte transformation induced by phytohaemagglutinin. Nature, (London) 219:751.

Biberfeld, G. (1977) Activation of human lymphocyte subpopulations by *Mycoplasma pneumoniae*. Scand. J. Immunol. 6:1145-1150.

Biberfeld, G., Biberfeld, P. and Sterner, G. (1974) Cell-mediated immune response following *Mycoplasma pneumoniae* infection in man. I. Lymphocyte stimulation. Clin. Exp. Immunol 17:29-41.

Biberfeld, G. and Gronowicz, E. (1976) *Mycoplasma pneumoniae* is a polyclonal B-cell activator. Nature 261:238-239.

Biberfeld, G. and Nilsson, E. (1978) Mitogenicity of *Mycoplasma fermentans* for human lymphocytes. Infect. Immun. 21:48-54.

Biberfeld, G., Arneborn, P., Forsgren, M., Von Stedingk, L. V. and Blomqvist, S. (1983) Non-specific polyclonal antibody response induced by *Mycoplasma pneumoniae in vitro* and *in vivo* . Yale J. Biol. & Med. 56: 639-642.

Brunner, H., Kahling, U., Rollberg, A., Beck, J. and Kirchner, H (1983) Effect of *Mycoplasma pneumoniae* and some of its fractions on host defense mechanisms. Yale J. Biol. & Med. 56:63-864.

Cassell, G. H. and Hill, A. (1979) Murine and other small animal mycoplasmas, in "The Mycoplasmas" Vol II. (Tully, J. G. and Whitcomb, R. F., Eds.), pp. 235-273, Academic Press, New York.

Cole, B. C., Golightly-Rowland, L. and Ward, J. R. (1975) Arthritis of mice induced by *Mycoplasma pulmonis*: humoral antibody and lymphocyte responses of CBA mice. Infect. Immun. 12:1083-1092.

Cole, B. C., Aldridge, K. E .and Ward, J. R. (1977) Mycoplasma-dependent activation of normal lymphocytes: Mitogenic potential of mycoplasmas for mouse lymphocytes. Infect. Immun. 18:393-399.

Cole, B. C., Aldridge, K. E., Sullivan, G. J. and Ward, J. R. (1980) Mycoplasma dependent activation of normal mouse lymphocytes: requirement for functional T-lymphocytes in the cytotoxicity reaction mediated by *Mycoplasma arthritidis*. Infect. Immun. 30:90-98.

Cole, B. C., Daynes, R. A. and Ward, J. R. (1981) Stimulation of lymphocytes by a mitogen derived from *Mycoplasma arthritidis*. I. Transformation is associated with an H-2 linked gene that maps to the I-E/I-C subregion. J. Immunol. 127:1931-1936.

Cole, B. C., Sullivan, G. J., Daynes, R. A., Sayed, I. A. and Ward, J. R. (1982) Stimulation of mouse lymphocytes by a mitogen derived from *Mycoplasma arthritidis*. II. Cellular requirements for T-cell transformation mediated by a soluble mycoplasma mitogen. J. Immunol. 128:2013-2018.

Cole, B. C., Naot, Y., Stanbridge, E. S. and Wise, K. S. (1985) Interactions of mycoplasmas and their products with lympoid cells *in vitro*, in "The Mycoplasmas" Vol. IV, (Razin, S. Barile, M. F., Eds.), pp. 203-257, Academic Press, New York.

Cole, B. C., Tuller, J. W. and Sullivan, G. J. (1987) Stimulation of mouse lymphocytes by a mitogen derived from *Mycoplasma arthritidis*. VI. Detection of a non-MHC gene(s) in the Eα bearing RIIIS mouse strain that is associated with a specific lack of T-cell responses to the *M. arthritidis* soluble mitogen. J. Immunol. 139:927-935.

Cole, B. C., Kartchner, D. R. and Wells, D. J. (1989) Stimulation of mouse lymphocytes by a mitogen derived from *Mycoplasma arthritidis*.. VII. Responsiveness is associated with expression of a product(s) of the gene family present on the T-cell receptor α/β for antigen J. Immunol. 142:4131-4137.

Cole, B. C., Kartchner, D. R. and Wells, D. J. (1990) Stimulation of mouse lymphocytes by a mitogen derived from *Mycoplasma arthritidis* (MAM). VIII. Selective activation of T-cells expressing distinct Vβ T-cell receptors from various strains of mice by the "Superantigen" MAM. J. Immunol. 144: 425-431.

Cole, B. C. and Wells, D. J. (1990) Immunosuppressive properties of the *Mycoplasma arthritidis* T-cell mitogen *in vivo*: inhibition of proliferative responses to T-cell mitogens. Infect. Immun. 58:228-236.

Copperman, R. and Morton, H. E. (1966) Reversible inhibition of mitosis in lymphocyte cultures by nonviable mycoplasma. Proc. Soc. Exp. Biol. Med. 123:790-795.

Davis, J. K., Thorp, R. B., Maddox, P. A. and Brown, M. B. (1982) Murine respiratory mycoplasmosis in F 344 and LEW rats: evolution of lesions and lung lymphoid cell populations. Infect. Immun. 36:720-729.

Davis, J. K., Simecka, J. W., Williamson, J. S. P., Ross, S. E., Juliana, M. M , Thorp, R. B. and Cassell, G. H. (1985) Non-specific lymphocyte responses in F 344 and LEW rats: susceptibility to murine respiratory mycoplasmosis and examination of cellular basis for strain differences. Infect. Immun. 49:152-158.

Gabridge, M. G. and Schneider, P. R. (1975) Cytotoxic effect of *Mycoplasma fermentans* on mouse thymocytes. Infect. Immun. 11:460-465.

Giebler, D., Brehm, G., Nicklas, W. and Kirchner, H. (1986) Activation of C57BL/6 spleen cells by the mitogenic principle derived from *Mycoplasma arthritidis.*. Immunol. 171:57

Ginsburg, H. and Nicolet, J. (1973) Extensive transformation of lymphocytes by a mycoplasma organism. Nature, (New Biol.) 246:143-146.

Ginsburg, H., Naot, Y. and Hollander, N. (1976) Lysis and necrosis: analysis of two cytotoxic phenomena mediated by lymphocytes. Israel J. Med. Sci. 12:435-453.

Kaklamanis, E. and Pavlatos, M. (1972) The immunosuppressive effect of mycoplasma infection. I. Effect on the humoral and cellular response. Immunology, 22:695-702.

Katz, R., Siman-Tov, R. and Naot, Y. (1983) Comparison of mitogens from *Mycoplasma pulmonis* and *Mycoplasma neurolyticum.* Yale J. Biol. and Med. 56:613-621

Keystone, E. C., Cunningham, A. J., Metcalf, A., Kennedy, M. and Quinn, P. A. (1982) Role of antibody in the protection of mice from arthritis induced by *Mycoplasma pulmonis.*. Clin. Exp. Immunol. 47:253-259.

Kirchner, H., Brunner, H. and Ruhl, H. (1977) Effect of *A. laidlawii* on murine and human lymphocyte cultures. Clin. Exp. Immunol. 29:176-180.

Kirchner, H., Giebler, D., Keyssner, K. and Nicklas, W. (1984) Lymphoproliferation induced in mouse spleen cells by *Mycoplasma arthritidis* mitogen reversal of the defect of nonresponder mice. Scand. J. Immunol. 20:133-139.

Lapidot, Z. and Naot, Y. (1990) Monoclonal antibodies inhibiting *Mycoplasma pulmonis* IOM Letts. 1:133.

Levin, D., Gershon, H. and Naot, Y. (1985) Production of Interleukin-2 by rat lymph node cells stimulated by *Mycoplasma pulmonis* membranes. J. Infect. Dis. 151:541-544.

Lynn, R. J. (1982) Modulation of the immune response with acholeplasmal lipoglycans. Rev. Infect. Dis. 4 suppl, S270.

Moritz, T., Giebler, D., Gunther, E., Nicklas, W. and Kirchner, H. (1984) Lymphoproliferative responses of spleen cells of inbred rat strains to *Mycoplasma arthritidis* mitogen. Scand. J. Immunol. 20:991-996.

Naot, Y., Tully, J. G. and Ginsburg, H. (1977) Lymphocyte activation by various Mycoplasma strains and species. Infect. Immun. 18:310-317.

Naot, Y. and Ginsburg, H. (1978) Activation of mouse B-lymphocytes by mycoplasma mitogen(s). Immunology, 34:715-720

Naot, Y., Siman-Tov, R. and Ginsburg, H. (1979a) Mitogenic activity of *Myco-plasma pulmonis*.   II. Studies on the biochemical nature of the mito-genic factor. Eur. J. Immunol. 9:149-154.

Naot, Y., Merchav, S., Ben-David, E. and Ginsburg, H. (1979b) Mitogenic acti-vity of *Mycoplasma pulmonis*.. I. Stimulation of rat B- and T-lympho-cytes. Immunol. 36:399-406.

Naot, Y., Davidson, S. and Lindenbaum, E. S. (1981) Mitogenicity and pathogen-icity of *Mycoplasma pulmonis* in rats. I. Atypical interstitial pneumonia induced by mitogenic mycoplasmal membranes. J. Infect. Dis. 143:55-62.

Simecka, J. W., Davis, J. K. and Cassell, G. H. (1989) Serum antibody does not account for differences in the severity of chronic respiratory disease caused by *Mycoplasma pulmonis* in LEW and F 344 rats. Infect. Immun. 57:3570-3575.

Smith, P. F. (1984) Lipoglycans from mycoplasmas. Critical Rev. Microbiol. 11:157-186.

Sugiyama, T., Smith, P. F., Langworthy, T. A. and Mayberry, W. R. (1974) Im-munological analysis of glycolipids and lipopolysaccharides derived from various mycoplasmas. Infect. Immun. 10:1273-1279.

Tumang, J. R., Posnett, D. N., Cole, B. C., Crow, M. K. and Friedman, S. M. (1990) Helper T-cell dependent human B-cell differentiation mediated by a mycoplasmal superantigen bridge. J. Exp. Med. 171:2153-2158.

Williamson, J. S. P., Davis, J. K. and Cassell, G. H. (1986) Polyclonal activation of rat splenic lymphocytes after *in vivo* administration of *Mycoplasma pulmonis* and its relation to *in vitro* response. Infect. Immun. 52:594-599.

MYCOPLASMA - ANIMAL PATHOGENS

Richard F. Ross

Veterinary Medical Research Institute
Iowa State University
Ames, Iowa 50011

MYCOPLASMAS OF CATTLE

Nine members of the genus *Mycoplasma* and one of the genus *Ureaplasma* have been shown to cause disease in cattle. *M. bovis* is a cause of septicemia, arthritis, mastitis, and pneumonia; *M. dispar* is a cause of pneumonia; *M. bovoculi* is a cause of conjunctivitis, along with *Moraxella bovis*; *M. bovigenitalium* is an occasional cause of seminal vesiculitis; and *M. mycoides* subsp. *mycoides* SC causes contagious bovine pleuropneumonia. *Ureaplasma diversum* is a cause of pneumonia, vulvovaginitis and infertility in cattle. Several species are known to be involved in mastitis in cattle, including *M. bovis, M. alkalescens, M. canadense, M. californicum, M. bovigenitalium*, and an unnamed mycoplasma known as Bovine Group 7. Other species isolated from cattle, but not specifically related to disease processes include *M. arginini, M. alvi, M. bovirhinis, M. verecundum*, and several species of acholeplasmas and anaeroplasmas. Useful references providing overviews of information about the bovine mycoplasmas and the associated diseases include those by Barile *et al.* (1985), Gourlay and Howard (1978), Gourlay and Howard (1979), Gourlay and Howard (1983), Jasper (1981), Nitzschke (1985), and Ross (1985a). Reference citations in this review will focus primarily on the latest information on bovine mycoplasmas.

Mycoplasma mycoides subsp. *mycoides* SC

Mycoplasma mycoides subsp. *mycoides* SC is the cause of a devastating chronic disease in cattle known as contagious bovine pleuropneumonia (CBPP). The disease, once spread throughout many countries in the world, still exists in Africa, India, Spain, Portugal, and France. Recently, fresh outbreaks of CBPP were reported in Italy. In addition to cattle, the organism causes disease in water buffalo, yak, reindeer, and bison.

Rapid Diagnosis of Mycoplasmas, Edited by I. Kahane
and A. Adoni, Plenum Press, New York, 1993

Clinical signs most often seen in CBPP include nasal discharge, dry cough, and progressive debilitation. The general course of the disease is 2 to 8 weeks in duration; affected animals often die, but may also recover gradually. Lesions seen in CBPP include a fibrinous pleuropneumonia with necrosis, marked accumulation of pleural exudate, and enlarged bronchial lymph nodes.

Transmission of *M. mycoides* is effected primarily by droplet, aerosol, and contact means. Finely dispersed bronchial secretions are expelled during coughing by diseased animals. In spite of the airborne mode of spread, CBPP generally is reputed to spread slowly. Once established in a herd of cattle, the disease persists in an endemic form.

Experimental pleuropneumonia can be induced by respiratory exposure to cultures. Following establishment in pulmonary lobules, there is fibrinous inflammation and spread via the lymphatics to other areas, including the pleura. Thrombosis of vessels leads to more severe damage, including necrosis. The organism has been shown recently to produce cytotoxic damage to cultured endothelial cells (Valdivieso-Garcia *et al.*, 1989). Necrotic lesions are encapsulated and sequestered. A galactan or surface glycocalyx produced by the organism may be an important invasin.

Small centered colonies (SC) are formed by this organism in contrast to the larger colonies formed by the virtually identical *M. mycoides* subsp. *mycoides* LC occurring in goats. The organism is relatively easy to isolate in mycoplasma media; glucose is fermented, but arginine and urea are not affected. The so-called "small colony" (SC) type fails to digest casein, will not liquify serum, and is less stable at 45°C than the LC type. In contrast, the "large colony" (LC) type found in goats digests casein, liquifies serum, and is more stable at 45°C. The SC and LC types have been distinguished utilizing one dimensional SDS-PAGE (Costas *et al.*, 1987). Typically, the organism is identified by means of MI, GI and EpiFA procedures; however, the unique distinguishing natures of the SC and LC types also need to be utilized. Poumarat (1990) reported the use of a dot immunobinding assay to distinguish organisms in the *M. mycoides* cluster.

Diagnosis of CBPP has been classically done for years on the basis of clinical signs and lesions of pleuropneumonia. The organism can be isolated easily in a variety of mycoplasma media. Ferronha *et al.* (1990) reported use of the peroxidase-antiperoxidase method for detection of *M. mycoides* in tissue. The intradermal skin test may be useful for detection of the infection and the complement fixation test is a very useful serodiagnostic procedure (Dannacher *et al.*, 1986; Poumarat *et al.*, 1989). An ELISA has also been reported for use in detection of antibodies to *M. mycoides* subsp. *mycoides* (LeGoff, 1986).

Strategies utilized for control and treatment of CBPP depend on the local policies or geographic situation. Variability in susceptibility has been reported among breeds and between individual animals; recovery from disease results in resistance to reinfection. Currently used vaccines in Africa consist of living attenuated cultures (T1) of *M. mycoides* (Miles, 1983). Inactivated vaccines have been only partially successful. According to Garba *et al.* (1986), vaccination with a killed Gladysdale strain of *M. mycoides* subsp. *mycoides* provided good protection in an experimental trial and was used in about 10,000 cattle in northern Nigeria. Other killed CBPP vaccines were reported to be effective in cattle (Gray *et al.*, 1986; Jeggo *et al.*, 1987). Therapy with antibiotics is generally not advocated; however tetracyclines or other antibiotics may be used if all animals in a herd are to be slaughtered directly or in order to control severe vaccine reactions.

Mycoplasma bovis

One of the most important species in cattle is *M. bovis*, a cause of pneumonia, arthritis, and mastitis. The organism has been isolated also from a variety of other sites, including the reproductive tract, aborted fetuses, and ocular secretions of cattle with keratoconjunctivitis. *M. bovis* has been isolated from cattle in a large number of countries. Once established in a herd, the organism persists and may become endemic, particularly the mastitis in dairy cattle. It is a frequent invader, along with other microbial agents, in respiratory disease of feed-lot cattle; however, its true impact in such disease is difficult to determine.

Mastitis occurring in dairy cattle may be caused by several different species of mycoplasmas; the most frequent appears to be *M. bovis*. Clinical signs vary from subclinical to very severe and from acute to chronic. Generally with overt disease, there is a sharp reduction in milk production, swelling and firmness of the mammary glands, and failure of antibiotic treatment (Pfutzner, 1990). The milk is described as watery with a sandy deposit; subsequently, a more purulent discharge is seen. The disease may persist for 2 to 8 weeks or longer.

Respiratory disease associated with *M. bovis* infection in calves is characterized by anorexia, apathy, coughing, dyspnea, and elevated temperatures. The organism generally occurs in mixed infections with other mycoplasmas, bacteria, and viruses. According to Pfutzner (1990), the incidence of pneumonia due to *M. bovis* can be as high as 100%.

Arthritis associated with *M. bovis* infection may be a sequela to the respiratory form of the disease, particularly in feedlot cattle (Radostits *et al.*, 1988; Pfutzner, 1990). There is lameness, swelling of joints, slight elevation of temperature, failure of antibiotic treatment and, if severe, reduced consumption of feed and debilitation.

Infertility has been associated with use of semen infected with *M. bovis*. The organism has been isolated from abortion and the disease has been produced experimentally (Bocklisch *et al.*, 1986). *In vitro* assessments revealed that *M. bovis* had no influence on development of bovine embryos (Bielanski *et al.*, 1989).

Lesions seen in the various forms of *M. bovis* disease include a purulent mastitis, involution of mammae, cranioventral consolidation of lungs with purple to grey coloration and fibrinopurulent synovitis and arthritis. Brys *et al.* (1989) demonstrated that septicemia commonly developed in young calves challenged intranasally with *M. bovis*.

Mycoplasma bovis forms typical centered colonies, growing on a variety of media, within 2 to 3 days. It does not ferment glucose or hydrolyze arginine or urea.

Transmission of *M. bovis* infection may occur by contact with contaminated mastitis treatment solutions and milking equipment and milkers' hands. Calves may become infected by suckling of cows with *M. bovis* mammary infections. Alternatively, the infection may be spread by aerosol.

M. bovis appears to be more invasive than most of the other bovine mycoplasmas and septicemia may occur. Invasion of the mammary gland appears primarily via the galactogenic route (Pfutzner, 1990). Evidence was presented that a toxin was produced which contributed to development of mastitis. In addition, cattle with acute mastitis have been shown to develop depressed lymphocyte stimulation and cell mediated responses. Unlike some mycoplasmas, *M. bovis* appears not to be mitogenic for bovine lymphocytes. In fact, the organism suppresses PHA induced stimulation of bovine lymphocytes (Finch and Howard, 1990; Thomas *et al.*, 1990) and mixed lymphocyte responses (Finch and Howard, 1990). Evidence has been obtained that *M. bovis* inhibits neutrophil respiratory burst (PMA induced chemiluminescence); thus, the organism may interfere with phagocyte function *in vivo* (Thomas *et al.*, 1991).

Diagnosis of *M. bovis* infection depends on the form of disease presented. The organism can be isolated easily in a variety of media. Brown *et al.* (1986) reported that SP4 medium was superior for isolation of mycoplasmas involved in mastitis. Gourlay *et al.* (1989) reported that characteristic microscopic lesions and demonstration of *M. bovis* by immunoperoxidase labelling were useful aids in diagnosis. The capture enzyme immunoassay has been used for detection of *M. bovis* in bull semen (Nielson *et al.*, 1987). An ELISA was also used to detect antibodies to *M. bovis* in cattle (Uhaa *et al.*, 1990). Hotzel *et al.* (1990) reported development of a DNA probe for detection of *M. bovis*.

Mastitis caused by *M. bovis* responds poorly to antibiotic therapy (Pfutzner, 1990); therefore, for control of this problem, it is best to detect carrier cows by culture of milk and to eliminate them from the herd (Fritzsch and Bornet, 1988) and/or segregate known infected cows and milk them separately (Brown *et al.*, 1986). Rigid sanitation procedures should be implemented to prevent transmission from infected to noninfected cows. For control of pneumonia and arthritis, management, sanitation, and environment should be improved. In addition, use of the all-in, all-out system of calf production in confinement rearing should help to reduce the severity of pneumonia problems. Alzieu *et al.* (1989) reported that spiramycin was useful for treatment of pneumonia associated with *M. bovis* and pasteurellae. Evidence that vaccines containing oil-adjuvant, *M. bovis* and other respiratory disease agents reduce the severity of calf pneumonia was presented by Stott *et al.* (1987) and Howard *et al.* (1990). However, Brys and Pfutzner (1989) reported that calves immunized passively with hyperimmune serum against *M. bovis* were not protected against intranasal challenge with the organism. In addition, vaccines did not prevent *M. bovis* mastitis (Boothby *et al.*, 1986; Boothby *et al.*, 1988) and seemed to increase the duration and severity of the disease (Boothby *et al.*, 1986).

Mycoplasma dispar

Mycoplasma dispar is a frequent isolate from normal and pneumonic lungs of calves. The organism is widespread in cattle, having been isolated from calves in England, Finland, Denmark, Japan and the U.S.. Gourlay *et al.* (1976) demonstrated that *M. dispar* was capable of inducing pneumonia, generally subclinical, experimentally. The organism is not known to occur in other animal species.

As indicated, *M. dispar* infection is most often subclinical. However, the organism also occurs in naturally occurring pneumonias along with other mycoplasmas, bacteria, and viruses. Under such circumstances, coughing, respiratory distress, and mortality may occur.

Lesions seen in *M. dispar* disease consist of purple to red consolidation in the cranioventral areas of the lung. Low passage isolates of the organism produce small, noncentered colonies, while higher passage cultures produce centered colonies. The organism grows slowly in broth, requiring 7 to 14 days. It ferments glucose, but does not hydrolyze arginine or urea.

Transmission of *M. dispar* is effected by respiratory secretions from infected cows or older calves to young calves. The air in calf houses is suspected to be an important source of *M. dispar* infection.

Pneumonia can be produced experimentally by inoculation of calves with cultures of *M. dispar* or lung homogenates containing the organism. It is thought to colonize on the lining epithelium of airways. Thomas *et al.* (1987 b) reported that *M. dispar* is ciliostatic and cytopathic for ciliated epithelial cells. Almeida and Rosenbusch (1990) confirmed by scanning electron microscopy that *M. dispar*-infected lungs had degeneration and destruction of ciliated epithelium in the distal bronchi and bronchioles. Furthermore, they found that calves with experimental *M. dispar* infection had reduced tracheobronchial clearance of bacteria in comparison to normal calves. Subsequently, Almeida and Rosenbusch (1991) demonstrated that antibodies against capsule from *M. dispar* were required for killing of the organism by bovine alveolar macrophages; in addition, the capsule was shown to impair killing of *Serratia marcescens* and *Staphylococcus aureus*. Finch and Howard (1990) reported that *M. dispar* inhibited the response of bovine lymphocytes to mitogens and mixed leucocyte responses *in vivo*. Calves less than 40 days of age develop an alveolitis, whereas calves over 40 days of age tend to develop the proliferative response (cuffing). Rosendal and Martin (1986), in a study of calves with respiratory disease in Ontario, found that calves with low antibody titers to *M. dispar* on arrival in the feedlot were at increased risk of being treated for respiratory disease.

For diagnosis, clinical signs are of little help since the infection often presents as a subclinical disease. The cranioventral consolidation and absence of acute inflammatory process may be indicative of *M. dispar*. The organism can be isolated in broth media such as those described by Gourlay and Leach (1970) and Friis (1979). The organism may also be detected by immunofluorescence procedures.

Little information has been presented on strategies for treatment or control of *M. dispar* pneumonia. Management, sanitation, and environmental factors should be optimized. All-in, all-out production in calf confinement systems should help to reduce frequency of spread from older calves and reduce the severity of pneumonia in newly stocked animals. Howard *et al.* (1987) reported that a combination vaccine containing killed respiratory syncytial virus, parainfluenza virus type 3, *M. bovis*, and *M. dispar* engendered protection against respiratory disease in a large beef rearing unit in England.

Mycoplasma bovoculi

Mycoplasma bovoculi is associated with conjunctivitis and keratoconjunctivitis in cattle and has been isolated in England, Africa, Canada, Denmark, Switzerland, and the U.S. The organism was a frequent isolate from eyes of 3 to 15 month old calves (Barber *et al.*, 1986).

Clinical signs seen in *M. bovoculi* disease include bilateral conjunctivitis, tearing, and photophobia. The disease can be produced experimentally by intraconjunctival inoculation of cultures of the organism. *M. bovoculi* appears to be an important predisposing infection for establishment of *Moraxella bovis* and other bacteria in the bovine eye (Rosenbusch and Ostle, 1986). *M. bovoculi* adheres to corneal and conjunctival epithelium without the aid of a specialized attachment tip (Salih and Rosenbusch, 1988).

M. bovoculi produces small centered colonies on agar media. The organism ferments glucose, but does not hydrolyze arginine or urea. Presumably, transmission of *M. bovoculi* is effected by close contact or by flies between acutely affected animals and normal cattle. Chronically infected animals are the principal reservoir of infection.

The widespread distribution of *M. bovoculi* and the clinical appearance of conjunctivitis in cattle are indicative of infection with this organism. The organism can be isolated in broth media such as those described by Gourlay and Leach (1970) and Friis (1979). Other mycoplasmas which can be isolated from cattle eyes include *M. bovis, M. bovirhinis, M. verecundum, A. laidlawii,* and *Ureaplasma diversum*. ELISA and MI tests are useful for serodiagnosis (Salih and Rosenbusch, 1986).

There is no information available on effective methods for control of *M. bovoculi* conjunctivitis. Salih *et al.* (1987) found that animals recovered from the infection resisted reinfection, but that experimental vaccination did not induce protection.

Ureaplasma diversum

Ureaplasma diversum is isolated from the female genital tract, prepuce and semen of bulls, pneumonic lungs of calves and feedlot cattle, and the eyes of cattle with keratoconjunctivitis. Isolations have been reported in England, the U.S., Japan, Denmark, and Canada. The organism is an important cause of granular vulvovaginitis, endometritis, salpingitis, early embryonic death, abortion, and birth of weak calves (Ruhnke and Miller, 1990).

As with *M. dispar* infection, respiratory tract disease is largely subclinical. Genital disease in the female is characterized by a purulent vulvar discharge, and inflamed, hyperemic vulvar mucosa with varying degrees of granularity. Up to 27% reduction in infertility may occur. In some field cases of conjunctivitis, ureaplasma may accompany *M. bovoculi* and *Moraxella bovis*. Conjunctivitis has been reproduced experimentally by intraconjunctival inoculation with ureaplasma.

Lesions seen in *U. diversum*-associated respiratory disease consist of purple to red consolidation in the cranioventral areas of the lung. As mentioned previously, gross lesions of granular vulvitis may be seen in the reproductive tract. Three serotypes of *U. diversum* have been described. Media for isolation of the organism include those reported by Taylor-Robinson *et al.* (1968), Livingston (1972), and Bitsch *et al.* (1976). *U. diversum* grows rapidly in broth, reaching peak titers in 32 h; however, viability declines rapidly.

Ureaplasmas appear to be very common in the pneumonic lungs of calves; occasionally, they are isolated from normal lungs. The principal reservoirs of ureaplasma infections in cattle are the respiratory tract and the urogenital tract. Spread of genital forms of the infection is facilitated by persistent infections in either the female or male genital tracts.

U. diversum has been shown to produce pneumonia, vulvitis, conjunctivitis, and mastitis experimentally. It apparently has no effect on semen quality, although semen is a vehicle for transmission of the organism. The organism may be a cause of endometritis and abortion. In addition, Ruhnke and Miller (1990) reported that seminal vesiculitis has been produced experimentally with *U. diversum* in bulls. Ruhnke *et al.* (1984) reported that aborted fetuses with *U. diversum* infection have microscopic lesions of alveolitis and placentitis. *U. diversum* has been shown to attach to the zona pellucida of bovine embryos (Britton *et al.*, 1989; Britton *et al.*, 1988 b). Quinn and Fortier (1990) reported that *U. diversum* adhered to epithelial, stromal, and gland cell cultures derived from bovine uteri.

Clinical signs of granular vulvitis should be considered suggestive of ureaplasma infection. Other signs, such as subclinical pneumonia or conjunctivitis, are less definitive. Diagnosis of abortion caused by *U. diversum* has been based on isolation of the organism and alveolitis and placentitis (Ruhnke and Miller, 1990). The organism can be isolated from the lesions using media described previously.

Little information is available on therapeutic strategies for control of *U. diversum* infection. Antibiotics with highest *in vitro* activity against the organism were tiamulin, erythromycin, tylosin, oxytetracycline, and chloramphenicol (Pilaszek and Truszczynsky, 1986). A mixture of gentamicin, tylosin, and lincomycin reduced numbers of ureaplasma in processed semen (Ruhnke and Miller, 1990). Caution needs to be exercised in embryo transplant work to avoid contamination of embryos with *U. diversum* (Britton *et al.*, 1988a). Culling of infected bulls has been utilized to stop transmission of *U. diversum* (Reid *et al.*, 1989b).

Mycoplasma bovigenitalium

Mycoplasma bovigenitalium was one of the first mycoplasmas characterized from cattle. The organism has been isolated from vaginal and semen samples, mastitis, pneumonia, and seminal vesiculitis. Although the organism is widespread in cattle, evidence that it is a major pathogen is lacking.

Overt clinical evidence of disease with *M. bovigenitalium* in cases of seminal vesiculitis may be inapparent or there may be pain on palpation of affected glands, pain on ejaculation, a slight febrile response, or uneasiness as evidenced by treading. *M. bovigenitalium* causes occasional cases of epididymitis, orchitis, and urethritis. Decreased viability of sperm may occur. Occasionally, the organism is involved in mastitis. Kreusel *et al.* (1989) reported that clinical disease did not develop in bulls inoculated intrapreputially with *M. bovigenitalium*. Similarly, Ball *et al.* (1990a) found no evidence of disease in cows inoculated into the uterus with this organism.

Affected seminal vesicles are enlarged, and when sectioned, brown with decreased secretions. Mastitic lesions are of a purulent character early followed by more prominence of the interstitial tissue. Respiratory disease associated with *M. bovigenitalium* consists of cranioventral consolidation of the lungs.

The organism can be grown easily on a variety of mycoplasma media, and it produces centered colonies often surrounded by the "film and spots" reaction. The organism does not ferment carbohydrates or hydrolyze arginine or urea.

M. bovigenitalium has been demonstrated in 16 to 94% of bull semen samples; incidence increases with increasing age. The organism is also present in up to 11% of samples of cervicovaginal mucus. Pfutzner (1989) found that nouroseothricin and lincomycin at 0.8 mg/ml could be used to eliminate *M. bovigenitalium, M. bovis,* or *A. laidlawii* from experimentally contaminated semen.

Media and methods for accurate detection of mycoplasmas in bull semen were reported by Richter *et al.* (1989) and Richter and Pfutznner (1989). Generally, a variety of media can be utilized for isolation of *M. bovigenitalium*. This organism should be considered in clinical cases of seminal vesiculitis or epididymitis and reduced sperm motility in bulls. Ahmed (1987) reported that growth inhibition, surface film inhibition, and growth precipitation procedures were useful for detection of antibodies in sera and milk whey from cows with *M. bovigenitalium* mastitis.

Mycoplasma alkalescens

This organism is an occasional isolate from respiratory samples, mastitis and arthritis and it has been implicated in an outbreak of arthritis with predisposing trauma to the joints. *M. alkalescens* hydrolyzes arginine, but has no effect on urea or glucose.

Mycoplasma bovirhinis

Mycoplasma bovirhinis has been isolated from respiratory tracts of cattle in England, Denmark, Japan, the U.S., Poland, and Czechoslovakia. While the organism is rather common in respiratory disease samples, it is apparently not a primary pathogen. *M. bovirhinis* grows well in a variety of media and forms centered colonies. It ferments glucose, but does not hydrolyze arginine or urea.

Mycoplasma californicum

Mycoplasma californicum is the second most common isolate from mastitis in cattle in California. It has also been isolated from cases of mastitis in England, Czechoslovakia, and Germany. Beer *et al.* (1986) reported isolation of the organism from arthritic joints of calves, and the lymph nodes, uterus, and lungs of cows. Pfutzner and Hofer (1989) evaluated several media formulations for efficiency of isolation of *M. californicum* from milk of mastitic cows. The organism has no effect on arginine, glucose or urea. ELISA has been used to detect antibodies to the organism in sera from infected cattle (Thomas *et al.*, 1987 a), In addition, Ball *et al.* (1990) found that an antigen capture ELISA with monoclonal antibodies was useful for detection of *M. californicum* in milk samples from infected cows. A combination of oxytetracycline and tylosin was beneficial when administered intramammarily in recently infected glands (Ball, 1989).

Mycoplasma canadense

Mycoplasma canadense has been isolated from mastitis, nasal mucus, vaginal mucus, semen, and synovial fluid of cattle. Ball *et al.* (1987) reported that the organism could be isolated from up to 40% of normal heifers after calving; however, they were unable to experimentally infect or induce disease in the bovine female reproductive tract. *M. canadense* hydrolyzes arginine, but has no effect on glucose or urea.

Mycoplasma Group 7

Group 7 organisms have been isolated from arthritis, mastitis, urogenital specimens, and aborted fetuses. It is reported to be associated with occasional outbreaks of respiratory disease and polyarthritis in calves. The organism ferments glucose, but does not hydrolyze arginine or urea. It crossreacts in serological tests with *M. capricolum* and the F38 mycoplasma from goats.

Mycoplasma alvi

Mycoplasma alvi is a flask-shaped mycoplasma isolated from the genital tract of cattle in England (Gourlay *et al.*, 1977). It has no known disease potential. The organism hydrolyzes arginine, but has no effect on glucose or urea.

Mycoplasma arginini

Mycoplasma arginini has been isolated from respiratory tracts of cattle in Switzerland, Germany, Romania, Czechoslovakia, the U.S., and Italy. The organism is apparently not a primary pathogen in cattle. *M. arginini* is a frequent isolate from bovine sera used in cell cultures and from cell cultures.

Acholeplasmas and Anaeroplasmas

Acholeplasma laidlawii has been isolated from mastitic milk, bulk tank milk, aborted fetuses, semen, preputial samples, nasal secretions, and pneumonic as well as normal lungs. Evidence that it is important as a pathogen has not been presented. The high prevalence of *A. laidlawii* and some other species of acholeplasmas in cattle make it essential that they be distinguished from mycoplasmas because they occur in the same tissue sites and grow more readily and more rapidly than mycoplasmas in media commonly used to isolate pathogenic mycoplasmas.

Anaeroplasmas are nonpathogenic anaerobic mycoplasmas from the rumen of cattle and other ruminant species. Some are sterol requiring, whereas others do not require sterols.

MYCOPLASMAS OF SHEEP AND GOATS

Mollicutes involved in disease in sheep and goats include 9 species of the genus *Mycoplasma* and one or more species of the genus *Ureaplasma*. Contagious agalactia of sheep and goats is caused by *M. agalactiae*; manifestations include septicemia, arthritis, and mastitis. *M. capri* is an occasional cause of pleuropneumonia in goats. Outbreaks of septicemia, arthritis, and mastitis are also occasionally caused by *M. capricolum* and *M. putrefaciens*. *M. conjunctivae* is a cause of conjunctivitis and keratoconjunctivitis in sheep and goats. *M. mycoides* subsp *mycoides* LC is a cause of septicemia, arthritis, mastitis, and pleuropneumonia in goats. *M. ovipneumoniae* is a cause of chronic subclinical pneumonia and is often involved in the more overt disease known as enzootic pneumonia in sheep and goats. Another organism, closely related to *M. capricolum,* known as the F38 mycoplasma, causes contagious caprine pleuropneumonia in goats. Ureaplasmas are also common in sheep and goats, causing infertility, abortion, granular vulvitis, and enhanced severity of urethral calculi in sheep. An unnamed taxon, group 11, also has been associated with granular vulvitis, and group G has been isolated from mastitis and arthritis (DaMassa *et al.*, 1990). Other species isolated from sheep or goats, which are apparently of no pathogenic significance, include *M. arginini, Acholeplasma* spp., and *Anaeroplasma* spp. Useful reviews of information on sheep and goat mycoplasmas and the diseases caused by them include those of Barile *et al.* (1985), Cottew (1979), Cottew (1983), McMartin *et al.* (1980) and Ross (1985 c). Reference citations in this review of sheep and goat mycoplasmas will focus on the most recent publications.

Mycoplasma agalactiae

Mycoplasma agalactiae is a cause of an important disease known as contagious agalactia in sheep and goats. This disease occurs mainly in many countries around the Mediterranean Sea and in Iran, Iraq, India, Mongolia, Portugal, Sudan, Switzerland, and the U.S.S.R.. Whether the organism has been isolated in all of these countries is not certain.

Clinically, the disease may present as acute, subacute, and chronic forms. Systemic signs in the acute disease include fever, inappetence, and lassitude. Mastitis presents as catarrhal to parenchymatous forms leading to fibrosis, involution, and loss of function. The milk from affected glands may be viscous and is yellow to blue. Swelling of joints, especially the tarsal and carpal joints, and lameness may be seen. Although conjunctivitis, keratitis, and corneal opacity have been reported, the direct role of *M. agalactiae* in eye disease is not clear.

Lesions seen include interstitial mastitis followed by fibrosis and abscessation. Affected joints evidence inflamed periarticular tissues, synovitis, and a caseous exudate within the joint cavity. *M. agalactiae* grows easily in a variety of mycoplasma media. It alkalinizes arginine, but has no effect on glucose or urea. Antigenic heterogeneity may occur among strains.

Transmission is effected by consumption of milk from affected mammae or by ocular discharges. The organism may be shed in the milk for many months. Initial invasion appears to be via the galactogenic route with septicemia occurring early during the course of the disease.

Lactational failure with mammary gland inflammation occurring post partum in endemic areas is highly suggestive of contagious agalactia. Accompanying arthritis is another indication. The organism can be isolated easily from mastitic milk or joint or ocular fluids. Media which have been used for isolation of the organism include those described by Turner *et al.* (1959) and Cottew *et al.* (1968).

Antibiotics reported to be useful for treatment of contagious agalactia include oxytetracycline, tylosin, spectinomycin, and erythromycin. Good management and sanitation, particularly prevention of suckling of infected dams by kids, should reduce spread of the disease. Vaccination has also been an aid in control. Erdag (1980) reported that both live and killed *M. agalactiae* vaccines are used successfully to control agalactia in sheep and goats in Turkey. Culture procedure has been useful for detection of chronically infected does; such animals should be culled for elimination of the carriers from an infected flock. Marino-Ode *et al.* (1984) and Levisohn *et al.* (1990a) reported use of ELISA for detection of antibodies to *M. agalactiae*. Vihan (1989) reported that N-acetyl-beta-D-glucosaminidase (NA-gase) activity was elevated in milk from goats with *M. agalactiae* mastitis.

Mycoplasma arginini

Mycoplasma arginini has been isolated from goats, sheep, cattle, and a variety of other hosts. It is isolated mainly from the respiratory tract and the upper gastrointestinal tract. Evidence that the organism is pathogenic for sheep or goats has not been presented.

Mycoplasma capricolum

Mycoplasma capricolum has been isolated from goats in Turkey, Australia, the U.S., and France, and from sheep in Zimbabwe and Morocco. It has been isolated from normal respiratory tracts and ears and from lesions of pneumonia and arthritis in goats. Severe outbreaks of systemic disease with mastitis and arthritis may occur in goats. In a study in Morocco, Taoudi *et al.* (1987) reported that it was the most frequently isolated mycoplasma from sheep pneumonia. The same workers reported that the organism produced mastitis in ewes. Schweighardt *et al.* (1989) isolated *M. capricolum* from alpine ibex in an animal reserve with disease characterized by septicemia, focal hepatic necrosis, and mortality.

Clinical features of overt *M. capricolum* disease include fever, depression, lameness, and joint swelling. At post mortem, animals with acute disease evidence lesions of septicemia. With a more prolonged course, there is arthritis, serositis, and meningitis. *M. capricolum* is grown easily in a variety of media. It forms typical centered colonies. Biochemically, it ferments glucose; some strains are reported to hydrolyze arginine. It should be noted that *M. capricolum* is closely related antigenically and by DNA homology to the F38 mycoplasma (Kibe *et al.*, 1985). Christiansen and Erno (1990) reported a comparison of RFLP patterns of rRNA genes in *M. capricolum* bovine group 7, and the F38 group; they concluded that RFLP patterns could be used to identify clinical isolates belonging to the F38 group.

Clinical features of overt *M. capricolum* disease include fever, depression, lameness, and joint swelling. At post mortem, animals with acute disease evidence lesions of septicemia. With a more prolonged course, there is arthritis, serositis, and meningitis. *M. capricolum* is grown easily in a variety of media. It forms typical centered colonies. Biochemically, it ferments glucose; some strains are reported to hydrolyze arginine. It should be noted that *M. capricolum* is closely related antigenically and by DNA homology to the F38 mycoplasma (Kibe *et al.*, 1985). Christiansen and Erno (1990) reported a comparison of RFLP patterns of rRNA genes in *M. capricolum*, bovine group 7, and the F38 group; they concluded that RFLP patterns could be used to identify clinical isolates belonging to the F38 group.

Relatively little information is available on the pathogenesis of *M. capricolum* disease; however, Sher *et al.* (1990) found that the organism has the potential to stimulate blast transformation of mouse lymphocytes, and membranes from the organism were found to stimulate bone marrow macrophages to secrete TNA-α and to kill tumor cells.

M. capricolum appears to be spread by poor milking practices and feeding of colostrum or milk from infected does to susceptible kids. Experimental infections resulted in septicemia followed by meningitis, serositis, and arthritis. Taoudi *et al.* (1988) confirmed the role of infected milk in transmission of *M. capricolum* to kids and demonstrated that adult animals inoculated intrabronchially developed only mild and transitory respiratory signs.

From the diagnostic standpoint, *M. capricolum* should be considered in any outbreak of septicemic disease in goats. As indicated, the organism can be isolated easily using a variety of media. Therapeutically, erythromycin, spiramycin, tetramycin and tylosin have been recommended.

Mycoplasma conjunctivae

Mycoplasma conjunctivae have been isolated from goats, sheep, and chamois with clinical keratoconjunctivitis. While the disease has been produced experimentally, the role of *M. conjunctivae* as a sole agent in field outbreaks of eye disease is not clear. Egwu *et al.* (1989), in a survey of microbiological flora in eyes of sheep, isolated *M. conjunctivae* from 92 of 240 (38%) with ovine infectious keratoconjunctivitis and 27 or 240 normal eyes (11%). Bacteria isolated more frequently from affected eyes included *Branhamella ovis*, *Escherichia coli*, and *Staphylococcus aureus*.

Clinically, there is lacrimation, inflammation of conjunctivae, and photophobia. The cornea becomes vascularized, clouded, and ulcerated. Abscessation and blindness may ensue.

M. conjunctivae may be isolated in media described by Barile *et al.* (1972), Nicolet and Freundt (1975), and Jones *et al.* (1976). The organism ferments dextrose, but does not utilize arginine or urea.

Keratoconjunctivitis with *M. conjunctivae* infection more commonly occurs during pasturing season, may be exacerbated by exposure to sunlight, and is commonly complicated with other agents. Hosie (1988) indicated that the disease occurred in Scotland most frequently in the fall and that blackface and Cheviot ewes were equally susceptible. For diagnosis, one should suspect *M. conjunctivae* involvement when keratoconjunctivitis is seen. Other mycoplasmas such as *M. agalactiae* or *M. mycoides* subsp. *mycoides* LC may be involved.

For control, topical application or parenteral administration (Hosie, 1989; Reid *et al.*, 1989a) of tetracyclines has been recommended. Limitation of sunlight exposure may also be important in flock control of the problem.

F38 Mycoplasma

Contagious caprine pleuropneumonia (CCPP) is caused by an organism known as the F38 mycoplasma (MacOwan, 1989). This disease, or a very similar one, has been reported from Libya, Sudan, Oman, Somalia, Chad, Kenya, Niger, Saudi Arabia, Yemen, Arab Republic, United Arab Emirates, Qatar, Bahrain, Kuwait, India, Turkey, U.S.S.R., South America, China, Italy, and Spain. It also occurs occasionally in Greece, Mexico, Portugal, and the U.S. However, clear evidence that the F38 mycoplasma is present in all of these countries has not been presented. CCPP may be the most serious disease occurring worldwide in goats.

Clinically, CCPP occurs in peracute, acute, and chronic forms. There is pyrexia, anorexia, coughing, dyspnea, and costal tenderness. Lesions seen at necropsy include fibrinous pneumonia, serofibrinous pleuritis, and occasionally pericarditis. Hematologic changes in goats with naturally occurring CCPP were characterized by Abdelsalam *et al.* (1988).

The F38 mycoplasma appears to grow best in medium containing up to 50% goat serum. It produces centered colonies, growing best under reduced oxygen, such as in a candle jar. It ferments glucose, but has no effect on urea or arginine.

The F38 mycoplasma is closely related antigenically and by DNA homology to *M. capricolum* (Kibe *et al.*, 1985). A polysaccharide-like antigen has been shown to be useful for serodiagnosis of F38 disease (Rurangirwa *et al.*, 1987 b).

F38 disease is assumed to be spread by contact and aerosol with chronic respiratory carriers playing a major role. Experimental disease has been produced by intratracheal inoculation of cultures.

Attenuated live culture or formalinized culture have been shown to be effective as vaccines for this disease (Rurangirwa *et al.*, 1987 a; King, 1988). King also reported that vaccines should not be administered until kids are 10 weeks of age or older in order to preclude maternal antibody interference with development of the active immune response. For therapy, tetracyclines or tylosin have been recommended.

Mycoplasma capri

Mycoplasma capri is an occasional isolate from pneumonia in goats; the organism has also been shown to cause pneumonia experimentally. Its significance in naturally occurring goat respiratory disease is not known. Widespread evidence of antibodies to *M. capri* was found in sera from goats in Oman (Jones and Wood, 1988). The organism can be isolated in a variety of media (Hayflick, 1965; Cottew, 1974). *M. capri* forms typical centered colonies on agar, and it ferments glucose but has no effect on arginine or urea.

Mycoplasma mycoides **subsp.** *mycoides LC*

Mycoplasma mycoides subsp. *mycoides* LC has been isolated in a variety of countries including Italy, Sweden, the U.S., Israel, and France from goats with systemic disease which may include arthritis and pneumonia. Clinical features of *M. mycoides* disease in goats include pyrexia, inappetence, dyspnea, lameness, swollen joints, mastitis, and keratoconjunctivitis. At necropsy, there is acute fibrinous pneumonia and pleuritis, suppurative polyarthritis, periarthritis, osteomyelitis, myocarditis, renal infarction, and lymphadenitis.

Mycoplasma mycoides subsp. *mycoides* LC grows rapidly in most media, forming typical centered colonies on agar. It ferments glucose, but does not hydrolyze arginine or urea. This so-called "large colony" (LC) type digests casein, liquifies serum, and is more stable at 45oC. The "small colony" (SC) type (contagious bovine pleuropneumonia) does not digest casein or liquify serum and is less stable at 45oC. The two types cannot be distinguished by use of the usual serologic procedures such as MI, GI, or EpiFA.

An important mode of transmission in some outbreaks in California was via the colostrum from infected mammary glands. A high proportion of kids consuming colostrum from infected dams developed disease. *M. mycoides* subsp. *mycoides* LC and other mycoplasmas have been isolated from the ear canal of goats (DaMassa and Brooks, 1991). Ear mites have been suspected as vectors for mycoplasmal disease in goats. DaMassa and Brooks (1991) demonstrated that *M. mycoides* could be cultured from the ear canal of goats, sheep, and pigs during mycoplasmemia. It is suspected that mycoplasmemia results in infection of the ear, and that the mites commonly found in the goat ear ingest the infected blood and transmit the organism to other goats. Recently, Nayak and Bhowmik (1990) reported experimental transmission of *M. mycoides* subsp. *mycoides* LC to susceptible kids by experimentally infected fleas of the order *Siphonaptera*.

The experimental disease can be induced by intratracheal or oral inoculation of the organism (DeMassa *et al.*, 1987). Evidence that the organism is often septicemic, in addition to causing pleuropneumonia, was presented by Rosendal (1981) and Bölske *et al.* (1989). Rosendal's group also presented evidence that *M. mycoides* is cytotoxic for (Valdivieso-Garcia *et al.*, 1989), and adheres to endothelial cells (Valdivieso-Garcia *et al.*, 1989b). In addition, a cytotoxic LC strain was shown to induce tumor necrosis factor *in vitro* and *in vivo* (Rosendal and Serebrin, 1990). Calves in contact with infected goats or inoculated directly with *M. mycoides* subsp. *mycoides* LC did not develop disease (Rosendal, 1983).

M. mycoides disease in young goats should be controlled by feeding of colostrum from normal does to those born from infected does. The infected does may be detected by culture of colostrum or milk and should be culled. Tylosin has been recommended for therapy; however, as with other severe mycoplasmoses, early therapy is essential. A formalin-killed vaccine provided protection against experimental challenge (Bar-Moshe *et al.*, 1984).

Levisohn *et al.*, (1990) reported use of the ELISA for diagnosis of *M. mycoides* subsp. *mycoides* LC disease in goats. Poumarat (1990) and Mitchelmore *et al.* (1990) reported use of dot immunobinding assay and computerized analysis of SDS-PAGE protein patterns, respectively, for investigation of the relationships between members of the *M. mycoides* cluster.

Mycoplasma ovipneumoniae

Mycoplasma ovipneumoniae is a widespread agent in sheep and goats. It has been isolated from sheep in Australia, New Zealand, the U.S., England, Scotland, Hungary, Oman, Mexico, Sudan, and Switzerland. The organism appears to be a cause of subclinical pneumonia which is often exacerbated by other agents such as *Pasteurella haemolytica* (enzootic pneumonia). The organism was isolated from 36% of 175 goats with respiratory disease (Goltz *et al.*, 1986). Brogden *et al.* (1988) isolated *M. ovipneumoniae* from the nasal secretions of 293 of 320 sheep in a ram test station; the organism was by far the most common of the mycoplasmas isolated. *M. ovipneumoniae* was strongly implicated as a major factor in an outbreak of pneumonia in captive Dall's sheep (Black *et al.*, 1988).

Clinically, naturally occurring *M. ovipneumoniae* associated disease presents with dry inspiratory rales, moist coughing, dyspnea, sneezing, and nasal discharge with moist inspiratory rales followed by a remission stage with occasional signs. Experimentally induced disease generally presents as a subclinical pneumonia. Evidence presented by Goltz *et al.* (1986) and Bocklisch *et al.* (1989) indicated that fever is an early clinical feature of experimentally induced *M. ovipneumoniae* disease. Pathology seen with *M. ovipneumoniae* disease consists of cranioventral pulmonary consolidation, resembling lesions of atelectasis. Pleuritis may also be seen (Goltz *et al.*, 1986).

M. ovipneumoniae is somewhat more fastidious, but can be isolated in several different media (see below). Colony development may be improved in a candle jar; colonies may be noncentered. The organism grows slowly in broth, produces slight opacity, and is improved by rotation in a slanted position during incubation. *M. ovipneumoniae* ferments glucose, but has no effect on arginine or urea. Using restriction endonuclease DNA analysis and SDS-PAGE of proteins, heterogeneity was detected among strains isolated from different flocks of sheep (Mew *et al.*, 1985). Comparison of 22 isolates using SDS-PAGE revealed marked heterogeneity (Thirkell *et al.*, 1990a). These workers identified 50 major polypeptides in one strain; 35 were shown to be antigenic using immunoblotting and membrane associated using radioimmune precipitation. Although considerable antigenic heterogeieity existed among isolates, at least 9 major antigens were conserved across all isolates. Further studies by the same group (Thirkell *et al.*, 1991) indicated significant cross-reactivity existed with ELISA and several other species of mycoplasmas. The specific crossreacting antigens were investigated utilizing immunoblotting.

Transmission of the organism is mediated primarily from reservoirs such as convalescent adult or older animals via contact or aerosol. Infection develops mainly following weaning (after 6-7 weeks of age) (Ionas *et al.*, 1985). Sequential nasal infections with different restriction enzyme types occurred within a single flock. The organism colonizes the nasal cavity transiently, then persists on the tracheobronchial epithelium. Jones *et al.* (1985) demonstrated that the organism produced ciliostasis and loss of cilia in tracheal organ cultures (Jones *et al.*, 1985). Experimental observations indicated that the organism may cause pleuritis in addition to pneumonia.

For diagnosis, the clinical features of a chronic enzootic pneumonia may be considered suggestive of *M. ovipneumoniae*. The organism can be isolated in broth media such as those described by Carmichael *et al.* (1972), Jones *et al.* (1976), Friis *et al.* (1976), or Frey *et al.* (1968) as modified by Clarke *et al.* (1974). The organisms can be detected in the airways of infected lung by immunofluorescence. ELISA appears to be useful for detection of antibodies to the organism (Thirkell *et al.*, 1990b).

Therapeutically, antibiotics have not been shown to be efficacious against the mycoplasmal component of this disease; however, appropriate therapy should be used for control of bacterial agents involved in the disease. Management, sanitation, and environment should be improved. All-in, all-out production in confinement systems should help to reduce severity of pneumonia. Vaccination has not been shown to be effective.

Mycoplasma putrefaciens

Mastitis and arthritis in dairy goats and polyarthritis in kids has been caused by *M. putrefaciens* (Da Massa *et al.*, 1987). Poor milking practices and feeding of raw, infected colostrum to kids were implicated in transmission of this organism. As with several other species of mycoplasmas, *M. putrefaciens* has been isolated from the ears of goats. The organism grows well in many media, forms centered colonies, and ferments glucose.

Ovine/Caprine Group 11 of Al-Aubaidi

The ovine/caprine group 11 organisms of Al-Aubaidi have been isolated from clinical cases of vulvovaginitis (Chima *et al.*, 1986). The organism crossreacts serologically with *M. bovigenitalium*.

Ovine and Caprine Ureaplasmas

Ureaplasmas are common in the urogenital tract of sheep and goats. They have been isolated from the respiratory tract only during rutting. Isolates from sheep have been classified into nine serogroups, one of which was associated with infertility, abortion, and granular vulvitis in sheep. The ureaplasmas have also been associated with urethral calculi in sheep. It appears that ureaplasma infection may influence the total amount of calculi and composition of calculi. Ball and McCaughey (1984) reported that treatment with tiamulin or oxytetracycline eliminated ureaplasmas from the urogenital tracts of some, but not all, infected sheep.

Acholeplasmas

Acholeplasmas isolated from sheep and goats include *A. laidawii*, *A. granularum*, and *A. oculi*. Their role in disease has not been established.

MYCOPLASMAL INFECTIONS OF SWINE

Three species of the genus *Mycoplasma* are known to cause disease in swine. *M. hyopneumoniae* causes chronic pneumonia in pigs 6 weeks of age or older, although occasionally the disease can be seen in younger pigs. *M. hyorhinis* causes polyserositis and arthritis in 3 to 10 week old pigs, and *M. hyosynoviae* causes arthritis in pigs 10 to 24 weeks of age. Other mycoplasmas isolated from swine include *M. flocculare*, *M. arginini*, *M. arthritidis*, *M. sualvi*, *M. hyopharyngis*, *Acholeplasma granularum*, and *A. laidlawii*. Binder and Kirchhoff (1988) recently reported isolation of anaerobic mycoplasmas from the intestines of swine. Useful reviews for information on swine mycoplasmas include those of Barile *et al.* (1985), Ross (1985d) Ross (1986), Whittlestone (1979), and Whittlestone (1983). The focus of this review will be on more recent information on swine mycoplasmas.

Mycoplasma hyopneumoniae

Mycoplasma hyopneumoniae is the cause of chronic pneumonia (Mycoplasmal Pneumonia of Swine or Enzootic Pneumonia) in swine characterized by a persistent, nonproductive cough, loss of condition, and growth retardation. Although *M. hyopneumoniae* initiates the disease, several microbial agents, as well as environmental factors are often involved.

Chronic pneumonia of swine is worldwide in distribution and occurs in virtually all herds. Surveys have indicated that from 30-80% of market swine have chronic pneumonia. Serologic surveys indicate that approximately 20% of breeding animals and 60% of herds have complement fixing antibodies to *M. hyopneumoniae* (Young *et al.*, 1983). Pointon *et al.* (1985) reported that rate of gain may be decreased as much as 16-30% and feed conversion by 14-20%. However, some studies have indicated no economic loss. The estimated average loss in U.S. swine production is $1.50 to $2.50 per pig marketed.

The incubation period is commonly 10 days to 3 weeks, although much longer intervals from suspected exposure to detection of clinically overt disease has been reported. The clinical signs include a sporadic, dry nonproductive cough, and an unthrifty appearance. Any febrile response is probably linked to involvement of secondary invaders. Generally, the disease is seen clinically after 5 to 7 weeks of age; it persists for 6 weeks or longer. Morbidity is generally high with low to moderate mortality, depending on the extent of involvement with other complicating factors. Some infections are clinically silent.

Typical lesions occurring in enzootic pneumonia consist of purple to tan or grey areas of cranioventral consolidation with varying degrees of firmness. The bronchi and bronchioles often contain catarrhal exudate, and the bronchial lymph nodes may be swollen and edematous. As mentioned, secondary invaders are common; therefore, many lesions have a mixed infection response. Lesions in uncomplicated *M. hyopneumoniae* disease may resolve within 6 weeks; however, lesions are often present 3 months after infection. When given intravenously, the organism may induce a chronic arthritis.

M. hyopneumoniae grows slowly in early passage from infected tissue. It can be isolated in media described by Friis (1975; 1979), Goodwin (1976), or Etheridge *et al.* (1979). The organism forms noncentered colonies on agar incubated in a candle jar. *M. hyopneumoniae* ferments glucose, but is inactive in arginine and urea.

Transmission of *M. hyopneumoniae* is assumed to be by droplet and contact means; however, breakdowns of enzootic pneumonia-free herds in close proximity to infected herds have been taken as evidence of airborne transmission (Goodwin, 1985; Jorsal and Thomsen, 1988).

Scanning (Mebus and Underdahl, 1977) and transmission (Blanchard *et al.*, 1990) electron microscopic examination have revealed a close association between the mycoplasma and cilia of infected porcine airways. Evidence has been presented that virulent strains have a thick glycocalyx (Tajima and Yagihashi, 1982; Tajima *et al.*, 1985; Huang *et al.*, 1986). Passage of the organism in swine may enhance virulence for pigs (Hannan *et al.*, 1984). Evidence has been presented that *M. hyopneumoniae* adheres to the ciliary tuft of ciliated epithelial cells from the swine trachea. The adherence is thought to be mediated by a combination of hydrophobic forces and ligand-type interactions (Zielinski and Ross, 1990; Zielinski, 1991). Epithelial damage seen in airways of infected swine has been simulated using tracheal organ cultures. The process was inhibited by convalescent serum (DeBey and Ross, 1990). Klinkert *et al.* (1985) reported cloning genes producing surface proteins from M. *hyopneumoniae*. Further molecular studies including assessment of the ribosomal RNA genes and analysis of transcription was reported (Taschke *et al.*, 1986); Taschke and Herrmann, 1986).

M. *hyopneumoniae* infection has been shown to induce suppression of antibody response in swine (Wannemuehler *et al.*, 1988) and, in combination with *Actinobacillus pleuropneumoniae*, to induce suppression of alveolar macrophage function (Caruso and Ross, 1990). M. *hyopneumoniae* infection increased severity of bacterial pneumonia such as caused by A. *pleuropneumoniae* (Yagihashi *et al.*, 1984; Ross, 1990) and *Pasteurella multocida* (Ciprian *et al.*, 1988).

Enzootic pneumonia may be suspected whenever there is widespread chronic coughing and poor growth and feed conversion in a herd. Necropsy findings of purple to gray cranioventral consolidation in the lungs is also suggestive of the disease; however, other infections also induce such lesions. M. *hyopneumoniae* can be detected in airways of lungs by direct (Amanfu *et al.*, 1984) or indirect immunofluorescence. Friis (1990) evaluated specificity of the indirect immunofluorescence procedure for detection of M. *hyopneumoniae* in swine lungs. Using lungs of swine infected with M. *flocculare*, he found little evidence of crossreactivity with M. *hyopneumoniae*. The organism can be detected in pneumonic lungs by use of an enzyme-linked immunoperoxidase technique (Bruggmann *et al.*, 1977; Doster and Lin, 1988), the polymerase chain reaction (Harasawa *et al.*, 1990), and capture ELISA (Pederson *et al.*, 1990). Stemke *et al.* (1987) reported development of a specific gene probe for M. *hyopneumoniae*.

The Tween 20 ELISA developed by Nicolet *et al.* (1980) and Bommeli and Nicolet (1983) appears to be the most useful serologic test for detection of antibodies to M. *hyopneumoniae* (Bölske *et al.*, 1990; Abiven *et al.*, 1990; Bereiter *et al.*, 1990). Using Tween 20 extracts of both M. *hyopneumoniae* and M. *flocculare*, Strasser and Nicolet (1990) and Bereiter *et al.* (1990) found that antibodies to these organisms in swine sera were specific and that reciprocal crossreactivity was minimal. Kazama *et al.* (1989) reported that specificity of the Tween 20 antigen could be improved by chromatography on Sepharyl S300. The Tween 20 ELISA has been used to survey for antibodies to M. *hyopneumoniae* in sow colostrum and milk (Zimmerman *et al.*, 1986; Nicolet, 1987). Feld *et al.* (1990) developed a competitive ELISA for detection of antibodies to M. *hyopneumoniae*. Detection was based on a biotinylated monoclonal antibody against a polypeptide of approximately 74 kDa.

Antibiotics such as the tetracyclines, lincomycin, and tiamulin have been recommended for treatment of enzootic pneumonia. While these drugs may be beneficial, especially for control of the bacterial agents involved, they appear not to be useful for control of the mycoplasma. Quinolone antibiotics appear to hold good promise for use in therapy of M. *hyopneumoniae* disease (Hannan *et al.*, 1989; Simon *et al.*, 1990; Ross *et al.*, 1990). Control strategies based on complete elimination of the organism such as by repopulation with SPF animals or derivation by way of the medicated early weaning program (Alexander *et al.*, 1990; Harris *et al.*, 1988) are the most effective; however, these strategies have limited potential for many herds because of the cost and risk of reinfection. Recently, new vaccines have been introduced for con-trol of *M. hyopneumoniae* disease (Dayalu and Ross, 1990; Peterson *et al.*, 1990). Kobisch *et al.*, (1987) reported development of a *M. hyopneumoniae* vaccine utilizing membranes of the organism. Protection was obtained by passive immunization (vaccination of pregnant sows) and by immunization of piglets (Kobisch *et al.*, 1990). These vaccines reduce severity of the lesions and may reduce the economic impact of the disease on growth.

Mycoplasma hyorhinis

Mycoplasma hyorhinis causes occasional cases of acute, subacute, and chronic polyserositis and arthritis in swine from 3 to 10 weeks of age. The disease is characterized by serofibrinous inflammation of the serous membranes and joints. It also occurs occasionally in highly susceptible (SPF) young adult swine.

Clinically, *M. hyorhinis* disease generally has a progressive onset, and there is labored breathing, a roughened hair coat, abdominal tenderness, lameness, decreased appetite, and elevated temperature. Gross lesions consist of serofibrinous inflammation of membranes lining the pericardial, pleural, and peritoneal cavities and serofibrinous to serosanguineous arthritis. In chronic stages, there are often adhesions in the body cavities and chronic arthritis.

M. hyorhinis may be isolated with a variety of mycoplasmal media. It forms centered colonies, ferments glucose, and does not utilize arginine or urea. Rosengarten and Wise (1990) demonstrated high frequency phase transitions in colony morphology and opacity and in expression of lipid-modified surface protein antigens of *M. hyorhinis*. This ability to switch phases may relate to ability of the organism to cause disease and persist in swine tissues.

Transmission is effected from adult carrier swine. The organism spreads rapidly in a litter of swine; many young pigs have clinically inapparent nasal and tracheobronchial infections. The organism is a frequent secondary invader in pneumonia caused by other agents.

Gross lesions of polyserositis and arthritis may be suggestive of *M. hyorhinis* infection; however, other causes such a *Haemophilus parasuis*, *Streptococcus suis*, and *Pasteurella multocida* also may cause these lesions. The organism can be isolated from typical acute and chronic lesions of polyserositis and arthritis. Serological methods, such as complement fixation and ELISA, are useful for detection of antibody to the organism, but are not generally available.

Affected animals generally do not respond well to antibiotic therapy. Treatment of clinically normal animals in contact with affected animals using tylosin, linomycin, tetracyclines, or quinolone antibiotics may be beneficial.

Mycoplasma hyosynoviae

Mycoplasma hyosynoviae causes an acute, subacute, and occasionally chronic, nonsuppurative arthritis in growing swine from 40 kg to slaughter weight and occasionally in young adult swine.

Clinically, signs in overt *M. hyosynoviae* disease consist of sudden onset of lameness, generally with little evidence of joint swelling. The acute stage persists for 3 to 10 days. Many animals recover and evidence no chronic lameness. At necropsy, affected joints often contain large amounts of sero-fibrinous to serosanguineous fluid and the synovial membranes are inflamed.

M. hyosynoviae can be isolated in most media. Growth is enhanced by mucin. The organism utilizes arginine and does not ferment glucose or utilize urea. *M. hyosynoviae* is carried in tonsils and pharyngeal secretions of many adult swine. It is intermittently shed in nasal secretions. Often, a few pigs are infected by weaning and these serve to spread the organism among penmates. Clinical expression of overt arthritis appears to depend on timing of exposure and enhancement of susceptibility by prior joint damage such as that caused by osteochondrosis.

For diagnosis, culture of synovial fluid samples from several acutely affected joints is optimal. Tylosin, lincocin, tiamulin, and probably, quinolone antibiotics are useful in therapy of acute *M. hyosynoviae* arthritis. Infection results in immunity to reinfection with the organism.

Mycoplasma flocculare

Mycoplasma flocculare has been isolated from the lungs and nasal cavities of normal swine and swine with respiratory disease. It is apparently not pathogenic (Abiven *et al.*, 1990), but is very similar genetically and antigenically to *M. hyopneumoniae*. While cross-reacting antibodies between *M. hyopneumoniae* and *M. flocculare* occur in swine sera, more recently developed serologic methods (ELISA) have obviated problems in distinguishing between infections caused by these two agents (Abiven *et al.*, 1990; Bereiter *et al.*, 1990). The organism can be grown in Friis medium. It often forms non-centered colonies and ferments glucose.

MYCOPLASMAS OF POULTRY

Mycoplasmas causing disease in chickens, turkeys, and ducks include the following species. *M. gallisepticum* is a cause of chronic respiratory disease in chickens and infectious sinusitis in turkeys. *M. meleagridis* is a cause of air-sacculitis in turkey poults. *M. synoviae* causes airsacculitis and synovitis in turkeys and chickens. *M. iowae* is a cause of airsacculitis and reduced hatchability of chicken eggs and, possibly, immunosuppression in turkey poults. *M. gallinarum* may be an important secondary invader in certain viral diseases. *M. anatis* is a cause of airsacculitis in ducklings. *M. anseris* and *M. cloacale* have been associated with reductions in egg production, infertility, inflammation of the cloaca and phallus, and lack of weight gain in hatched goslings (Bradbury *et al.*, 1988; Stipkovits *et al.*, 1986). Several other species of mycoplasmas have been isolated from poultry; however, their relationship to disease has not been clearly demonstrated. Useful reviews on poultry mycoplasmas include those by Barile *et al.* (1985), Jordan (1979), Jordan (1983), and Yoder (1991). Citations in this review will be primarily for advances made subsequent to the previous reviews on poultry mycoplasmas.

Mycoplasma gallisepticum

Mycoplasma gallisepticum is a cause of chronic respiratory disease (CRD) of chickens and infectious sinusitis of turkeys. The agent is distributed world-wide in poultry populations, except where rigorous control measures have been implemented. When present in a flock, *M. gallisepticum* is often a cause of major economic loss. Condemnations at slaughter account for a major part of the economic loss. In addition, there is poor production efficiency (growth and egg laying), and medication costs. Mycoplasmas isolated from geese and ducks in France were shown to be closely related to *M. gallisepticum* (Dupiellet *et al.*, 1990).

Signs of *M. gallisepticum* infection include respiratory rales, coughing, nasal discharge, and, frequently, sinusitis in turkeys. Onset of the disease is often slow and the disease is often chronic.

Media for isolation of *M. gallisepticum* include those described by Hall (1962), Vardaman (1967), Frey *et al.* (1968), and Jordan (1983). An evaluation of media and methods for accurate detection of mycoplasmas in turkeys was reported recently by Rott *et al.* (1989). The authors recommended culture of palatine, cloacle, and semen samples for detection of low level infections. *M. gallisepticum* forms centered colonies and ferments glucose. Levisohn *et al.* (1989) reported development of a gene probe for detection of *M. gallisepticum* in tissue specimens and for rapid identification of the organism in enrichment cultures from primary clinical specimens. The probe detected the organism during early stages of infection more rapidly than by culture method; success rates for detection were comparable to those obtained by culture. Biotinylated gene probes for the organism have been developed by Geary *et al* (1990) and Levisohn *et al.* (1990 b). An immunobinding assay in 96-well filtration manifold was used by Sharp *et al.* (1991) for differentiation of avian mycoplasmas. According to the authors, the assay detected 50 ng of mycoplasmal protein, approximately 3×10^4 colony forming units, in mixed or pure cultures. The polymerase chain reaction was applied with very high sensitivity in detection of *M. gallisepticum* DNA by Nascimento *et al.* (1991).

Recently, Goll (1989) reported that a national survey in the U.S. revealed good uniformity among laboratories in reporting of serological test results for mycoplasmosis in chickens and turkeys. Tests evaluated were the serum plate agglutination test and the hemagglutination inhibition test, both widely used in diagnosis of avian mycoplasmoses. In a comparison of various serological tests for detection of antibodies to *M. gallisepticum*, Avakian and Kleven (1990) found that the serum plate agglutination test was most sensitive and the hemagglutination inhibition test had the highest specificity. False positive reactions were obtained with ELISA tests; however, results obtained using immunoblotting suggested that several species-specific polypeptides had potential to be utilized as improved ELISA antigens. Kleven and Avakian

(1990) and Megahed *et al.* (1990) also identified polypeptides which have potential as specific antigens for use in the *M. gallisepticum* ELISA. Panangala *et al.* (1990) utilized capture ELISA with monoclonal antibodies to detect antbodies to *M. gallisepticum* and *M. synoviae* in sera from experimentally immunized birds and commercial flock sera. Immunobinding assays (Shimizu *et al.*, 1990; Cummins *et al.*, 1990) have also been used for detection of antibodies to *M. gallisepticum.* Brown and Butcher (1990) found that egg yolks could be utilized to screen flocks for presence of antibody to *M. gallisepticum.* Shimizu *et al.* (1990) reported use of an adhesion-hemadsorption inhibition test for detection of antibody in sera of chickens infected with *M. gallisepticum.* The test was based on inhibition of adsorption of chicken or sheep red blood cells to *M. gallisepticum* which were adhered to plastic surfaces.

Transmission of *M. gallisepticum* may occur by contact, aerosol, and droplet means from infected carrier chickens or turkeys. Another very important mode of transmission is via venereal and egg transmission. The organism is frequently carried in the oviduct and on male genitalia. Kleven (1990) also found that RFLP analysis was useful for epidemiologic studies on *M. gallisepticum.* RFLP patterns obtained with several strains associated with clinical outbreaks of disease were different from that of the F-strain used for vaccination. Strain variability in virulence of *M. gallisepticum* field isolates was reported by Ley *et al.* (1990)

The incubation period appears to vary from 6 to 21 days experimentally. Stress factors may precipitate clinical outbreaks. As with many other respiratory pathogenic mycoplasmas, attachment of respiratory epithelial cells is an initial event in the pathogenesis of *M. gallisepticum* disease. The organism has been shown to have a specialized attachment moiety. A hemagglutinin was purified and shown by Forsyth *et al.* (1990) to be a highly immunogenic protein in *M. gallisepticum.*

A variety of antibiotics have been used as injectable or feed medications for treatment of CRD. Of these, the tetracycline antibiotics, tylosin, tiamulin, and lincomycin combined with spectinomycin have been more effective. Recently, a quinolone antibiotic, danofloxacin, was shown to reduce mortality and airsac lesions in experimentally infected chicks (Kempf *et al.*, 1990 a).

Several strategies have been proven effective for control of *M. gallisepticum* infections in poultry. Carriers can be detected by use of serologic methods such as the HI test. Serologically negative adults are used as a source of eggs for hatching to establish *M. gallisepticum*-free populations. Another strategy is to immunize layer chickens with an avirulent strain, such as the F-strain, in order to prevent overt disease. Yamamoto *et al.* (1990) reported that continuous use of the F-strain vaccine in replacement layer flocks results in displacement of the original field strain of *M. gallisepticum.* Strain specific DNA probes were used to track prevalence of wild-type and vaccine strains. Similarly, Dovc *et al.* (1990) reported use of RFLP analysis to differentiate strains of *M. gallisepticum* or *M. gallinarum* in epidemiological studies. The avirulent F-strain is too virulent for use in turkeys. An inactivated oil emulsion bacterin has also been utilized. Neither vaccine prevents infection of the upper respiratory tract in the face of a heavy challenge; however, improved egg production, egg size and grade, and feed conversion may be obtained by

91

using vaccines. Talkington and Kleven (1985) and Cummings and Kleven (1986) found that the F-strain induced better protection against tracheal infection with *M. gallisepticum* than the killed vaccine. Temperature sensitive mutants may also be used to induce protection. Other alternatives for control of *M. gallisepticum* include dipping of fertile eggs in solutions of antibiotics such as tylosin or erythromycin, injecting lincomycin into the fertile eggs, or heating of fertile eggs to prevent transmission of the organism; all of these strategies are applied prior to incubation of fertile eggs.

Mycoplasma synoviae

Mycoplasma synoviae is a cause of infectious synovitis and airsacculitis in turkeys and chickens. The organism has been isolated primarily in the U.S. However, Molokwu *et al.* (1987) reported isolation of the organism from chickens with CRD in Nigeria and Morrow *et al.*, (1990 a) from Australia. In a chronological study of experimental *M. synoviae* infection, Levisohn *et al.* (1986) found progressive changes in the trachea including edema, deciliation, and some desquamation of epithelia. Epithelium began regenerating from 15 days PI onward. Evidence of a specialized attachment organelle was not detected in *M. synoviae*.

Restriction endonuclease analysis of *M. synoviae* strains revealed that strains could be grouped and that electrophoretic patterns obtained were fairly stable (Morrow *et al.*, 1990 b). It was proposed that genotypic heterogeneity identified by REA may be useful for epidemiological studies on *M. synoviae*. *M. synoviae* has been shown to possess immunoglobulin Fc receptors (Lauerman and Reynolds-Vaughn, 1991).

As with many other mycoplasmas, contact and aerosol are important modes of transmission for *M. synoviae*. However, egg transmission appears to be the principal mode of transmission.

M. synoviae disease is an acute generalized process manifesting primarily as airsacculitis or arthritis. Synovitis occurring in the joints, keel bursae, and tendons is also seen. In a study of experimentally induced *M. synoviae* infection, tracheae of turkeys and chickens evidenced focal loss of cilia, and hyperplasia of goblet and basal cells (Kempf *et al.*, 1990 a). In addition, decreased ciliary activity was seen in tracheal rings established *in vitro* from infected birds. Zhao and Yamamoto (1990 b) reported development of recombinant DNA probes for identification of *M. synoviae*. Immunobinding (Shimizu *et al.*, 1990; Cummins *et al.*, 1990) and microimmunofluorescence assays (Bradbury *et al.*, 1990) have been used for detection of antibodies to *M. synoviae*. Ley and Avakian (1990) reported use of RFLP analysis to differentiate strains of *M. synoviae*. Control measures include immersion of fertile eggs in antibio-tics, or heating of the fertile eggs prior to incubation. Chlortetracycline has been administered in the feed to layers to reduce the impact of *M. synoviae* infection.

Mycoplasma meleagridis

Mycoplasma meleagridis causes airsacculitis in turkeys. The disease became evident with the elimination of *M. gallisepticum* from many flocks; it was found that up to 50% of progeny were infected with *M. meleagridis*. Lesions are commonly seen under such circumstances in the day old poult. Rott *et al.* (1989 a) isolated *M. meleagridis* from a high percentage of palatine and cloacal swabs from turkey hens and toms. Isolation of the organism from embryonated eggs varied from 50 to 100% with the duration of laying.

M. meleagridis is transmitted primarily from the infected oviduct of the hen to the egg. Spread among newly hatched poults occurs as well. Infection of the reproductive tract may occur as a consequence of insemination with contaminated semen. Egg transmission is minimal in hens if the infection is restricted to the upper respiratory tract and if clean semen is used.

The organism can be isolated in media described by Jordan (1983) and Rott *et al.* (1989 b). As with other poultry mycoplasmas, the organism can be controlled by dipping of fertile eggs in antibiotic solutions or by injection of antibiotics into the eggs. Sanitation is important in semen collection and insemination.

Mycoplasma iowae

Mycoplasma iowae is a cause of reduced hatchability of chicken embryos, airsacculitis, arthritis, tenosynovitis, and rupture of the digital flexor tendon. Bradbury and Kelly (1991) recently reported that infection of broiler chicks at one day of age resulted in stunting and poor feathering, as well as rupture of the digital flexor tendon, tenosynovitis, tendon fibrosis, and arthritis. Shareef *et al.* (1990) reported use of immunogold labelling to detect *M. iowae* in the cloaca and secondary folds of the turkey vagina. Evidence has been obtained that *M. iowae* infection in young turkeys may damage the bursa of Fabricius and cause immunosuppression. The organism has been shown to be capable of colonizing in the gastrointestinal tract of turkey poults (Sha-Majid and Rosendal, 1987b). In further work, the same authors (Sha-Majid and Rosendal (1987 a) found that the strains of *M. iowae* could be grown on medium containing 0.05% bile, a property which has potential value in selective media as well as in distinguishing the organism from other avian mycoplasmas. A species-specific DNA probe for *M. iowae* was reported by Zhao and Yamamoto (1990).

Mycoplasma gallinarum

Mycoplasma gallinarum is another agent isolated from chickens, turkeys, and other fowl. The organism is generally considered to be nonpathogenic. However, it has been shown to exacerbate respiratory disease when mixed infections with infectious bronchitis virus occur.

MYCOPLASMAS OF HORSES

Mycoplasmas isolated from horses include *M. equirhinis*, *M. fastidiosum*, *M. equigenitalium*, *M. felis*, and *M. subdolum*. The only ones for which there is evidence of pathogenicity are *M. felis* and *M. equigenitalium*. Several species of acholeplasmas have also been isolated from horses. Reviews containing information on equine mycoplasmas include those by Lemcke (1979), Poland and Lemcke (1978), and Ross (1985b).

Mycoplasma equigenitalium

Mycoplasma equigenitalium has been isolated from cervical mucus of mares, stallion semen, and an aborted equine fetus. The organism has been reported from Canada, Germany, and Yugoslavia. A survey of samples from various sites in mares and stallions on 6 farms in Ontario revealed that *M. equigenitalium* and *M. subdolum* were the most frequently isolated (Bermudez *et al.*, 1987). Isolations were made from samples collected from the clitoral fossa in the mare and the urethra of the stallion. Bermudez *et al.* (1990a) found that the organism attached to equine uterine tube ciliated cells and caused cytopathology and decreased ciliary movement. In subsequent work, the same authors (Bermudez *et al.*, 1990 b) reported an association between epithelial cell injury in oviductal explants, attachment of the organism, and calmodulin release. *M. equigenitalium* can be isolated in medium described by Kirchhoff (1978). It forms typical centered colonies and ferments glucose.

Mycoplasma equirhinis

Mycoplasma equirhinis has been isolated from the trachea, nasopharynx, and tonsils of both normal horses and horses with respiratory disease. Initial reports were from England and Germany. The pathogenic significance of *M. equirhinis* has not been determined; it spreads by contact among experimental ponies and CF antibodies develop in their sera. *M. equirhinis* can be isolated in medium described by Poland and Lemcke (1978). It forms typical centered colonies on agar and hydrolyzes urea.

Mycoplasma fastidiosum

Another organism isolated from the nasopharynx of horses is *M. fastidiosum*. Its pathogenic significance has not been determined. The organism is fastidious and is recovered only when other more rapidly growing mycoplasmas are not present. A medium described by Lemcke and Poland (1980) has been useful for isolation of the organism.

Mycoplasma felis

Mycoplasma felis is the most common glycolytic mycoplasma in the equine respiratory tract. It has been isolated in England, Germany and Canada. Rosendal *et al.* (1986) reported that it is involved in pleuritis in foals. Useful media for isolation of *M. felis* include those of Allam and Lemcke (1975) and Poland and Lemcke (1978). The organism ferments glucose, but is inactive in arginine and urea. Brown et al. (1990) reported development of an immuno-binding assay for identification of *M. felis*.

Mycoplasma subdolum

Mycoplasma subdolum is occasionally isolated from cervical mucus and aborted equine fetuses; however, it has not been shown to be a pathogen. The organism may be isolated in media described by Krabisch *et al.* (1973) and Poland and Lemcke (1978). *M. subdolum* hydrolyzes arginine, but is inactive in glucose and urea.

ACKNOWLEDGEMENT

Appreciation is expressed to Barbara Erickson, Janet Read, Janet Reese, and Kevin Timmerman for their assistance in preparation of this manuscript.

REFERENCES

Abdelsalam, E. B., Goraish, I.A. and Tartour, G. (1988) Clinico-pathological aspects of naturally-occuring contagious caprine pleuropneumonia in the Sudan. Rev. Elev. Med. Pays Trop. 41:52-54.

Abiven, P., Strasser, M., Kobisch, M. and Nicolet, J. (1990) Antibody response of swine experimentally infected with *Mycoplasma hyopneumoniae* and *Mycoplasma flocculare*. Zbl. Bakt. Suppl. 20:8177-818.

Ahmed, A.A. (1987) An outbreak of *Mycoplasma bovigenitalium* mastitis in Egypt. Egypt J. Vet. Sci. 24:45-53.

Alexander, T. J. L., Thornton, K., Boon, G., Lysons, R.J. and Gush, A. F. (1980) Medicated early weaning to obtain pigs free from pathogens endemic in the herd of origin. Vet. Rec. 106:114-119.

Allam, N. M. and Lemcke, R. M. (1975) Mycoplasmas isolated from the respiratory tract of horses. J. Hyg. 74:385-408.

Almeida, R. and Rosenbusch, R. (1990) Impaired function of the mucociliary apparatus of calves infected with *Mycoplasma dispar*. IOM Letters 1:310.

Almeida, R. and Rosenbusch R. (1991) Interaction between capsulated *Mycoplasma dispar* and bovine alveolar macrophages. Proc. 91 Gen. Mtg. Am. Soc. Microbiol. Abst. G-40.

Alzieu, J. P., Bichet, H. J., Levrier, B., Van Gool, F., Bayle, R., Libersa, M. and Espinasse, J. (1989) Efficacy and long-lasting activity of spiramycin in young beef cattle with infectious enzootic bronchopneumonia (I.E.B.P.). Bov. Pract. 24:38-41.

Amanfu, W., Weng, C.N., Ross, R.F. and Barnes, H.J. (1984) Diagnosis of myco-plasmal pneumonia of swine: sequential study of direct immunofluo-rescence. Am. J. Vet. Res. 45:1349-1352.

Avakian, A. P. and Kleven, S. H. (1990) The humoral immune response of chickens to *Mycoplasma gallisepticum* and potential causes of false positive reactions in avian mycoplasma serology. Zbl. Bakt. Suppl 20:500-512.

Ball, J. H. and Campbell, J. N. (1989) Antibiotic treatment of experimental *Mycoplasma californicum* mastitis. Vet. Rec.   125:377-378.

Ball, H.J. and McCaughey, W.J. (1984) Investigating into the elimination of ureaplasmas from the urogenital tract of ewes. Brit. Vet. J. 140:292-299.

Ball, H. J., Armstrong, D., McCaughey, W. J. and Kennedy, S. (1987) Experimental intrauterine inoculation of cows at oestrus with *Mycoplasma canadense*. Vet. Rec. 120:370.

Ball, H. J., Armstrong, D. Kennedy, S. and McCaughey, W. J. (1990a) Experimental intrauterine inoculation of cows at oestrus with *Mycoplasma bovigenitalium*. Vet. Rec. 12:486.

Ball, H. J., Armstrong, D. Kennedy, S. and McCaughey, W. J. (1990a) Experimental intrauterine inoculation of cows at oestrus with *Mycoplasma bovigenitalium*. Vet. Rec. 12:486.

Ball, H. J., Mackie, D. P., Finlay, D., McNair, J. and Pollack, D. A. (1990b) An antigen capture ELISA test using monoclonal antibodies for the detection of *Mycoplasma californicum* in milk. Vet. Immunol. Immunopathol. 25:269-278.

Barber, D. M. L., Jones, G. E., and Wood, A. (1986) Microbial flora of the eyes of cattle. Vet. Rec. 118:204-206.

Barile, M. F., DelGuidice, R. and Tully, J. G. (1972) Isolation and characterization of *Mycoplasma conjunctivae* sp.n. from sheep and goats with keratoconjunctivitis. Infect. Immun. 5:70-76.

Barile, M. F., Bové, J. M., Bradbury, J. M., Cassell, G. H., Clyde Jr., W. A., Cottew, G. S. and Whittlestone, P. (1985) Current status on control of mycoplasmal diseases of man, animals, plants and insects. Bull. Inst. Past. 83:339-373.

Bar-Moshe, B., Rapoport, E. and Brenner, J. (1984) Vaccination trials against *Mycoplasma mycoides* subsp. *mycoides* (large-colony-type) infection in goats. Isr. J. Med. Sci. 20:972-974.

Beer, K., Durrung, H. and Pfutzner, H. (1986) Untersuchungen zur Organmanifestation von *Mycoplasma californicum* beim Rind. Arch. Exp. Vet. Med. 40:S63-66.

Bereiter, M., Young, T., Joo, H. S. and Ross, R. F. (1990) Evaluation of the ELISA and comparison to the complement fixation test and radial immunodiffusion enzyme assay for detection of antibodies against *Mycoplasma hyopneumoniae* in swine serum. Vet. Microbiol. 25:177-192.

Bermudez, V., Miller, R., Johnson, W., Rosendal, S. and Ruhnke, L. (1987) Recovery of *Mycoplasma* spp. from the reproductive tract of the mare during the estrous cycle. Can. Vet. J. 28:519-522.

Bermudez, V., Miller, R., Rosendal, S. and Johnson, W. (1990a) *In vitro* cytopathic effect of *Mycoplasma equigenitalium* on the equine uterine tube. Zbl. Bakt. Suppl. 20:419-428.

Bermudez, V., Miller, R. B., Rosendal, S., Johnson, W. and Fernando, A. (1990b) Peroxidation as a mechanism of virulence of *Mycoplasma equigenitalium* causing cell injury measured by calmodulin levels and ciliary activity using equine uterine tube explants. IOM Letters 1:311-312.

Bielanski, A., Eaglesome, M. D., Ruhnke, H. L. and Hare, W. C. D. (1989) Isolation of *Mycoplasma bovis* from intact and microinjected preimplantation bovine embryos washed or treated with trypsin or antibiotics. J. Vitro Fert. Embryo Trans. 6:236-241.

Binder, A. and Kirchhoff, H. (1988) Isolation of anaerobic mollicutes from the intestine of swine. Vet. Microbiol. 17:151-158.

Bitsch, V., Friis, N. F. and Krogh, H. V. (1976) A microbiological study of pneumonic calf lungs. Acta Vet. Scand. 17:32-42.

Black, S. R., Barker, I. K., Mehren, K. G., Crawshaw, G. J., Rosendal, S., Ruhnke, L., Thorsen, J. and Carman, S.P. (1988) An epizootic of *Mycoplasma ovipneumoniae* infection in captive Dall's sheep (*Ovis dalli dalli*). J. Wild. Dis. 24:627-635.

Blanchard, B., Cavalier, A., LeLannic, J. and Kobisch, M. (1990) Electron microscopic observation of respiratory tract from gnotobiotic piglets inoculated with *Mycoplasma hyopneumoniae*. IOM Letters 1:480-481.

Bocklisch, H., Pfutzner, H., Martin, J., Templin, G. and Kreusel, S. (1986) *Mycoplasma-bovis*-Aborte bei Kuhen nach experimenteller Infektion. Arch. Exper. Vet. Med. 40:S48-55.

Bocklisch, H., Pfutzner, H. and Zepezauer, V. (1989) Naturliche und experimentelle infektionen von schaflammern mit *Mycoplasma ovipneumoniae*. Arch. Exper. Vet. Med. 43:S755-761.

Bölske, G., Engvall, A., Renstrom, L. H. M. and Wierup, M. (1989) Experimental infections of goats with *Mycoplasma mycoides* subspecies *mycoides*, LC type. Res. Vet. Sci. 46:247-252.

Bölske, G., Johansson, K.-E., Strandberg, M.-L. and Bergstrom, K. (1990) Comparison of the cross-reactions to different *Mycoplasma hyopneumoniae* antigen preparations in ELISA. Zbl. Bakt. Suppl. 20:832-834.

Bommeli, W. R. and Nicolet, J. (1983) A method for the evaluation of enzyme-linked immunoassay results for diagnosing enzootic pneumonia in pig herds. Proc. 3rd Int. Symp. World Assoc. Vet. Lab. Diagnost. 2:439-442.

Boothby, J. T., Jasper, D. E. and Thomas, C. B. (1986 a) Experimental intramammary inoculation with *Mycoplasma bovis* in vaccinated and unvaccinated cows: effect on milk production and milk quality. Can. J. Vet. Res. 50: 200-204.

Boothby, J. T., Jasper, D. E. and Thomas, C. B. (1986 b) Experimental intramammary inoculation with *Mycoplasma bovis* in vaccinated and unvaccinated cows: effect on the mycoplasma infection and cellular inflammatory response. Cornell Vet. 76:188-197.

Boothby, J. T., Suhore, C. E., Jasper, D. E., Osburn, B. I. and Thomas, C. B. (1988) Immune responses to *Mycoplasma bovis* vaccination and experimental infection in the bovine mammary gland. Can. J. Vet. Res. 52:355-359.

Bradbury, J. M. and Kelly, D. F. (1991) *Mycoplasma iowae* infection in broiler breeders. Avian Path. 20:67-78.

Bradbury, J. M., Loughanane, J. P. and Jordan, F. T. W. (1990) Microimmunofluorescence for the detection of antibodies to avian mycoplasmas. IOM Letters 1:168-169.

Britton, A. P., Miller, R. B., Ruhnke, H. L., and Johnson, W. H. (1988a) The recovery of ureaplasmas from bovine embryos following *in vitro* exposure and ten washes. Theriogenol. 30:997-1003.

Britton, A. P., Ruhnke, H. L., Miller, R .B. and Johnson, W. H. (1988b) Adherence of *Ureaplasma diversum* to the bovine zona pellucida. Theriogenol. 29:229.

Britton, A. P., Miller, R. B., Ruhnke, H. L. and Johnson, W. M. (1989) Protein a gold identification of ureaplasmas on the bovine zona pellucida. Can. J. Vet. Res. 53:172-175.

Brogden, K. A., Rose, D., Cutlip, R. C., Lehmkuhl, H. D. and Tully, J. G. (1988)

Isolation and identification of mycoplasmas from the nasal cavity of sheep. Am. J. Vet. Res. 49:1669-1872.

Brown, M. B. and Butcher, G. D. (1990) Comparison of egg yolk and serum samples for detection of antibodies to *Mycoplasma gallisepticum*. IOM Letters 1:166-167.

Brown, M. B., Reed, P. A. and Shearer, J. K. (1986) Comparison of media for isolation of bovine mycoplasmas from milk. 6th Int. Congr. IOM Abst. PII-120.

Brown, M. B., Gionet, P. and Senior, D. F.(1990) Identification of *Mycoplasma felis* and *Mycoplasma gatae* by an immunobinding assay. J. Clin. Microbiol. 28:1870-1873.

Bruggmann, S., Engberg, B. and Ehrensperger, F. (1977) Demonstration of *M. suipneumoniae* in pig lungs by the enzyme-linked immunoproxidase technique. Vet. Rec. 101:137.

Brys, A. and Pfutzner, H. (1989) Prufung eines Hyperimmun-serums bei intranasal mit *Mycoplasma bovis* infizierten Kalbern. Arch. Exp. Vet. Med. 43: S677-683.

Caruso, J. P. and Ross, R. F. (1990) Effects of *Mycoplasma hyopneumoniae* and *Actinobacillus (Haemophilus) pleuropneumoniae* infections on alveolar macrophage functions in swine. Am. J. Vet. Res. 51:227-231.

Chima, J. C., Erno, H. and Ojo, M. O. (1986) Characterization and identification of caprine, genital mycoplasmas. Acta Vet. Scand. 27:531-539.

Christiansen, G. and Erno, H. (1990) RFLP in rRNA genes of *Mycoplasma capricolum*, the caprine F38-like group and the bovine serogroup 7. Zbl. Bakt. Suppl 20:479-488.

Ciprian, A., Pijoan, C., Cruz, T., Camacho, J., Tortora, J., Colmenares, G., Lopez-Revilla, R. and de la Garza, M. (1988) *Mycoplasma hyopneumoniae* increases the susceptibility of pigs to experimental *Pasteurella multocida* pneumonia. Can. J. Vet. Res. 52:434-438.

Clarke, J. K., Brown, V. G. and Alley, M. R. (1974) Isolation and identification of mycoplasmas from the respiratory tract of sheep in New Zealand. N.Z. Vet. J. 22:117-121.

Costas, M., Leach, R. H. and Mitchelmore, D. L. (1987) Numerical analysis of PAGE protein patterns and the taxonomic relationships within the 'Mycoplasma mycoides cluster'. J. Gen. Microbiol. 133:3319-3329.

Cottew, G. S. (1974) The mycoplasmas of sheep and goats INSERM. 33, 357-362.

Cottew, G. S. (1979) Caprine-ovine mycoplasmas, in "The Mycoplasmas" Vol. II, (Tully, J. G. and Whitcomb, R. F.,Eds.), pp. 103-132. Academic Press, New York.

Cottew, G. S. (1983) Recovery and identification of caprine and ovine mycoplasmas, in "Methods in Mycoplasmology" Vol. II, (Tully, J. G. and Whittlestone, R. J., Eds.), pp. 91-104. Academic Press, New York.

Cottew, G. S., Watson, W. A., Arisory, F., Erdag, O. and Buckley, L.S. (1968) Differentiation of *Mycoplasma agalactiae* from other mycoplasmas of sheep and goats. J. Comp. Path. 78:275-282.

Cummings, T. S. and Kleven, S. H. (1986) Evaluation of protection against *Mycoplasma gallisepticum* infection in chickens vaccinated with the F strain of *M. gallisepticum*. Avian Dis. 30:169-171.

Cummins, D. R., Reynolds, D. L. and Rhoades, K. R. (1990) An avidin-biotin enhanced dot-immunobinding assay for the detection of *Mycoplasma gallisepticum* and *M. synoviae* serum antibodies in chickens. Avian Dis. 34:36-43.

DaMassa, A. J. and Brooks, D .L. (1991) The external ear canal of goats and other animals as a mycoplasma habitat. Sm. Rum. Res. 4:85-93.

DaMassa, A. J., Brooks, D. L., Holmberg, C. A. and Moe, A. I. (1987) Caprine mycoplasmosis: an outbreak of mastitis and arthritis requiring the destruction of 700 goats. Vet. Rec. 120:409-413.

DaMassa. A. J., Nascimento, E. R., Khan, M. I., Yamamoto, R. and Brooks, D. L. (1990) An unusual mycoplasma isolated from caprine mastitis and arthritis with possible systematic manifestions. IOM Letters 1:485.

Dannacher, G., Perrin, M., Martel, J. L., Perreau, P. (in memorium) and LeGoff, C. (1986) Report on evaluation of the European comparative trial concerning complement fixation test for diagnosis of contagious bovine pleuropneumonia. Ann. Rech. Vet. 17:107-114.

Dayalu, K. I. and Ross, R. F. (1990) Evaluation of experimental vaccines for control of porcine pneumonia induced by *Mycoplasma hyopneumoniae*. Proc. 11th Int. Congr. Pig Vet. Soc. Lausanne, Switzerland, 11:83.

Debey, M. C. and Ross, R. F. (1990) Ciliostatic and cytotoxic effect of *Mycoplasma hyopneumoniae in vitro*. IOM Letters 1:315-316.

Doster, A. R. and Lin, B. C. (1988) Identification of *Mycoplasma hyopneumoniae* in formalin-fixed porcine lung, using an indirect immunoperoxidase method. Am. J. Vet. Res. 49:1719-1721.

Dovc, P., Bencina, D. and Zajc, I. (1990) DNA analysis for *Mycoplasma gallinarum* epidemiology. IOM Letters. 1:528-529.

Dupiellet, J. P., Vuillaume, A., Rousselot, D., Bové, J. M. and Bradbury, J. M. (1990) Serological and molecular studies on *Mycoplasma gallisepticum* strains. Zbl. Bakt. Suppl. 20:859-864.

Edson, R. K., Yamamoto, R. and Farver, T. B. (1986) *Mycoplasma meleagridis* of turkeys: probability of eliminating egg-borne infection. Avian Dis. 31:264-271.

Egwu, G. O., Faull, W. B., Bradbury, J. M. and Clarkson, M. J. (1989) Ovine infectious keratoconjunctivitis: a micro-biological study of clinically unaffected and affected sheep's eyes with special reference to *Mycoplasma conjunctivae*. Vet. Rec. 125:253-256.

Erdag, O. (1989) Investigations on the preparation and application of vaccine against contagious *Mycoplasma agalactia* or sheep and goats in Turkey. Proc. Int. Symp. Mycoplasma. Theiler pp. 20-22.

Etheridge, J. R., Cottew, G. S. and Lloyd, L. C. (1979) Isolation of *Mycoplasma hyopneumoniae* from lesions in experimentally infected pigs. Aust. Vet. J. 55:356-359.

Feld, N. C., Qvist, P., Ahrens, P., Friis, N. F. and Meyling, A. (1990) A monoclonal blocking ELISA detecting serum antibodies to *Mycoplasma hyopneumoniae*. IOM Letters 1:375-376.

Ferronha, M. H., Ferreira, H. S. and Correia, I. (1990) Visualization of *Mycoplasma mycoides* subsp. *mycoides* (SC) and its immunoreactive sites in lung lesions. IOM Letters 1:488.

Finch, J. M. and Howard, C. J. (1990) Inhibitory effect of *M. dispar* and *M. bovis* on bovine immune responses *in vitro*. Zbl. Bakt. Suppl. 20:563-569.

Forsyth, M., Tourtellotte, M. and Geary, S. (1990) Characterization of a hemagglutinin from *Mycoplasma gallisepticum*. IOM Letters 1:530.

Frey, M. L., Hanson, R. P. and Anderson, D. P. (1968) A medium for the isolation of avian mycoplasmas. Am. J. Vet. Res. 29:2163-2171.

Friis, N. F. (1975) Some recommendations concerning primary isolation of *Mycoplasma suipneumoniae* and *Mycoplasma flocculare*. Nord. Vet. Med. 27:337-339.

Friis, N. F. (1979) Selective isolation of slowly growing acidifying mycoplasmas from swine and cattle. Acta Vet. Scand. 20:607-609.

Friis, N. F. (1990) Demonstration of *M. flocculare* by immunofluorescent staining in lungs of swine. Zbl. Bakt. Suppl. 20:835-836.

Friis, N. F., Palsson, P. A. and Petursson, G. (1976) *Mycoplasma ovipneumoniae* demonstrated in Icelandic sheep. Acta Vet. Scand. 17:255-257.

Fritzsch, V. M. and Bornet, G. (198) Okonomische Aspekte bei der Bekampfung der durch *Mycoplasma bovis* hervorgerufenen Mastitis des Rindes. Mh. Vet. Med. 43:120-125.

Garba, S. A., Ajayi, A., Challa, L. D., Bello, M. K., Gazama, J. N. Z., Gimba, H., Ngbede, J., Bitrus, B. and Adegboye A.O. (1986) Field trial of inactivated oil-adjuvant Gladysdale strain vaccine for contagious bovine pleuropneumonia. Vet. Rec. 119:376-377.

Geary, S. J., Gladd, M. F. and Gabridge, M. G. (1990) Species-specific biotinylated DNA probe for *M. gallisepticum*. Zbl. Bakt. Suppl. 20:864-866.

Goll, F. (1989) National survey to determine uniformity of serological test results for avian mycoplasmosis. Avian Dis. 33:760-763.

Goltz, J. P., Rosendal, S., McGraw, B. M. and Ruhnke, H. L. (1986) Experimental studies on the pathogenicity of *Mycoplasma ovipneumoniae* and *Mycoplasma arginini* for the respiratory tract of goats. Can. J. Vet. Res. 50:59-67.

Goodwin, R. F. W. (1976) An improved medium for the isolation of *Mycoplasma suipneumoniae*. Vet. Rec. 98:260-261.

Goodwin, R. F. W. (1985) Apparent reinfection of enzootic-pneumonia-free pig herds: search for possible causes. Vet. Rec. 116:690-694.

Gourlay, R. N. and Howard, C. J. (1978) Isolation and pathogenicity of mycoplasmas from the respiratory tract of calves, in: "Respiratory Diseases of Cattle Current Topics in Veterinary Medicine", Vol. 3, (Nijhoff, M., Ed.) pp. 295-304. The Hague.

Gourlay, R. N. and Howard, C. J. (1979) Bovine mycoplasmas, in "The Mycoplasmas" Vol. II (Tully, J. G. and Whitcomb, R F., Eds.), pp. 49-102. Academic Press. New York.

Gourlay, R. N. and Howard, C. J. (1983) Recovery and identification of bovine mycoplasmas, in "Methods in Mycoplasmology" Vol. II, (Tully, J. G. and Razin, S., Eds.), pp. 81-89. Academic Press, New York.

Gourlay, R. N. and Leach R. H. (1970) A new mycoplasma species isolated from pneumonic lungs of calves (*Mycoplasma dispar* sp. *nov.*) J. Med. Microbiol. 3:111-123.

Gourlay, R. N., Howard, C. J., Thomas, L. H. and Stott, E. J. (1976) Experimentally produced calf pneumonia. Res. Vet. Science 20:167-173.

Gourlay, R. M., Wyld, S. G. and Leach, R. H. (1977) *Mycoplasma alvi* a new species from bovine intestinal and urogenital tracts. Int. J. Sust. Bact. 27:86-96.

Gourlay, R. N., Thomas, L. H. and Wyld, S. G. (1989) Increased severity of calf pneumonia associated with the appearance of *Mycoplasma bovis* in a rearing herd. Vet. Rec. 124:420-422.

Gray, M. A., Simam, P. and Smith, G. R. (1986) Observations on experimental inactivated vaccines for contagious bovine pleuropneumonia. J. Hyg. 97:305-315.

Hall, C. F. (1962) *Mycoplasma gallisepticum* antigen production. Avian Dis. 6:359-362.

Hannan, P. C. T., Banks, R. M., Bhogal, B. S., Blanchflower, S. E., Donald, A. C., Fish, J. P., and Smith, D. (1984) Reproducible pneumonia in gnotobiotic piglets induced with broth cultures of *Mycoplasma hyopneumoniae* and the effect of animal passage on virulence. Res. Vet. Sci. 36:153-163.

Hannan, P. C.T., O'Hanlon, P. J. and Rogers, N. H. (1989) *In vitro* evaluation of various quinolon antibacterial agents against veterinary mycoplasmas and porcine respiratory bacterial pathogens. Res. Vet. Sci. 46:202-211.

Harasawa, R., Koshimizu, K. and Asada, K. (1990) Species-specific detection of *Mycoplasma hyopneumoniae* by using polymerase chain reaction (PCR). IOM Letters 1:83.

Harris, D. L., Wiseman, B. S., Platt, K. B., Hill, H. T., Armbrecht, P. J. and Anderson, L. A. (1988) Continuous-flow procedure for deriving PRV-free pigs from a PRV infected herd. Proc. Conf. Res. Workers Anim. Dis. 69:69.

Hayflick, L. (1965) Tissue cultures and mycoplasmas. Tex. Rep. Biol. Med. 23:285-303.

Hosie, B. D. (1988) Keratoconjunctivitis in a hill sheep flock. Vet. Rec. 122:40-43.

Hosie, B. D. (1989) Infectious keratoconjunctivitis in sheep and goats. Vet. Ann. 29:93-97.

Hotzel H., Sachse, K. and Pfutzner, H. (1990) DNA probes for the detection of *Mycoplasma bovis* and *Mycoplasma bovigenitalium*. IOM Letts. 1:384-385.

Howard, C. J., Stott, E. J., Thomas, L. H., Gourlay, R. N. and Taylor, G. (1987) Protection against respiratory disease in calves induced by vaccines containing respiratory syncytial virus, parainfluenza type 3 virus, *Mycoplasma bovis* and *M. dispar*. Vet. Rec. 121:372-376.

Howard, C. J., Stott, E. H., Thomas, L. H., Gourlay, R. N. and Taylor, G. (1990) Vaccination against natural outbreaks of respiratory disease in calves associated with *Mycoplasma bovis, M. dispar*, and respiratory syncytial virus infection. Zbl. Bakt. Suppl. 20:400-405.

Huang, F., Wu, Y., Li., Y. and Wen, D. (1986) The ultrastructure of the cells and cell membranes of *Mycoplasma suipneumoniae*. Acta Vet. Zootech. Sin. 17:184-187.

Ionas, G., Mew, A.J ., Alley, M. R., Clark, J. K., Robinson, A. J. and Marshall, R. B. (1985) Colonization of the respiratory tract of lambs by strains of *Mycoplasma ovipneumoniae*. Vet. Microbiol. 10: 533-539.

Jasper, D. E. (1981) Bovine mycoplasma mastitis. Advances Vet. Sci. 25:121-159.

Jeggo, M. H., Wardley, R. C. and Corteyn, A. H. (1987) A reassessment of the dual vaccine against rinderpest and contagious bovine pleuropneumoniae. Vet. Rec. 120:131-135.

Jones, G. E. and Wood, A. R. (1988) Microbiological and serological studies on caprine pneumonias in Oman. Res. Vet. Sci. 44:125-131.

Jones, G. E., Foggie, A., Moulo, D. L. and Livitt, S. (1976) The comparison and characterization of glycolytic mycoplasmas isolated from the respiratory tract of sheep. J. Med. Microbiol. 9:39-52.

Jones, G. E., Keir, W. A. and Gilmour, J. S. (1985) The pathogenicity of *Mycoplasma ovipneumoniae* and *Mycoplasma arginini* in ovine and caprine tracheal organ cultures. J. Comp. Path. 95:477-487.

Jordan, F. T. W. (1983) Recovery and identification of avian mycoplasmas, in "Methods in Mycoplasmology" Vol. II, (Tully, J. G. and Razin, S., Eds.) pp. 69-79. Academic Press, New York.

Jorsal, S. E. and Thomsen, B. L. (1988) A cox regression analysis of risk factors related to *Mycoplasma suipneumoniae* reinfection in Danish SPF-herds. Acta Vet. Scand. Suppl. 29:436-438.

Kazama, S. Yagihashi, T. and Seto, K. (1989) Preparation of *Mycoplasma hyopneumoniae* antigen for the enzyme-linked immunosorbent assay. Can. J. Vet. Res. 53:176-181.

Kempf, I., Gesbert, G., Guillet, M., Bennejean, G. and Cooper, A.C. (1990a) Efficiency of danofloxacin in the control of mycoplasmosis following experimental infection with *Mycoplasma gallisepticum*. IOM Letts. 1:532.

Kempf, I., Olivier, C., Morin, M., Guittet, M. and Bennejean, G. (1990 b) Pathological models of *Mycoplasma synoviae* infection in broilers and turkeys. Zbl. Bakt. Suppl. 20:700-702.

Kibe, M. K., Bidwell, D., Turp, P. and Smith, G. R. (1985) Demonstration of cross-reacting antigens in F38 and related mycoplasmas by enzyme-linked immunosorbent assay (ELISA) and immunoblotting. J. Hyg. 95:95-106.

King, G. L. (1988) Optimum age to vaccinate for contagious caprine pleuropneumonia. Vet. Rec. 123:572-573.

Kirchhoff, H. (1978) *Mycoplasma equigenitalium*, a new species from the cervix region of mares. Int. J. Syst.Bact. 28:496-502.

Kleven, S. (1990) Epidemiological studies of *Mycoplasma gallisepticum* using restriction endonuclease analysis. Zbl. Bakt. Suppl. 20:494-499.

Kleven, S. H. and Avakian, A. P. (1990) Use of purified *M. gallisepticum* and *M. synoviae* polypeptides as diagnostic antigens. IOM Letters 1:172-173.

Kleven, S. H., Rowland, G. N. and Olson, N. O. (1991) *Mycoplasma synoviae*, in "Diseases of Poultry" 9th edition (Calnek, B. W., Barnes, H. J., Beard, C. W., Reid, W. M. and Yoder, H. W., Eds.) pp. 223-231. IA State Univ. Press, Ames.

Klinkert, M.-Q., Hermann, R. and Schaller, H. (1985) Surface proteins of *Mycoplasma hyopneumoniae* identified from an *Escherichia coli* expression plasmid library. Infect. Immun. 49:329-335.

Kobisch, M., Quillien, L., Tillon, J. P. and Wroblewski, H. (1987) The *Mycoplasma hyopneumoniae* plasma membrane as a vaccine against porcine enzootic pneumonia. Ann. Inst. Pasteur/Immunol. 138:693-705.

Kobisch, M., Milward, F., Desmettre, Ph. and Morvan, P. (1990) Prevention of *Mycoplasma hyopneumoniae* experimental infection by vaccination: active and passive protection. IOM Letters 1:125-126.

Krabisch, P., Kirchhoff, H. and Lepel, J. F. (1973) Nachweis von Mycoplasmen au Genitalschleimhauten von Stuten. Dtsch. Tierarztl. Wschr. 80:493-495.

Kreusel, S., Bocklisch, H., Pfutzner, H., Brys, A., Leirer, R. and Ziecienhals, U. (1989) Experimentelle Infectionen von Bullen mit *Mycoplasma (M.) bovis* and *M. bovigenitalium*. Arch. Exp. Vet. Med. 43:S705-712.

Lauerman, L. H. and Reynolds-Vaughn, R. A. (1991) Immunoglobulin G. Fc receptors of *Mycoplasma synoviae*. Avian Dis. 35, 135-138.

LeGoff, C. (1986) Technique immunoenzymatique appliquee au diagnostic serologique de la peripneumoniae. Note preliminaire. Rev. Elev. Med. 39:171-173.

Lemcke, R. M. (1979) Equine mycoplasmas, in "The Mycoplasmas" Vol. II, (Tully, J. G. and Whitcomb, R. F., Eds.), pp. 178-189. Academic Press, New York.

Lemcke, R. M. and Poland, J. (1980) *Mycoplasma fastidiosum*: a new species from horses. Int. J. Syst. Bact. 30:151-162.

Levisohn, S., Yegana, Y., Dykstra, M. J. and Hod, I. (1986) Electron microscope studies of the interaction of *Mycoplasma synoviae* with the chicken tracheal epithelium. 6th Int. Congr. IOM, Abst, PI-53.

Levisohn, S., Hyman, H., Perlman, D. and Razin, S. (1989) The use of a specific DNA probe for detection of *Mycoplasma gallisepticum* in field outbreaks. Avian Path. 18:535-541.

Levisohn, S., Davidson, I., Cara Vergara, M.-R. and Rapport, E. (1990 a) Application of an ELISA test for diagnosis of caprine mycoplasmosis. IOM Letters 1:499-500.

Levisohn, S., Hyman, H. and Razin, S. (1990 b) Differential diagnosis of *M. gallisepticum* and *M. synoviae* in mixed infection of chicken flocks using ^{32}P and biotin-labeled gene products. IOM Letters 1:536-537.

Ley, D. H. and Avakian, A. P. (1990) Comparison of *Mycoplasma synoviae* strains. IOM Letters 1:538-539.

Ley, D. H., McLaren, J.M., Dingfelder, R. S. and McBride, M. A. T. (1990) Pathogenicity, transmissibility and immunogenicity of atypical *Mycoplasma gallisepticum* isolates from turkeys. Zbl. Bakt. Suppl. 20:868-870.

Livingston, C. W. (1972) Isolation of T-strain of mycoplasma from Texas feedlot cattle. Am. J. Vet. Res. 33:1925-1929.

MacOwan, K. J. (1989) Contagious caprine pleuropneumonia (CCPP). Proc. Int. Symp. Mycoplasm. Theiler. pp. 31-41.

Marino-Ode, U., Postizzi, S. and Nicolet, J. (1984) Epidemiologische Untersuchungen uber die Verbreitung der infektiosen Agalaktie der Ziegen im Kanto Tessin. Schweiz. Arch. Tierheilk. 126:111-119.

McMartin, D. A., MacOwen, K. J. and Swift, L. L. (1980) A century of classical contagious caprine pleuropneumonia: from original description to aetiology. Br. Vet. J. 136:507-515.

Mebus, C. A. and Underdahl, N. R. (1977) Scanning electron microscopy of trachea and bronchi from gnotobiotic pigs inoculated with *Mycoplasma hyopneumoniae*. Am. J. Vet. Res. 38:1249-1254.

Megahed, M., Forsyth, M., Tourtellotte, M. and Geary, S. (1990) Antigens responsible for *Mycoplasma gallisepticum* specificity and cross reactivity within ELISA and western blots. IOM Letters 1:540.

Mew, A. J., Ionas, G., Clarke, J. K., Robinson, A. J. and Marshall, R.B. (1985) Comparison of *Mycoplasma ovipneumoniae* isolates using bacterial restriction endonuclease DNA analysis and SDS-PAGE. Vet. Microbiol. 10:541-548.

Miles, R. J. (1983) Effect of some cultural factors on T_1 broth vaccine for contagious bovine pleuropneumonia. Trop. An. Hlth. Prod. 15:144-148.

Mitchelmore, D. L., Leach, R. H., Connolly, K. R. and Costas, M. (1990) Computer analysis of SDS-PAGE protein patterns of mycoplasmas: an aid to classification and identification? IOM Letters 1:174-175.

Molokwu, J. U., Adegboye, D. S. and Emejuaiwe, S. O. (1987) Studies on chronic respiratory disease of poultry in Nigeria. III. Documentation of *Mycoplasma synoviae* infection and other recently reported avian mycoplasma species by culture and serology. Bull. Anim. Hlth. Prod. Afr. 35:340-343.

Morrow, C. J., Bell, I. G., Walker, S. B., Markham, P. F. , Thorp, B.H. and Whitear, K. G. (199 a) Isolation of *Mycoplasma synoviae* from infectious synovitis of chickens. Aust. Vet. J. 67:121-124.

Morrow, C. J., Whitear, K. G. and Kleven, S. J. (1990 b) Restriction endonuclease analysis of *Mycoplasma synoviae* strains. Avian Dis. 34:611-616.

Nascimento, C. R., Yamamoto, R., Herrick, K. R. and Tait, R. C. (1991) Polymerase chain reaction for detection of *Mycoplasma gallisepticum*. Avian. Dis. 35:62-69.

Nayak, N. C. and Bhowmik, M. K. (1990) Goat flea (Order *Siphonaptera*) as a possible vector for the transmission of caprine mycoplasma polyarthritis with septicaemia. Prev. Vet. Med. 9:259-266.

Nicolet, J. (1987) Current status of the serodiagnosis of enzootic pneumonia in swine. Isr. J. Med. Sci. 23:650-653.

Nicolet, J. and Freundt, E. A. (1975) Isolation of *Mycoplasma conjunctivae* from chamois and sheep affected with keratoconjunctivitis. Zbl. Vet. Med. 22:302-307.

Nicolet, J., Paroz, P. and Bruggmann, S. (1980) Tween 20 soluble proteins of *Mycoplasma hyopneumoniae* as antigen for an enzyme linked immunosorbent assay. Res. Vet. Sci. 29:305-309.

Nielsen, K. H., Stewart, R. B., Garcia, M. M. and Eaglesome, M. D. (1987) Enzyme immunoassay for detection of *Mycoplasma bovis* antigens in bull semen and preputial washings. Vet. Red. 120:596-598.

Nitzsche, E. (1985) *Mycoplasma mycoides* subsp. *mycoides,* in "Handbuch der Bakteriellen Infektionen bei Tieren" Vol. V, (Blobel, H. and Schliesser, T., Eds.), pp. 413-446. Gustav Fischer, Jena.

Panangala, V. S., Hwang, M. Y., Lauerman, L. H., Kleven, S. H., Giambrone, J. J., Gresham, M. and Mitra, A. (1990) Immunoenzymatic test with monoclonal antibodies for detection of avian *Mycoplasma gallisepticum* and *M. synoviae* antibodies. Zbl. Bakt. Suppl. 20:517-525.

Pedersen, M. W., Friis, N. F. and Ahrens, P. (1990) Detection of *Mycoplasma hyopneumoniae* in pneumonic pig lungs by an ELISA using monoclonal antibodies. IOM Letters 1:399-400.

Petersen, G., Weiss, D., Egan, J., Korshus, J., Peters, R. and Miron, M. (1990) Response to *Mycoplasma hyopneumoniae* vaccination in nursing piglets. Proc. 11th Int. Congr. Pig Vet. Soc. Lausanne, Switzerland. 11:84.

Pfutzner, H. (1989) Untersuchungen zur *in-vitro*-wirkung von Antibiotika auf Mykoplasmen unter den Bedingungen der Aufbereitung von Bullensperma. Arch. Exp. Vet. Med. 43:S725-728.

Pfutzner, H. (1990) Epizootiology of the *Mycoplasma bovis* infection of cattle. Zbl. Bakt. Suppl. 20:394-399.

Pfutzner, H. and Hofer, M. (1989) Vergleichende Prufung der Eignung verschiedener Nahrboden zur Isolierung von *Mycoplasma californicum* aus Milchproben. Arch. Exp. Vet. Med. 43:S699-704.

Pilaszek, J. and Truszczynski, M. (1986) Antibiotikasensibilitat der Ureaplasmen vom Rind. Arch. Exp. Vet. Med. 40:S88-93.

Pointon, A. M., Byrt, D. and Heap, P. (1985) Effect of enzootic pneumonia of pigs on growth performance. Aust. Vet. J. 62:13-18.

Poland, J. and Lemcke, R. (1978) Mycoplasmas of the respiratory tract of horses and their significance in upper respiratory tract disease. J. Eq. Med. Surg. S1:437-446.

Poumarat, F. (1990) Taxonomic relationships with "*M. mycoides* cluster" and within ruminant mycoplasmas "glucose arginine negative cluster" indicated by dot immunobinding on membrane filtration (MF dot). IOM Letts 1:401-402.

Poumarat, F., Perrin, M., Belli, P. and Martel, J. L. (1989) Correlation entre l'excretion des mycoplasmes et les cinetiques des anticorps mis en evidence par fixation du complement, hemagglutination passive et seroagglutination rapide, au course d'une infection experimentale de bovins par *Mycoplasma mycoides* subsp. *mycoides* SC. Revue Elev. Med. Vet. Pays. Trop. 42:357-364.

Quinn, P. A. and Fortier, M. A. (1990) Growth and attachment of *Ureaplasma diversum* in co-culture with bovine endometrial cells. IOM Letts. 1:337-338.

Radostits, O. M., Janzen, E. and Doige, C. (1988) *Mycoplasma arthritis* in feedlot cattle. Can. Vet. J. 29:531.

Reid, S. W., Madill, D. G. and Vreugdenhil, A. H. (1989 a) An outbreak of keratoconjunctivitis (pinkeye) in sheep. Can. Vet. J. 30:180.

Reid, S. W., Madill, D. G. and Vreugdenhil, A. H. (1989 b) Ureaplasmal vulvo-vaginitis and infertility in eight southern Ontario dairy herds. Can Vet. J. 30:255.

Rhoades, K. R. (1984) Comparison of strains of *Mycoplasma iowae*. Avian Dis. 28:710-717.

Richter, A. and Pfutzner, H. (1989) Nachweis von Mykoplasmen in experi-mentell infiziertem Bullensperma. Arch. Exp. Vet. Med. 43:S721-724.

Richter, A., Pfutzner, H. and Jacob W. K. (1989) Untersuchungen zur Nach-weissicherheit der Kontamination von Bullensperma mit Mykoplas-men. Arch. Exp. Vet. Med. 43:S713-720.

Rosenbusch, R. F. and Ostle, A. G. (1986) *Mycoplasma bovoculi* infection in-creases ocular colonization by *Moraxella ovis* in calves. Am. J. Vet. Res. 47:1214-1224.

Rosendal, S. (1981) Experimental infection of goats, sheep, and calves with the large colony type of *Mycoplasma mycoides* subsp. *mycoides*. Vet. Pathol. 18:71-81.

Rosendal, S. (1983) Susceptibility of goats and calves after experimental inocu-lation or contact exposure to a Canadian strain of *Mycoplasma mycoides* subsp. *mycoides* isolated from a goat. Can. J. Comp. Med. 47:484-490.

Rosendal, S. and Martin, S. W. (1986) The association between serological evidence of mycoplasma infection and respiratory disease in feedlot cattle. Can. J. Vet. Res. 50:179-183.

Rosendal, S. and Serebin, S. (1990) Induction of tumor necrosis factor by the large colony variant of *Mycoplasma mycoides* subsp. *mycoides*. IOM Letters 1:507.

Rosendal, S., Blackwell, T. E., Lumsden, J. H., Physick-Sheard, P.W., Viel, L., Watson, S. and Woods, P. (1986) Detection of antibodies to *Mycoplasma felis in horses*. J. Am. Vet. Med. Assoc. 188:292-294.

Rosengarten, R. and Wise, K. S. (1990) Phenotypic switching in mycoplasmas: phase variation of diverse surface lipoproteins. Sci. 247:315-320.

Ross, R. F. (1985a) Mycoplasmas in cattle, in "Handbuch der Bakteriellen In-fektionen bei Tieren" Vol. V, (Blobel, H. and Schliesser, T., Eds.), pp. 314-344. Gustav Fischer, Jena.

Ross, R. F. (1985b) Mycoplasmas in horses, in "Handbuch der Bakteriellen Infektionen bei Tieren" Vol. V, (Blobel, H. and Schliesser, T., Eds.), pp. 406-412. Gustav Fischer, Jena.

Ross, R. F. (1985c) Mycoplasmas of sheep and goats, in "Handbuch der akteri-ellen Infektionen bei Tieren" Vol. V, (Blobel, H. and Schliesser, T., Eds.), pp. 345-373. Gustav Fischer, Jena.

Ross, R. F. (1985d) Mycoplasmas of swine, in "Handbuch der akteriellen Infek-tionen bei Tieren" Vol. V, (Blobel, H. and Schliesser, T., Eds.), pp. 374-406. Gustav Fischer, Jena.

Ross, R. F. (1986) Mycoplasma diseases, in "Diseases of Swine" 6th edition, (Leman, A. D., Straw, B., Glock, R. D., Mengeling, W. L., Penny, R. H. C. and Scholl, E. Eds.), pp. 469-483. IA State Univ. Press, Ames.

Ross, R. F. (1990) Enhancement of bacterial pneumonia in swine by *Mycoplasma hyopneumoniae*. IOM Letts. 1:127-128.

Ross, R. F. and Whittlestone, P. (1983) Recovery of, identification of, and serological response to porcine mycoplasmas, in "Methods in Mycoplas-

Rott, M., Pfutzner, H., Gigas, H. and Rott, G. (1989 b) Diagnostische Erfahrugen bei der routinemasigen Uber-wachung von Putenbestanden auf Mykoplasmen infektionen. Arch. Exper. Vet. Med. 43:S743-746.

Ruhnke, H. L. and Miller, R. B. (1990) Effect of *Ureaplasma diversum* on bovine reproduction: epidemiological and experimental aspects. IOM Letters 1:64-65.

Ruhnke, H. L., Palmer, N. C., Doig, P. A. and Miller, R. B. (1984) Bovine abortion and neonatal death associated with *Ureaplasma diversum*. Theriogenol. 21:295-301.

Rurangiriwa, F. R., McGuire, T. C., Kibor, A. and Chema, S. (1987a) An inactivated vaccine for contagious caprine pleuropneumonia. Vet. Rec. 121:397-402.

Rurangiriwa, F. R., McGuire, T. C. and Magnuson, N. S. (1987b) Composition of a polysaccharide from mycoplasma (F-38) recognized by antibodies from goats with contagious pleuropneumonia. Res. Vet. Sci. 42:175-178.

Salih, B. A. and Rosenbusch, R. G. (1986) Antibody response in calves experimentally or naturally exposed to *Mycoplasma bovoculi.*. Vet Microbiol. 11:93-102.

Salih, B. A. and Rosenbusch, R. F. (1988) Attachment of *Mycoplasma bovoculi* to bovine conjunctival epithelium and lung fibroblasts. Am. J. Vet. Res. 49:1661-1664.

Salih, B. A., Ostle, A. G. and Rosenbusch, R. F. (1987) Vaccination of cattle with *Mycoplasma bovoculi* antigens: evidence for field immunity. Comp. Immun. Microbiol. Infect. 10, 109-116.

Schweighhardt, H., Pechan, P. Lahermann, E. and Krassing, G. (1989) *Mycoplasma capricolum* - Infektion beim Alpensteinbock (*Capra ibex ibex*) - eine Fallbeschreibung. Kleintierpraxis. 34:S297-299.

Shah-Majid, M. and Rosendahl, S. (1987 a) Evaluation of growth of avian mycoplasmas on bile salt agar and in bile broth. Res. Vet. Sci. 43:188-190.

Shah-Majid, M. and Rosendahl, S. (1987 b) Oral challenge of turkey poults with *Mycoplasma iowae*. Avian. Dis. 31:365-369.

Shareef, J.M., Willcox, J. and Kumar, P. (1990) Immunogold electron microscopy for identification of *Mycoplasma iowae* in infected turkey tissues. Zbl. Bakt. Suppl. 20:875-877.

Sharp, P., Van Ess, P., Ji, B. and Thomas, C. G. (1991) Immunobinding assay for the speciation of avian mycoplasmas adapted for use with a 96-well filtration manifold. Avian Dis. 35:332-336

Sher, T., Yamin, A., Rottem, S. and Gallily, R. (1990) Induction of blast transformation and TNF secretion by *Mycoplasma capricolum* membranes. Zbl. Bakt. Suppl. 20:578-583.

Shimizu, T., Nagamoto, H. and Takahata, T. (1990) A hemadsorption inhibition test for detecting antibodies to avian mycoplasmas. IOM Letts. 1:170-171.

Simon, F., Semjen, G., Dobos-Kovacs, M. Laczay, P., and Cserep, T. (1990) Efficacy of enrofloxacin against enzootic pneumonia in swine. Proc. 11th Int. Congr. Pig Vet. Soc. Lausanne, Switzerland, 11:96.

Stemke, G. W., Nordal, R. A., Robertson, J. A., Doran, J. L. and Roy, K. L. (1987) Construction of a species-specific gene probe for *Mycoplasma hyopneumoniae.* Proc. Am. Soc. Microbiol. 122.

Simon, F., Semjen, G., Dobos-Kovacs, M. Laczay, P., and Cserep, T. (1990) Efficacy of enrofloxacin against enzootic pneumonia in swine. Proc. 11th Int. Congr. Pig Vet. Soc. Lausanne, Switzerland, 11:96.

Stemke, G. W., Nordal, R. A., Robertson, J. A., Doran, J. L. and Roy, K. L. (1987) Construction of a species-specific gene probe for *Mycoplasma hyopneumoniae.* Proc. Am. Soc. Microbiol. 122.

Stipkovitz, L., Brown, P. A., Glavits, A. and Zajer, J. (1986) Significance of ureaplasma infection in infertility of turkeys. Arch. Exper. Vet. Med. 40:103-104.

Stott, E. J., Thomas, L. H., Howard, C. J. and Gourlay, R. N. (1987) Field trial of a quadrivalent vaccine against calf respiratory disease. Vet. Red. 121:342-347.

Strasser, M. and Nicolet, J. (1990) Evaluation of an ELISA for *Mycoplasma flocculare.* Zbl. Bakt. Suppl. 20: 848-851.

Tajima, M. and Yagihashi, T. (1982) Interaction of *Mycoplasma hyopneumoniae* with the porcine respiratory epithelium as observed by electron microscopy. Infect. Immun. 37:1162-1169.

Tajima, M., Yagihashi, T. and Nunoya, T. (1985) Ultrastructure of mycoplasmal capsules as revealed by stabilization with antiserum and staining with ruthenium red. Jpn. J. Vet. Sci. 47:217-223.

Talkington, F. D. and Kleven, S. H. (1985) Evaluation of protection against colonization of the chicken trachea following administration of *Mycoplasma gallisepticum* bacterin. Avian Dis. 29:998-1003.

Taoudi, A., Johnson, D.W. and Kheyyali,D. (1987) Pathogenicity of *Mycoplasma capricolum* in sheep after experimental infection. Vet. Microbiol. 14:137-144.

Taoudi, A., Karib, H., Johnson, D. W. and Fassi-Fehri, M. M. (1988) Comparison ou pouvoir pathogene de trois souches de *Mycoplasma capricolum* pour la chevre et le chevreau nouveau-ne. Revue Elev. Med. Vet., Pays Trop. 41:353-358.

Taschke, C. and Herrmann, R. (1986) Analysis of transcription and processing signals of the 16S-23S rRNA operon of *Mycoplasma hyopneumoniae.* Mol. Gen. Genet. 205:434-441.

Taschke, C., Klinkert, M.-Q., Wolters, J. and Herrmann, R. (1986) Organization of the ribosomal RNA genes in *Mycoplasma hyopneumoniae*: the 5S rRNA gene is separated from the 16S and 23S rRNA genes. Mol. Gen. Genet. 205:428-433.

Taylor-Robinson, D., Williams, M. H. and Haig, D. A. (1968) The isolation and comparative biological and physical characteristics of T-mycoplasmas of cattle. J. Gen. Microbiol. 54:33-46.

Thirkell, D., Spooner, R. K., Jones, G. E. and Russell, W. C. (1990a) Polypeptide and antigenic variability among strains of *Mycoplasma ovipneumoniae* demonstrated by SDS-PAGE and immunoblotting. Vet. Microbiol. 21:241-254.

Thirkell, D., Spooner, R. K., Jones, G. E. and Russell, W. C. (1990b) The humoral immune response of lambs experimentally infected with *Mycoplasma ovipneumoniae.* Vet. Microbiol. 24:143-153.

Thirkell, D., Spooner, R. K., Jones, G. E., Russell, W. C. and Voice, M. W. (1991) Cross-reacting antigens between *Mycoplasma ovipneumoniae* and other species of mycoplasma of animal origin, shown by ELISA and immunoblotting with reference antisera. Vet. Microbiol. 26:249--261.

Thomas, C. B., Jasper, D. E., Boothby, J. T. and Dellinger, J. D. (1987a) Enzyme-linked immunosorbent assay detection of *Mycoplasma californicum*-specific antibody in bovine serum: optimization of assay determinants and control of serologic cross reactions. Am. J. Vet. Res. 48:590-595.

Thomas, C. B., Mettler, J., Sharp, P., Jensen-Kostenbader, J. and Schultz, R. D. (1990) *Mycoplasma bovis* suppression of bovine lymphocyte response to phytohemagglutinin. Vet. Immunol. Immunopathol. 26:143-155.

Thomas, C. B., Van Ess, P., Wolfgram, L. J., Riebe, J., Sharp, P. and Schultz, R. D. (1991) Adherence to bovine neutrophils and suppression of neutrophil chemiluminescence by *Mycoplasma bovis*. Vet. Immunol. Immunopathol. 27:365-381.

Thomas, L. H., Howard, C. J., Parsons, K. R. and Anger, H. S. (1987b) Growth of *Mycoplasma bovis* in organ cultures of bovine foetal trachea and comparison with *Mycoplasma dispar*. Vet. Microbiol. 13:189-200.

Turner, A.W., Stableforth, A. W. and Galloway, I. A. (1959) Pleuropneumonia group of diseases. Infect. Dis. An. 2:437-480.

Uhaa, I. J., Riemann, H. P., Thurmond, M. C. and Franti, C. E. (1990) The use of the enzyme-linked immunosorbent assay (ELISA) in serological diagnosis of *Mycoplasma bovis* in dairy cattle. Vet. Res. Commun. 14:279-285.

Valdivieso-Garcia, A., Rosendal, S., Allen, O. B., Thompson, C. M. and Watson, S. (1989) Cytotoxicity of *Mycoplasma mycoides* subspecies *mycoides* for cultured endothelial cells. Zbl. Bakt. 272:202-209.

Valdivieso-Garcia, A., Rosendal, S. and Serebrin, S. (1989b) Adherence of *Mycoplasma mycoides* subspecies *mycoides* for cultured endothelial cells. Zbl. Bakt. 272:210-215.

Vardaman, T.H. (1967) A culture medium for the production of *Mycoplasma gallisepticum* antigen. Avian Dis. 11:123-129.

Vihan, V. S. (1989) Determination of Na-gase activity in milk for diagnosis of subclinical caprine mastitis. Sm. Rum. Res. 2:359-356.

Wannemuehler, M. J., Minion, F. C. and Ross, R. F. (1988) Immune suppression of *Mycoplasma hyopneumoniae* infected swine. 7th Int. Congr. IOM Mtg. Abst. 70.

Whittlestone, P. (1979) Porcine mycoplasmas, in "The Mycoplasmas" Vol. II, (Tully, J. G. and Whitcomb, R. F., Eds.), pp. 133-176. Academic Press, New York.

Yagihashi, T., Nunoya, T., Mitui, T., and Tajima, M. (1984) Effect of *Mycoplasma hyopneumoniae* infection on the development of *Haemophilus pleuropneumoniae* pneumonia in pigs. Jpn. J. Vet. Sci. 46:705-713.

Yamamoto, R. (1991) *Mycoplasma meleagridis* infection, in "Diseases of Poultry" 9th edition, (Calnek, B. W., Barnes, H. J., Beard, C. W., Reid, W. M. and Yoder, H. W., Eds.), pp. 212-113. IA State Univ. Press, Ames.

Yamamoto, R., Kleven, S. H., Khan, M. I. and Zhao, S. (1990) *Mycoplasma gallisepticum* strain and species-specific recombinant DNA probes in disease investigations. IOM Letts. 1:123-124.

Yoder, H. W. (1984) Avian mycoplasmosis in "Diseases of Poultry" 8th edition, (Hofstad, M. S., Calnek, B. W., Helmboldt, C. F., Reid, W. M, and Yoder, H. W., Eds.), pp. 187-220. IA State Univ. Press, Ames.

Yoder, H. W. (1991) *Mycoplasma gallisepticum* infection, in"Diseases of Poultry" 9th edition, (Calnek, B. W., Barnes, H. J., Beard, C. W., Reid, W. M. and Yoder, H. W., Eds.), pp. 198-212. IA State Univ. Press, Ames.

Young, T. F., Ross, R. F. and Drisko, J. (1983) Prevalence of antibodies to *Mycoplasma hyopneumoniae*. Am. J. Vet. Res. 44:1946-1948.

Zhao, S. and Yamamoto, R. (1990 a) *Mycoplasma iowae* species-specific DNA probe. IOM Letts. 1:405-406.

Zhao, S. and Yamamoto, R. (1990 b) Recombinant DNA probes for Mycoplasma synoviae. Avian Dis. 34:709-716.

Zielinski, G. C. (1991) Adherence to host tissues, surface hydrophobicity, and pathogenic and phenotypic characteristics of *Mycoplasma hyopneumoniae*. Ph.D. Thesis.

Zielinski, G. C. and Ross, R. F. Morphology and hydrophobicity of the cell surface of *Mycoplasma hyopneumoniae*. Am. J. Vet. Res., accepted 1990.

Zimmermann, W., Tschudi, P. and Nicolet, J. (1986) ELISA-serologie in Blut und Kolostralmilch: eine Moglichkeit zur Uberwachung der enzootischen Pneumonie (EP) in Schweine-bestanden. Schweiz. Arch. Tierheilk. 128:299-306.

DETECTION OF ADHERENCE OF *UREAPLASMA UREALYTICUM* TO BOVINE MUCOSA FALLOPIAN TUBE CELLS IN CULTURE

A. Saada[1], E. Rahamim[2], I. Kahane[1] and Y. Beyth[3]

Department of Membrane & Ultrastructure Research[1]
Interdepartmental unit, Electron Microscopy Laboratory[2],
The Hebrew University-Hadassah Medical School;
Department of Obstetrics and Gynecology[3]
Hadassah University Hospital, Jerusalem, Israel

INTRODUCTION

Ureaplasma urealyticum is the most commonly isolated mycoplasma from the human urogenital tract and is associated with various clinical conditions, such as nonogonococcal urethritis, infertility, amnionitis, and spontaneous abortions (Taylor-Robinson, D. and McCormack, W. M., 1979). The mechanisms of *U. urealyticum* pathogenicity are yet unknown. However, its adherence to urethral epithelial cells, spermatozoa, and other cells, has been documented (Busolo *et al.*, 1984; Shepard, M. C. and Masover, G. K., 1979; Kotani, H. and McGarrity, G. J., 1986; McGarrity, G. J. and Kotani, H., 1986). The speculation about the linkage between the adherence and pathogenicity is relevant, since it was found to be a prerequisite for pathogenicty of other mycoplasmas *e.g., Mycoplasma pneumoniae* (Hu, P.-C. *et al.*, 1977). However, the few studies conducted on the interaction of various *U. urealyticum* strains with HeLa, 3T6, CV1, WI 38 cell cultures (Kotani, H. and McGarrity, G. J., 1986; Taylor-Robinson, D. and Carney, F. E., 1974), and bovine oviductal organ cultures (Stalheim, O. H. V. *et al.*, 1976; Taylor-Robinson, D. and Carney, F. E., 1974), did not provide a clear answer. In some studies, the *U. urealyticum* did not seem to cause any cell damage (Taylor-Robinson, D. and Carney, F. E., 1974), while in others, cytopathic effects (Stalheim *et al.*, 1976) and cell death (Kotani, H. and McGarrity, G. J., 1986) were reported. Since urea is an essential growth factor for *U. urealyticum* (Shepard, M. C. and Masover, G. K., 1979), in most studies it was added to the culture medium in order to establish infections. The urea in the medium is degraded to ammonia and carbon dioxide by the highly active ureaplasmal urease (Shepard, M. C. and Masover, G. K., 1979). The ammonia may act as a cell damaging factor due to the toxicity of the ammonium ion or by alkalinizating the medium. This was indicated in experiments by Stalheim *et al.* (1977), in which Jack bean urease added to bovine

Rapid Diagnosis of Mycoplasmas, Edited by I. Kahane
and A. Adoni, Plenum Press, New York, 1993

oviductal organ cultures was shown to mimic the effect of *U. urealyticum* infection. The involvement of urease may be elucidated by additional experiments using organ or cell cultures. For these, cell cultures are preferred, since adherence and ultrastructural damage are more readily assessed. Since, at present, a satisfactory human, ciliated, cell culture model from the female upper genital tract is lacking, we studied these parameters on a similar bovine model, bovine Fallopian tube mucosa cells in culture (FTMCC), which is a primary cell culture mainly consisting of epithelial-ciliated cells (Beyth, Y. *et al.*, 1988)

MATERIALS AND METHODS

U. urealyticum, Growth and Metabolic Labelling

U. urealyticum Serotypes 3 and 8 (obtained from Professor E. A. Freundt Aarhus, Denmark), were grown in PPLO broth supplemented with horse serum (10%), fresh yeast extract, phenol red, and urea (Bloomster, T. G. and Lynn, R. J., 1981) until the late logarithmic phase when the pH reached 7.8.

In order to label the *Ureaplasmas*, organisms from one liter medium were harvested by centrifugation and washed twice in 0.25 M NaCl as described (Saada and Kahane, 1988). The pellet was resuspended in 0.8 ml Hanks buffered salt solution, from which sulfate containing salts were omitted, and replaced with NaCl (HBSS-M). Subsequently, a mixture of L-amino acids (Sigma Chemicals), to the concentrations recommended by Dawis *et al.*. (1980), and 0.5 mCi L[^{35}S] methionine (Amersham, England) were added. The suspension was divided into 4 aliquots and incubated for 2 h at 37°C, then 1 ml HBSS-M containing 0.33 mM methionine (Sigma Chemicals) was added. After 10 min chase, the suspension was centrifuged for 10 min at 15000 rpm at 4°C in a microfuge (Hettich, Germany). The supernatant was discarded. The pellet was washed twice in methionine containing HBSS-M and was suspended to a concentration of 0.05 mg/ml protein in Ham F10 medium.

Cell Cultures

Bovine Fallopian tube mucosa cells were cultured according to Beyth *et al.* (1987): Bovine salpingectomy specimens were collected and transported in Leibowitz L-15 medium (Beit Haemek, Israel) with glutamine, antibiotics (penicillin 75 µg/ml, streptomycin 75 µg/ml, gentamycin 80 µg/ml, Fungizone 0.5 µg/ml) and bovine fetal serum (10%). The Fallopian tubes were cut open and the epithelium was gently scraped off and suspended in Ham F10 medium (Beit Haemek, Israel), supplemented with glutamine, antibiotics (penicillin 75 µg/ml, streptomycin 75 µg/ml), and lactic acid (1 mM), sodium carbonate (20 mM), and 10% bovine fetal serum. The resulting small tissue segments and cell aggregates were seeded onto 35-mm tissue culture dishes coated with extracellular matrix (Vlodovsky, I., 1980). Cultures were incubated at 37°C in a 5.5% CO_2 humidified incubator for 4-7 days before use. All cultures were screened for mycoplasmas and ureaplasmas and were found negative. Prior to all experiments, the cultures were washed 3 times with supplemented Ham F10 medium without antibiotics.

Adherence of *U. urealyticum* to FTMCC

The adherence was assessed by incubating 2 ml of suspension of labelled *U. urealyticum* with each dish of FTMCC. After incubation at 37°C, the dishes were washed five times with phosphate buffered saline and the cells were gently scraped off with a rubber policeman. After solubilization with 0.5% sodiumdodecylsulfate (30 min at 37°C) the remaining radioactivity was determined by liquid scintillation.

Infection of FTMCC with *U. urealtyicum*

2 ml medium without antibiotics and 20 µl (2x10⁵ CCU) logarithmic *U. urealyticum* culture were added to each dish. In control dishes, 20 µl *U. urealyticum* growth medium titered to pH 7.8 with ammonium carbonate were added. The effect of ammonia was studied by adding ammonium carbonate to uninfected culture (as a 20 mM solution) to the same concentration as determined in infected cultures, with intervals of 6-8 h. The cultures were maintained at 37°C in 5.5% CO_2. When the urease inhibitor Flurofamide (Norwich Eaton Pharmaceuticals, Norwich, NY, USA) was used, 10 µl of a 2 mM aqueous solution were added to each dish.

Protein Determination

The protein content of the *Ureaplasma* suspension and the solubilized cell cultures was determined by the method of Bradford (1974) using bovine serum albumin (Sigma Chemicals) as standard.

Determination of urea and ammonia concentration

In order to determine the urea content in cell culture supernatants, Jack bean urease (5 units) (Sigma Chemicals, Israel) was added to 5 µl medium and incubated for 30 min at 37°C. The ammonia concentration was determined by a modified Berthelot reaction using 2 mM ammonium carbonate as standard (Wong, B. L. and Shobe, C. R., 1973).

Scanning Electron Microscopy (SEM)

The cell cultures were washed 3 times with phosphate buffered saline (0.1 M pH 7.2) (PBS) before fixation with 2.5% glutaraldehyde in PBS for 1 h at 4°C. Following several rinses in the same buffer, the cells were post-fixed in 1% osmium tetroxide for 1 h. Dehydration was carried out through a graded series of ethanol and subsequently dried by a graded series of Freon 113 in absolute ethanol. After triple rinsing in 100% freon, the specimens were vigorously shaken in the air for a few seconds. The culture dishes were coated with gold and examined under Philips 505 SEM at 30 KV.

Transmission Electron Microscopy (TEM)

The cells were washed and dehydrated as described for SEM, then washed twice in propylene oxide and embedded in Epon epoxy resin. Thin sections cut with an LKB III 8802A ultra-microtome were contrasted with uranyl acetate (10% in 50% methanol) and lead citrate (4%). The sections were examined under Philips TEM 300 at 60 KV.

RESULTS

The quantitative assessment of the adherence of *U. urealyticum* to FTMCC was feasible upon the achievement of a procedure by which we obtained labelled ureaplasmas with a high specific radioactivity. The organisms, which were metabolically labelled with L-[^{35}S] methionine, adhered to FTMCC in an almost linear fashion during the experiment (Fig. 1). After 3 h, about 5% of the ureaplasmas were adhering to the host cells.

In early stages of infection (3-6 hrs), *U. urealyticum* were detected on the cell surface and adhering to the cilia as observed by TEM (Fig. 2), while no structural damage to the FTMCC was seen. Later, 24-48 h following the infection, ureaplasma-like particles were detected in intracellular vesicles (Fig. 3). Vesicles of this type were not observed in uninfected control cultures.

After 48 h, cell damage was extensive; clumped cilia (Fig. 4b), exfoliation (Fig. 4c), and bleb-like protrusions (Fig. 4d) were observed by SEM. In control cultures, none of the aforementioned observations were seen (Fig. 4a).

In order to evaluate the role of ureaplasmal urease in the observed cytopathic effects, its activity was assayed by monitoring the ammonia liberated in infected cultures. The ammonia levels were found elevated in the infected cell cultures, irrespective of urea supplementation in the culture medium (Fig. 5) indicating that urea was produced locally by FTMCC. Indeed, this was confirmed in uninfected cultures, by the finding that these produced 10.0 ± 2.0 mM urea during 48 h.

The involvement of the ureaplasmal urease in the ammonia production was proven by the finding that Flurofamide, a potent urease inhibitor (Saada and Kahane, 1988), almost completely inhibited ammonia production in infected cultures (Fig. 5). These specimens were not examined by electron microscopy, since Flurofamide also induced some structural changes of the uninfected controls.

Another approach to investigating the possible role of ammonia produced by the ureaplasmal urease was by adding ammonium carbonate to uninfected FTMCC at approximately the same rate and concentration as ammonia was produced in infected cultures. Cell cultures from these experiments examined by SEM showed only the effect of clumped cilia (Fig. 4b).

All the experiments were conducted on *U. urealyticum* serotype 8 and were also examined using *U. urealyticum* serotype 3 in at least two experiments. No significant difference in adherence, ammonia production or ultrastructural damage to FTMCC was detected between serotypes 3 and 8.

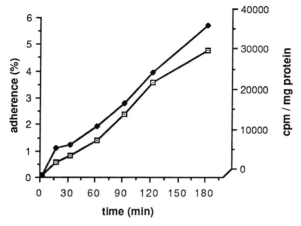

Figure 1. Adherence of *U. urealyticum* to FTMCC

U. urealyticum labelled with L-[35S] methionine was incubated with FTMCC. After repeated washings, the remaining radioactivity was determined and was also expressed as a percentage of the initial radioactivity added.

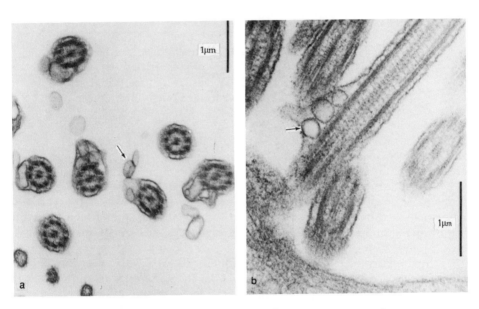

Figure 2(a-b). Transmission electron micrographs (TEM) of *U. urealyticum* infected FTMCC.

FTMCC was infected with *U. urealyticum* for 6 h, washed and prepared for TEM. Note ureaplasma-like particles (arrows) on the cilia, cross section (2a), longitudinal section (2b). Bar=1 μm.

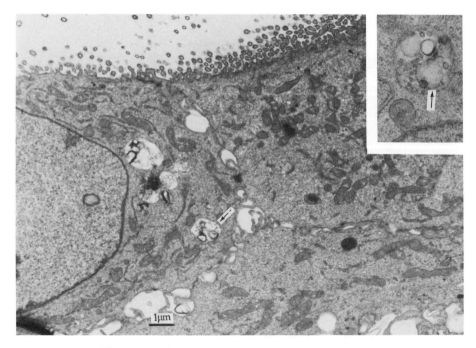

Figure 3. Transmission electron micrograph (TEM) of *U. urealyticum* infected FTMCC.

FTMCC was infected with *U. urealyticum* for 24 hrs. Partially digested ureaplasma-like particles (arrows) were seen in intracellular vesicles. Insert: higher magnification of an intracellular vesicle. Bar=1 μm.

DISCUSSION AND CONCLUSIONS

Our studies provide further evidence for the adherence and cytopatic effects of *U. urealyticum* to host cells. The high specific radioactivity, which can be achieved by metabolic labelling of the organisms, should lead to further insight of the molecular aspects of the *Ureaplasmas'* adherence mechanism.

In the current experiments, the adherence to FTMCC was found to be rapid, linear, and reached the same level as the adherence to human erythrocytes (Saada *et al.*, 1991). These results resemble the adherence of other pathogenic *Mycoplasmas, e.g., M. gallisepticum* and *M. pulmonis,* to host cells (Glasgow, L. R. and Hill, R. L., 1980; Minion, F. C. *et al.*, 1984).

The observations by electron microscopy added another dimension of the interaction of *U. urealyticum* with the host cells. The association with cilia is particularly interesting, since other mycoplasmas, *e.g., M. pneumoniae*, adhere only to the cell surface when infecting epithelial cells (Kahane, I., 1984).

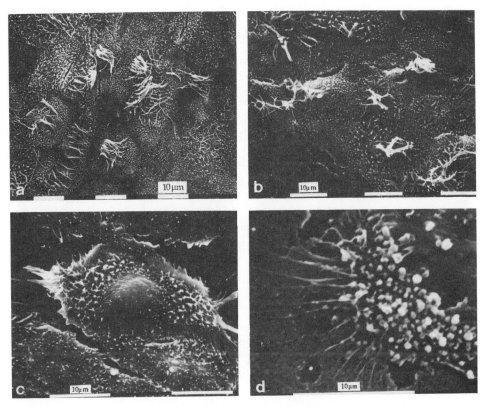

Figure 4(a-d). Scanning electron micrographs (SEM) of *U. urealyticum* infected FTMCC

Uninfected FTMCC (4a) and infected with *U. urea-lyticum* for 48 h (b-d) were washed and prepared for SEM as described. Notice the clumped cilia (4b), exfoliation (4c), and bleb-like protrusions (4d) of the infected cells. Bar=10 μm.

However, in recent studies, *M. equigenitalium* has also been reported to adhere to cilia of the equine uterine tube (Bermudez, V. *et al.*, 1988). These findings may suggest the occurrence of receptors on cilia to some mycoplasmas, but not to others. The nature of such receptors is yet to be elucidated.

The ultrastructural damage observed, especially at the later stages of infection, can be attributed to the direct effect of the *Ureaplasmas* present and not to depletion of medium components, since the organisms did not multiply during the experiments. Similar conclusions were reached by Chen *et al.* (1988) when studying *M. pneumoniae* infection of HeLa cells under restrictive medium conditions.

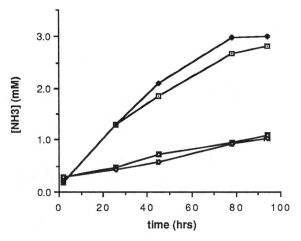

Figure 5. Ammonia production in *U. urealyticum* infected FTMCC.

Ammonia production was monitored in the supernatant of uninfected FTMCC and cell cultures infected with *U.urealyticum* in the absence of exogenous urea. In addition, the ammonia produced in infected cultures in the presence of (10 μg/ml) urea or in the presence of (50 μM) Flurofamide was determined.

Since FTMCC are nonphagocytic cells, the observation of intracellular vesicles at the later stages of infection suggest the induction of a phagocytic process of the host cells by the *Ureaplasmas*. This observation resembles the findings of Stalheim *et al.* (1974), with bovine oviductal organ cultures (Stalheim *et al.*, 1974), and of Collier (1972) for *M. pneumoniae* infection of human fetal trachea (Collier, A. M., 1972).

The presence of *U. urealyticum* caused an elevation of the ammonia content in FTMCC supernatant. This was shown to be due to the highly active ureaplasmal urease which hydrolyzed urea produced by the cell culture. Inhibition of this enzyme by Flurofamide abolished the ammonia production in infected cultures. Ammonia was suggested to be a pathogenic factor in *U. urealyticum* infection (Stalheim *et al.*, 1977). Our study supports this speculation, since the addition of ammonium carbonate to uninfected cultures caused ultrastructural changes such as cilia clumping. However, since *U. urealyticum* infected cultures exhibited more severe cell damage, it is suggested that additional mechanisms of pathogenicity play a role in this process, among them may be the production of oxygen radicals, as was indicated for *M. pneumoniae* (Almagor *et al.*, 1984) and other mycoplasmas (Kahane, unpublished results). This possibility has yet to be examined.

ACKNOWLEDGEMENTS

We thank D. Pickholtz for skilled technical assistance and I. Vlodovsky for supplying coated culture dishes.

REFERENCES

Almagor, M., Kahane, I., and Yatziv, S. (1984) The role of superoxide anion in host cell injury induced by *Mycoplasma pneumoniae* infection: Study in normal and trisomy 21 cells. J. Clin. Invest. 73:842-847.

Bermudez, V., Miller, R., Rosendal, S., and Johnson, W. (1988) *In vitro* cytopathic effect of *Mycoplasma equigenitalium* on the equine uterine tube. Proc. 7th Intl. IOM Congress, p. 127 Baden, Austria.

Beyth, Y., Nachum, R., Horowitz, A., Ron, N., and Vlodovsky I. (1987) Development of tissue culture model of Fallopian tube mucosa. Proc. 43rd Annu. Meet. Amer. Fertil. Soc., p. 22, Reno, NE, USA.

Bloomster, T. G. and Lynn, R. J. (1981) Effect of antibiotics on the dynamics of color change in *Ureaplasma urealyticum* cultures. J. Clin. Microbiol. 13:598-600.

Bradford M. (1974) A rapid and sensitive method for the quantitation of microgram quantities of protein, utilizing the principle of protein dye binding. Anal. Biochem. 72:248-254.

Busolo, F., Zanchetta, R., and Bertoloni, G. (1984) Mycoplasmic localization patterns on spermatozoa from infertile men. Fertil. Steril. 42:412-416.

Chen, Y. and Krause, D. C. (1988) Parasitism of hamster trachea epithelial cells by *Mycoplasma pneumoniae*. Infect. Immun. 56:570-576.

Collier, A. M. (1972) Pathogenesis of *Mycoplasma pneumoniae* infection as studied in the human fetal trachea in organ culture, in: "Pathogenic Mycoplasmas" (A Ciba Foundation Symposium., Ed.) Amsterdam, London, N.Y. pp. 307-327. Elsevier Excerpta Medica. North-Holland.

Dawis, R. W, Botstein, D. and Roth, J. (1980) Advanced bacterial genetics, Cold Spring Harbor, N.Y., Cold Spring Harbor Laboratory.

Glasgow, L. R. and Hill, R. L. (1980) Interaction of *Mycoplasma gallisepticum* with sialyl glycoproteins. Infect. Immun. 30:353-361.

Hu, P.-C., Collier, A. M., and Baseman, J. B. (1984) Surface parasitism by *Mycoplasma pneumoniae* of respiratory epithelium. J. Exp. Med. 145:1328-1343.

Kahane, I. (1984) *In vitro* studies on the mechanism of adherence and pathogenicity of mycoplasmas. Isr. J. Med. Sci. 20:874-877.

Kotani, H. and McGarrity, G. J. (1086) Ureaplasma infection of cell cultures. Infect. Immun. 52:437-444.

McGarrity, G.J. and Kotani, H. (1986) Ureaplasma-eukaryotic cell interaction *in vitro*. Pediatr. Infect. Dis. 5, s316-s318.

Minion, F. C., Cassell, G. H., Pnini, S., and Kahane I. (1984) Multiphasic interactions of *Mycoplasma pulmonis* with red blood cells defined by adherence and hemagglutination. Infect. Immun. 44:394-400.

Saada, A. and Kahane, I. (1988) Purification and characterization of urease from *Ureaplasma urealyticum*. Zbl. Bakt. Hyg. A. 269:160-167.

Saada, A., Terespolsky, Y., Adoni, A., and Kahane, I. (1991) Adherence of *Ureaplasma urealyticum* to human erythrocytes. Infect. Immun. 59:467-469.

Shepard, M. C., Masover, G. K. (1979) Special features of ureaplasmas. in: "The Mycoplasmas", Vol. 1. (Barile M. F. and Razin, S. Eds.) pp. 451-494. Academic Press, New York.

Stalheim, O. H. V. and Gallagher, J. E. (1977) Ureaplasmal epithelial lesions related to ammonia. Infect. Immun. 15:995-996.

Stalheim, O.H.V., Proctor, S.J., Gallagher J.E. (1976) Growth and effects of *Ureaplasmas* (T mycoplasmas) in bovine oviductal organ cultures. Infect. Immun. 13:915-925.

Taylor-Robinson, D. and Carney, F. E. (1974) Growth and effect of mycoplasmas in Fallopian tube organ cultures. Br. J. Vener. Dis. 50:212- 215.

Taylor-Robinson, D., McCormack, W. M. (1979) Mycoplasmas in human genitourinary infections, in: "The Mycoplasmas" Vol. III (Tully, J. G. and Whitcomb, R. F. Eds.) Academic Press, New York.

Vlodovsky, I., Lui, G.M., and Gospodariwicz, D. (1980) Morphological appearance, growth behavior and migratory activity of human tumor cells maintained on matrix vs. plastic. Cell 1a:607.

Wong, B. L. and Shobe, C. R. (1973) Single step purification of urease by affinity chromatography. Can. J. Microbiol. 20:623-630.

SEROLOGICAL IDENTIFICATION OF MOLLICUTES

Joseph G. Tully

Mycoplasma Section, National Institute of Allergy & Infectious
Diseases, National Institutes of Health, Frederick, MD, USA

INTRODUCTION

Mollicutes are bacteria without cell walls, flagella, pili, or other structural components commonly found in other prokaryotes. In addition, the
mollicute genome is the smallest among all other self-replicating organisms.
As a consequence of these characteristics, mollicutes possess limited biosyn-
thetic capabilities and are devoid of many of the chemical components that
form the antigenic mosaic of prokaryotes.

Serologic analysis of mollicutes is, therefore, fairly well dependent upon
membrane (including adhesins) and cytoplasmic antigens. These antigens are
usually proteins or glycoprotein-lipoprotein complexes, and less often of a
pure carbohydrate nature.

Over 138 species have now been described within the class *Mollicutes*,
and more than 30 additional isolates are purported candidates for species designations. Since genetic probes or gene amplification techniques, as well as
other means of identification, are unavailable for the majority of these organisms, conventional serologic tests still play a very important role in laboratory
identification at the species level. These tests are necessary for identification
of all mollicutes regardless of host origin (human, other animals, or plant/ insect), and are also frequently applied to assaying host immune responses to the
organisms.

This presentation will focus on the advantages and disadvantages of
four specific serologic tests currently employed in species identification of unknown mollicute isolates. These include the growth inhibition, agar plate immunofluorescence, metabolism inhibition, and spiroplasma deformation
tests. Finally, brief comments will be offered on two current problems in serologic identification, those involving laboratory techniques for the differenti-

Rapid Diagnosis of Mycoplasmas, Edited by I. Kahane
and A. Adoni, Plenum Press, New York, 1993

ation of *Mycoplasma pneumoniae* and *M. genitalium* and problems in commercial availability of type-specific antisera to mollicutes.

Application of the enzyme-linked immunosorbent assay (ELISA) and immunoblotting technique to serologic identification of mollicutes will be covered in another presentation in this volume.

MODIFICATIONS IN PREPARATION OF MOLLICUTE ANTISERA

A necessary component in serologic identification of mollicutes is the availability of a battery of type-specific immune sera of adequate potency. Basic methodology in preparation of antiserum in rabbits has been presented earlier (Senterfit, 1983a), and only minor modifications in procedure are now being recommended.

Because antigen purity is of the highest priority, only recognized type strains obtained directly from recognized culture collections (American Type Culture Collection, Rockville, MD, USA; National Collection of Type Cultures, London, UK) should be employed as antigens. Antiserum being made to putative new species should always utilize strains purified by conventional filtration- cloning techniques (Tully, 1983).

Standard procedures for preparing antiserum of adequate potency in the rabbit has always involved mixing antigen with an adjuvant. The most common adjuvant in use has been one combining various chemical components of the tubercule bacillus with non-metabolizable paraffin oil (Freund's Complete Adjuvant). Recently, more purified bacterial components or immunoadjuvants have been developed, which are combined with metabolizable oils (such as squalene) as the depot agent (Ribi adjuvant system, Ribi Immuno-Chem Res. Inc., Hamilton, MT, USA; TiterMax, CytRx Corp., Atlanta, GA, USA). In test comparisons in rabbits in our laboratory, we found that the Ribi adjuvant was effective in stimulating satisfactory growth inhibiting antibody to various mollicutes while significantly reducing local tissue reactions (sterile abscesses) at the injection site.

GROWTH INHIBITION TEST

The agar growth inhibition (GI) test is based upon some early observations of Derrick Edward and colleagues (Nicol and Edward, 1953; Edward and Fitzgerald, 1954) that incorporation of specific immune serum into an agar medium would inhibit mollicute growth. Huijsmans-Evers and Ruys (1956) first described application of a disc modification to the procedure, and Clyde (1964) later extended the technique to other mollicutes and defined the practical value of the test in species identification. Current methodology has been given in detail (Clyde, 1983a).

The advantages of the test include few required materials, a minimal amount of antiserum (25 µl) applied to each paper disc, and a single agar plate can be used to screen 3-4 different antisera. The disadvantages involve a required battery of type-specific antisera; the organism to be serotyped must be purified by filtration-cloning procedures; some mollicute species exhibiting serologic strain variation (*M. hominis, M. hyorhinis, M. arginini, M. iowae, etc.*) may not be inhibited by a single antiserum; and the test organism must grow on an agar medium.

Perhaps the most critical factor in the GI test is the number of organisms inoculated onto the agar plate. An inoculum of approximately 1,000 to 100,000 organisms per ml of broth culture is best. Larger inocula will usually overwhelm the inhibitory activity of most antisera, and smaller inocula may prevent visualization of appropriate zones of inhibition.

The test system, originally designed for *Mycoplasma* or *Acholeplasma* species, has been slightly modified for the identification of ureaplasma serovars or biovars (Black, 1973; Piot, 1977; Shepard and Lunceford, 1978), and for *Spiroplasma* species or serogroups (Whitcomb *et al.*, 1982; Williamson and Whitcomb, 1983). For specific application of the procedure to serotyping various animal- derived mollicutes, one should consult the following: avian, (Jordan, 1983); bovine, (Gourlay and Howard, 1983); caprine-ovine, (Cottew, 1983); canine, (Ogata, 1983); swine, (Ross and Whittlestone, 1983); murine, (Cassell, Davidson, Davis and Lindsey, 1983); and other laboratory animals, (Hill, 1983).

The GI test is not recommended for measurement of specific host immune responses, primarily because of low sensitivity and absence of any quantitative evaluation for the test. Recommended serologic techniques for detection of mollicute antibody in human or animal hosts have been presented earlier (Clyde and Senterfit, 1983).

AGAR PLATE IMMUNOFLUORESCENCE TEST

The development of an immunofluorescence test on agar colonies of mollicutes was first described by DelGiudice and colleagues (DelGiudice *et al.*, 1967). The technique is based upon the staining of these colonies with a type-specific conjugated antiserum and examination of stained colonies under fluorescence microscopy and incident illumination. Currently, this test is probably the most rapid and widely used procedure for specific identification of mollicutes (Gardella *et al.*, 1983).

Aside from the rapid and specific identification of mollicutes, the test also has other advantages: purified (cloned) isolates are not required, so primary or early-passage isolates can be identified with appropriate conjugates; serologic strain heterogeneity is less a problem than in the growth inhibition test; and agar colonies can repeatedly be treated with individual conjugates until a positive reaction is observed.

The test as originally described was performed as a direct immunofluorescence procedure, requiring a battery of fluorescein-conjugated antisera. However, an indirect test system can be used, involving initial treatment of colonies with individual, unconjugated antiserum, which is then followed by application of a fluorescein-conjugated antiglobulin (usually anti-rabbit) appropriate for the type-specific antiserum employed.

Further modifications have been suggested that reduce the amount of conjugate or antiserum employed, frequently involving the staining of small agar blocks containing several colonies. These and other techniques are described or referenced in the recommended methodology (Gardella *et al.*, 1983). Further information and references on the use of the direct or indirect immunofluorescence test to specific groups of mollicutes can be found in the following reports: ureaplasmas (Black and Krogsgaard-Jensen, 1974; Piot, 1977; Taylor-Robinson, 1983b); for various animal mollicutes, see list of references in growth inhibition technique above.

The indirect immunofluorescence method has also been used to measure reactive immunoglobulins in host serum and, with appropriate labeled antiglobulin reagents, can measure class-specific antibodies. While this technique has generally been superseded by the ELISA in assaying antibodies to mollicutes in man and animals, it remains useful in some research applications (Furr and Taylor-Robinson, 1984).

METABOLISM INHIBITION TEST

The metabolism inhibition (MI) test is essentially a growth inhibition test performed in liquid media (Purcell *et al.*, 1966a, b; Taylor-Robinson *et al.*, 1966). The test utilizes organisms growing in a broth medium containing a specific metabolizable substrate (glucose, arginine, or urea) and an appropriate pH indicator. Specific antibody inhibits metabolism and consequently prevents the changes in the pH of the culture medium from occurring. The most recent version of standard MI methodology can be found in Taylor-Robinson (1983a). A modification of the test system for mollicutes that are able to reduce 2, 3, 5 triphenyltetrazolium chloride has also been described (Senterfit, 1983b).

As noted earlier, the antigen concentration in this test should also be carefully standardized to the recommended level (100 to 1,000 color changing units/ ml). Concentrated test antigen can be prepared and frozen at -70°C, and then titrated in broth to assess the proper dilution of antigen for the MI test.

Application of the MI test to serologic identification of mollicutes is most useful in situations were the organism does not grow well enough on agar to facilitate testing by growth inhibition. This occurs frequently with freshly isolated ureaplasmas or spiroplasmas. Modifications in the test for ureaplasmas were suggested by Robertson and Stemke (1979). The MI test was first applied to spiroplasmas in 1979 (Williamson *et al.*, 1979), and has become the most useful procedure for definitive species characterization of these organisms (Williamson, 1983; Tully *et al.*, 1987).

Again, the MI technique has generally been superseded by the ELISA in assaying antibodies to mollicutes in man and animals, but it does have its usefulness in certain research applications. Serum containing various broad-spectrum antibiotics or other inhibitory substances (hemoglobin, *etc.*) may give false-positive MI titers.

SPIROPLASMA DEFORMATION TEST

The spiroplasma deformation (DF) test was originally developed to study serologic relatedness of various helical spiroplasmas (Williamson *et al.*, 1978, 1979) and was based upon the concept observed earlier that specific antiserum would inhibit cellular motility of some spirochetes. With spiroplasmas, specific antiserum not only affected motility, but produced major alterations in helical structure and, eventually, cellular lysis. A standardized methodology has been defined (Williamson, 1983), as well as a technique where both the DF and MI tests can be performed in a single microtiter plate (Williamson, 1983; Williamson and Whitcomb, 1983; Williamson *et al.*, 1979).

The DF test is a rapid serotyping procedure for spiroplasmas and requires few materials other than an actively growing broth culture of organisms, test antisera, and the proper equipment for dark-field microscopy. However, current recommendations suggest that the MI test be used as a final definitive confirmation of serotyping results obtained by DF.

Antigen concentration is also an important factor in this test, with approximately 25-50 helices per microscopic field (1250 X) the maximum number for proper visualization. Prefiltration (220 nm) of the broth medium to be used for cultivation of viable antigen will remove background material that may impede detection of deformed helices.

LABORATORY DIFFERENTIATION OF *MYCOPLASMA GENITALIUM* AND *MYCOPLASMA PNEUMONIAE*

Some patients with respiratory disease have been found to be colonized with both *Mycoplasma pneumoniae* and *Mycoplasma genitalium* (Baseman *et al.*, 1989). Although it is clearly established that *M. pneumoniae* plays a direct role in acute respiratory disease, the role that *M. genitalium* may have in this or other human diseases is still uncertain. Mixed cultures of these two organisms have also been identified in isolates obtained from joint fluids of a patient with pneumonia and polyarthritis (Davis *et al.*, 1988; J. G. Tully and J. B. Baseman, unpublished data).

These two mycoplasmas share a number of very important features, including fastidious growth requirements, similar metabolic activities (including glucose fermentation), cytopathogenicity, possession of a terminal attachment structure with associated adhesin proteins, and considerable serologic cross-reactivity. Although some of the latter cross-reactivity may be due to common amino acid sequences in their respective adhesin proteins, most shared reactivity comes from the similar glycolipids (complement-fixing) and other antigens in the membranes of the two organisms. Since the complement-fixation test, which is employed frequently for measuring *M. pneumoniae* antibody in clinical infections, is based upon glycolipid antigens, this test is essentially invalid for distinguishing between infections with either organism (Tully and Baseman, 1991). Further details of the cross-reactions noted in conventional serologic tests have been recorded (Taylor-Robinson *et al.*, 1983; Lind *et al.*, 1984).

Table 1. Identification of *Mycoplasma genitalium* and *Mycoplasma pneumoniae* by plate immunofluorescence test.

Antigens (agar colonies)	M. pneumoniae			M. genitalium		
	1:32	1:256	1:1024	1:16	1:64	1:25
M. pneumoniae	4+	2+	±	3+	Neg	Neg
M. genitalium	3-4	Neg	Neg	4+	1+	±

Antigens treated with indicated dilutions of each specific conjugated antiserum: (Fluorescence of agar colonies of two organisms when treated with indicated dilutions of each specific conjugated antiserum)

As a consequence of these observations, laboratory differentiation of *M. genitalium* from *M. pneumoniae*, and eventual determination of the role of the former in disease, pose difficult diagnostic problems. Several techniques that can differentiate the two organisms are described briefly.

The agar plate immunofluorescence test is perhaps the most rapid technique for detection of both mycoplasmas. Primary throat specimens cultivated in SP-4 broth medium and showing appropriate color shifts in the pH indicator (toward acid pH), should be diluted about 1:1000 in fresh broth and plated to two SP-4 agar plates. This dilution should yield, after incubation, about 200-300 colonies of the potentially mixed mycoplasmas on each plate. The col-onies on each plate should be stained with an appropriate dilution of one of the specific conjugated antiserum. The dilution selected should be chosen after pretesting the conjugate on hand to establish that it will stain only the homologous organism (Table 1). In the case depicted, the *M. pneumoniae* conjugate at a dilution of 1:256 will only stain *M. pneumoniae*, while the *M. genitalium* conjugate diluted 1:64 will stain only that species.

Table 2 shows the results when a mixed but uncloned throat specimen (TW 10-5) containing both mycoplasmas is evaluated by the MI and GI serologic tests. Significant cross-reactions will be seen in the MI test because of shared membrane antigens between the two organisms. However, in the GI test, no significant growth inhibition is observed with either antiserum, primarily because it allows at least one of the mycoplasmas in the mixture to grow up to the antiserum disc. Results obtained with a cloned TW 10-5 throat isolate, yielding either pure *M. pneumoniae* (P) or *M. genitalium* (G) strains, and control type strains of each organism, are also shown in the table.

AVAILABILITY OF TYPE-SPECIFIC ANTISERUM TO MOLLICUTES

As noted above, there are approximately 138 currently established species in the class *Mollicutes* and more than 30 additional unclassified strains that are candidates for species descriptions. Without adding other new species that may come along in years ahead, laboratories involved in species identifica-

Table 2.   Serologic tests for separation of *Mycoplasma pneumoniae* and *Mycoplasma genitalium* strains isolated from human oropharynx.

Strains or isolates or as antigens	Serologic test results in metabolism inhibition (MI) tests or growth inhibition (GI) with antiserum to:[a]			
	M. pneumoniae (FH)		*M. genitalium* (G37)	
	MI	GI	MI	GI
Controls				
M. pneumoniae (FH)	10,240	6	80	0
M. genitalium (G37)	80	0	1,280	6
Throat specimens				
TW 10-5 uncloned	10,240	0	640	0
TW 10-5P (cloned)	5,120	6	80	2
TW 10-5G (cloned)	80	1	1,280	5

[a]MI titers measured as reciprocal of serum dilution showing inhibition of growth in broth medium; GI titers expressed as millimeters of inhibition around paper discs saturated with specific immune sera.

tion are facing a current situation where more than 170 type-specific antisera are required for adequate testing and identification. It is quite likely that this number will reach 200 before the year 2000. This represents an awesome challenge both to current and future mollicutologists to maintain a repository of required and appropriate antisera.

   To compound this situation, there appears to be no current commercial source with an extensive repertoire of typing sera, or even any apparent commercial interest in such materials. If serologic identification is to continue to be an important diagnostic endeavor, and evidence now on hand would argue against molecular or genetic techniques fulfilling this need, then the community of investigators working with these organisms must consider alternate solutions. Some international cooperative effort now seems imperative to meet this current and future need. Perhaps the International Organization for Mycoplasmology can become the stimulus and organizer of such efforts.

REFERENCES

Baseman, J. B., Dallo, S. F., Tully, J. G. and Rose, D. L. (1988) Isolation and characterization of *Mycoplasma genitalium* strains from the human respiratory tract. J. Clin. Microbiol. 26:2266-2269.

Black, F. T. (1973) Modification of the growth inhibition test and its application to human T-mycoplasmas. Appl. Microbiol. 25:528-533.

Black, F. T. and Krogsgaard-Jensen, A. (1974) Application of indirect immunofluorescence, indirect haemagglutination and polyacrylamide-gel electrophoresis to human T-mycoplasmas. Acta Pathol. Microbiol. Scand., Sec. B, 82:345-353.

Cassell, G. H., Davidson, M. K., Davis, J. K. and Lindsey, J. R. (1983) Recovery and identification of murine mycoplasmas, in: "Methods in Mycoplasmology" (Tully, J. G. and Razin, S., Eds.), Vol. II, pp. 129-142. Academic Press, New York.

Clyde, W. A., Jr. (1964) Mycoplasma species identification based upon growth inhibition by specific antisera. J. Immunol. 92:958-965.

Clyde, W. A., Jr. (1983) Growth inhibition tests, in: "Methods in Mycoplasmology" (Razin, S. and Tully, J. G., Eds.), Vol. I, pp. 405-410. Academic Press, New York.

Clyde, W. A., Jr. and Senterfit, L. B. (1983) Serological identification of mycplasmas from humans, in: "Methods in Mycoplasmology" (Tully, J. G. and Razin, S., Eds.), Vol. II, pp. 37-45. Academic Press, New York.

Cottew, G. S. (1983) Recovery and identification of caprine and ovine mycoplasmas, in: "Methods in Mycoplasmology" (Tully, J. G. and Razin, S., Eds.), Vol. II, pp. 91-104. Academic Press, New York.

Davis, C. P., Cochran, S., Lisse, J., Buck, G., DiNuzzo, A. R., Weber, T. and Reinarz, J. A. (1988) Isolation of *Mycoplasma pneumoniae* from synovial fluid samples in a patient with pneumonia and polyarthritis. Arch. Int. Med. 148:969-970.

DelGiudice, R. A., Robillard, N. F. and Carski, T. R. (1967) Immunofluorescence identification of mycoplasma on agar by use of incident illumination. J. Bacteriol. 93:1205-1209.

Edward, D. G. ff. and Fitzgerald, W. A. (1954) Inhibition of growth of pleuropneumonia-like organisms by antibody. J. Pathol. Bacteriol. 68:23-30.

Furr, P. M. and Taylor-Robinson, D. (1984) Micro-immunofluorescence technique for detection of antibody to *Mycoplasma genitalium*. J. Clin. Pathol. 37:1072-1074.

Gardella, R. S., DelGiudice, R. A. and Tully, J. G. (1983) Immunofluorescence, in: "Methods in Mycoplasmology" (Razin, S., and Tully, J. G., Eds.), Vol. I, pp. 431-439. Academic Press, New York.

Gourlay, R. N. and Howard, C. J. (1983) Recovery and identification of bovine mycoplasmas, in: "Methods in Mycoplasmology" (Tully, J. G. and Razin, S., Eds.), Vol. II, pp. 81-89. Academic Press, New York.

Hill, A. C. (1983) Recovery and identification of mycoplasmas from other laboratory animals (including primates), in: "Methods in Mycoplasmology" (Tully, J. G. and Razin, S., Eds.), Vol. II, pp. 143-147. Academic Press, New York.

Huijsmans-Evers, A. G. M. and Ruys, A. C. (1956) Microorganisms of the pleuropneumonia group (family *Mycoplasmataceae*) in man. II. Serological identification and discussion of pathogenicity. Ant. van Leeuwenhoek J. Serol. 22:377-384.

Jordan, F. T. W. (1983) Recovery and identification of avian mycoplasmas, in: "Methods in Mycoplasmology" (Tully, J. G. and Razin, S., Eds.), Vol. II, pp. 69-79. Academic Press, New York.

Lind, K., Lindhardt, B. O., Schutten, H. J., Blom, J. and Christiansen, C. (1984) Serological cross-reactions between *Mycoplasma genitalium* and *Mycoplasma pneumoniae*. J. Clin. Microbiol. 20:1036-1043.

Nicol, C. S. and Edward, D. G. ff. (1953) Role of organisms of the pleuropneumonia group in human genital infections. Brit. J. Vener. Dis. 29:141-150.

Ogata, M. (1983) Recovery and identification of canine and feline mycoplasmas, in: "Methods in Mycoplasmology" (Tully, J. G. and Razin, S., Eds.), Vol. II, pp.105-113. Academic Press, New York.

Piot, P. (1977) Comparison of growth inhibition and immunofluorescence tests in serotyping clinical isolates of *Ureaplasma urealyticum*. Brit. J. Vener. Dis. 53:186-189.

Purcell, R. H., Taylor-Robinson, D., Wong, D. and Chanock, R. M. (1966a) Color test for the measurement of antibody to T-strain mycoplasmas. J. Bacteriol. 92:6-12.

Purcell, R. H., Taylor-Robinson, D., Wong, D. and Chanock, R. M. (1966b) A color test for the measurement of antibody to the non-acid forming human mycoplasma species. Amer. J. Epidemiol. 84:51-66.

Robertson, J. A. and Stemke, G. W. (1979) Modified metabolic inhibition test for serotyping strains of *Ureaplasma urealyticum*. J. Clin. Microbiol. 9:673-676.

Ross, R. F., and Whittlestone, P. (1983) Recovery of, identification of, and serological response to porcine mycoplasmas, in: "Methods in Mycoplasmology" (Tully, J. G. and Razin, S., Eds.), Vol. II, pp. 115-127. Academic Press, New York.

Senterfit, L. B. (1983a) Preparation of antigens and antisera, in: "Methods in Mycoplasmology" (Razin, S. and Tully, J. G., Eds.), Vol. I, pp. 401-404. Academic Press, New York.

Senterfit, L. B. (1983b) Tetrazolium reduction inhibition, in: "Methods in Mycoplasmology" (Razin, S. and Tully, J. G., Eds.), Vol. I, pp. 419-421. Academic Press, New York.

Shepard, M. C., and Lunceford, C. D. (1978) Serological typing of *Ureaplasma urealyticum* isolates from urethritis patients by an agar growth inhibition method. J. Clin. Microbiol. 8:566-574.

Taylor-Robinson, D. (1983a) Metabolism inhibition tests, in: "Methods in Mycoplasmology" (Razin, S. and Tully, J. G., Eds.), Vol. I, pp. 411-417. Academic Press, New York.

Taylor-Robinson, D. (1983b) Serological identification of ureaplasmas from humans, in: "Methods in Mycoplasmology" (Tully, J. G. and Razin, S., Eds.), Vol. II, pp. 57-63. Academic Press, New York.

Taylor-Robinson, D., Purcell, R. H., Wong, D. C. and Chanock, R. M. (1966) A colour test for the measurement of antibody in certain mycoplasma species based upon the inhibition of acid production. J. Hyg. 64:91-104.

Taylor-Robinson, D., Furr, P. M. and Tully, J. G. (1983) Serological cross-reactions between *Mycoplasma genitalium* and *M. pneumoniae*. Lancet i: 527.

Tully, J. G. (1983) Cloning and filtration techniques for mycoplasmas, in: "Methods in Mycoplasmology" (Razin, S. and Tully, J. G., Eds.), Vol. I, pp. 173-177. Academic Press, New York.

Tully, J. G. and Baseman, J. B. (1991) Mycoplasma. Lancet, 337:1296.

Tully, J. G., Rose, D. L., Clark, E., Carle, P., Bové, J. M., Henegar, R. B., Whitcomb, R. F., Colflesh, D. E. and Williamson, D. L. (1987) Revised group classification of the genus *Spiroplasma* (class *Mollicutes*), with proposed new groups XII to XXIII. Int. J. Syst. Bacteriol. 37:357-364.

Whitcomb, R. F., Tully, J. G., McCawley, P. and Rose, D. L. (1982). Application of the growth inhibition test to *Spiroplasma* taxonomy. Int. J. Syst. Bacteriol. 32:387-394.

Williamson, D. L. (1983) The combined deformation metabolism inhibition test, in: "Methods in Mycoplasmology" (Razin, S. and Tully, J. G., Eds.), Vol. I, pp. 477-483. Academic Press, New York.

Williamson, D. L. and Whitcomb, R. F. (1983) Special serological tests for spiroplasma identification, in: "Methods in Mycoplasmology", (Tully, J. G. and Razin, S., Eds.), Vol. II, pp. 249-259.

Williamson, D. L., Whitcomb, R. F. and Tully, J. G. (1978) The spiroplasma deformation test, a new serological method. Curr. Microbiol. 1:203-207.

Williamson, D. L., Tully, J. G. and Whitcomb, R. F. (1979) Serological relationships of spiroplasma as shown by combined deformation and metabolism inhibition tests. Int. J. Syst. Bacteriol. 29:345-351.

RAPID DETECTION OF PHLOEM-RESTRICTED MOLLICUTES

Monique Garnier, Leyla Zreik, Colette Saillard
and Joseph-Marie Bové

Laboratoire de Biologie Cellulaire et Moleculaire
INRA et Universite de Bordeaux II
Domaine de la Grande Ferrade - B.P. 81
33883 Villenave d'Ornon Cedex, France

INTRODUCTION

Spiroplasmas, Mycoplasma-like organisms (MLOs) and Bacteria-like organisms (BLOs)

Three different types of pathogenic prokaryotes (spiroplasmas, MLOs, and BLOs) can be found in the phloem of plants. They are more precisely localized in the sieve tubes of the phloem tissue, *i.e.* the vessels in which the photosynthetically-enriched sap circulates. Spiroplasmas are helical mollicutes which have been obtained in pure culture as early as 1971 (Saglio *et al.*, 1971) and fully characterized (Saglio *et al.*, 1973; Whitcomb *et al.*, 1986; Saillard *et al.*, 1987). They are responsible for three plant diseases: citrus stubborn disease, corn stunt disease, and Syrian periwinkle yellows, respectively caused by *S. citri*, *S. kunkelii* and *S. phoeniceum*. As pure cultures of spiroplasmas were available, polyclonal antibodies were produced as early as 1971 for the serological detection of *S. citri*. Later, monoclonal antibodies (MA) as well as DNA probes were prepared.

MLOs were first observed in 1967 (Doi *et al.*, 1967) and have been found associated with more than 300 diseases of plants, but they have not been obtained in culture to date. Therefore, the study of these prokaryotes was difficult. Indeed, the lack of a culture made it difficult to produce specific reagents. In 1985, MAs directed against the MLO associated with aster yellows disease were obtained (Lin and Chen, 1985). Since then, MAs specific for other MLOs have been produced. DNA probes are also available for certain MLOs since 1987 (Kirkpatrick *et al.*, 1987).

Rapid Diagnosis of Mycoplasmas, Edited by I. Kahane
and A. Adoni, Plenum Press, New York, 1993

BLOs are also phloem-restricted prokaryotes and, like MLOs, they have not been obtained in culture. However they differ from the MLOs (and from the spiroplasmas) by the presence of a cell wall of the gram negative type, and thus are not mollicutes.

In nature, spiroplasmas, MLOs, and BLOs are transmitted from plant to plant by insect vectors (leafhoppers or psyllids).

MLOs were thought to be mollicutes on the basis of their ultrastructure. Indeed, as other human, animal, or plant mollicutes, they were surrounded by a single unit membrane. It is only very recently that MLOs were shown to be true mollicutes on the basis of their genomic and phylogenetic properties (Lin and Sears, 1989 and 1991). The genome size of some MLOs was analyzed by pulse field gel electrophoresis and shown to range between 630 and 1200 kbp. The GC content of their DNA was 23-29.5%. These values are characteristic of the mollicutes. In addition, phylogenetic studies based on the sequence of 16S rRNA have shown that MLO 16S rRNA was typical of mollicutes and more precisely of the anaeroplasma-acholeplasma group. Their relation to the acholeplasma group is also shown by the fact that the UGA codon is a stop codon in MLOs, as it is in *Acholeplasma*, while in *Mycoplasma* and *Spiroplasma*, UGA codes for tryptophan (Yamao *et al.*, 1985; Renaudin *et al.*, 1986).

DETECTION BY ELECTRON MICROSCOPY

Electron microscopy was the first technique used to detect phloem-restricted prokaryotes in plants. The helical morphology of spiroplasmas is easily seen when relatively thick sections (250 nm) are cut through leaf midribs of infected plants. On the contrary, MLOs are pleiomorphic. Spiroplasmas and MLOs can be distinguished from BLOs because they are surrounded by a single, 100 nm thick unit membrane while BLOs possess a cell wall and, therefore, the thickness of their envelope is 250 nm.

Electron microscopy is a time consuming technique and has been replaced by other detection methods (serology, DNA-DNA hybridization) in the case of spiroplasma and a few MLO diseases. However, electron microscopy is still used when an MLO etiology has to be established, or when other detection methods are not available.

DETECTION OF MLOs BY SEROLOGY

Production of Monoclonal Antibodies

In 1986, MLO-specific MAs were produced for the first time by using partially purified MLO preparations from aster yellows-MLO infected leafhoppers (Lin and Chen, 1985). However, as the insect vectors of many MLO diseases are unknown, we have developed a general method for the production of MLO specific MAs by using infected plant material as the immunogen (Martin-Gros *et al.*, 1987). Indeed, MLOs can be easily transmitted to periwinkle plants (*Catharantus roseus*) by dodder (*Cuscuta campestris*), and the MLO-titers are generally higher in periwinkle plants than in primary hosts. Hence, MLO enriched preparations can be produced by purification of phloem tissue from infected periwinkle plants after elimination of the parenchyma tissue with pectinase and cellulase. For immunization, the MLO-enriched preparation is injected intraperitoneally into a mouse in the presence of a mouse immunoserum prepared against phloem purified from healthy periwinkle plants. Screening of MLO- specific MAs was achieved by two methods, a differential avidin biotin ELISA in which each hybridoma supernatant was tested against vascular tissue purified from healthy or infected periwinkle plants and differential immunofluorescence (IF) on leaf midrib sections from healthy and infected periwinkle plants. Using these methods, MAs specific for the MLOs of tomato stolbur, clover phyllody, and witches' broom disease of lime trees were produced.

Application to the detection of the tomato stolbur MLO.

Stolbur is a severe disease of solanaceous plants resulting in flower sterility and therefore no fruit production. By using the previously described method, MAs specific for the tomato stolbur MLO were produced (Garnier et al., 1990). MA 2A10 was selected for the detection of the tomato stolbur MLO as it gave high optical densities (OD) in double antibody sandwich ELISA (DAS-ELISA) as well as strong IF reactions in the phloem of stolbur infected periwinkle plants. Specificity of MA 2A10 for the tomato stolbur MLO was determined by testing by IF and DAS-ELISA periwinkle plants infected with various MLOs or spiroplasmas. No positive reactions were observed with plant mollicutes other than the stolbur MLO. The epidemiology of tomato stolbur was studied. Detection of the tomato stolbur MLO in various solanaceous plants was achieved by IF and DAS-ELISA. The tomato stolbur MLO could be detected in tomato, eggplant, sweet pepper, and tobacco. IF proved to be a more reliable technique than DAS-ELISA as inhibitors of ELISA reactions seemed to be present in homogenates of some solanaceae. The tomato stolbur MLO could also be detected in non-solanaceous plants such as celery affected by porcelain disease, strawberries with yellowing and flower virescence, and in bindweed (*Convolvulus arvensis*), a pereneous wild plant very often found in or near stolbur affected tomato fields. Bindweed is thus likely to be a reservoir plant of the stolbur MLO. The insect vector of the disease was identified using MA 2A10. Indeed, hoppers were captured with a D-VAC aspirator, separated into species and tested by DAS-ELISA for the presence of the stolbur MLO. One species, *Hyalestes obsoletus* (*Cixiideae*), gave very high OD (>2). *Hyalestes obsoletus* individuals were captured and put individually on tomato, eggplant or periwinkle plants for transmission. Successful transmission of the tomato stolbur MLO in those three plant species were obtained with these leafhoppers, naturally infected with the stolbur MLO.

Application to the MLO of witches' broom disease

Witches' broom disease of lime (WBDL) trees is a very recent disease which was described for the first time in 1986 in the Sultanate of Oman (Bové, 1986). It is one of the most severe diseases of citrus. Its spread is very rapidly; first restricted to the coastal plain, the disease has reached the interior regions of the Sultanate in 1987 and the United Arab Emirates in 1989. We showed, by electron microscopy, that witches' broom disease of lime was of MLO etiology. The MLO was transmitted to periwinkle plants via dodder (Garnier et al.,

1991). Eighteen MAs specific for the WBDL-MLO have been produced. All of them gave good IF reactions in the phloem of infected periwinkle plants or lime trees. Some MAs have been selected for DAS-ELISA detection of the WBDL-MLO in plant and insects.

DETECTION OF MLOs BY DNA HYBRIDIZATION

Apple Proliferation MLO

Apple proliferation affects apple trees in Europe and results in poor quality of fruit and reduced productivity of the trees.

MLO-DNA Preparation. A fraction enriched in MLO-DNA has been obtained by ultracentrifugation of total DNA extracted from infected periwinkle plants onto a cesium chloride gradient in the presence of bisbenzimide (Kollar et al., 1990). Bisbenzimide is a DNA stain which binds to A and T bases in the DNA. This results in a decrease of the DNA density. As MLOs are characterized by a high content of A and T bases in their DNA, they can fix a lot of bisbenzimide molecules on the many A and T bases. Plant DNA, containing less AT bases, will fix less bisbenzimide and thus will have a higher density than MLO-DNA. By repeated centrifugations in the presence of bisbenzimide, partially purified apple proliferation MLO-DNA has been obtained.

MLO-DNA Cloning. The MLO-enriched DNA preparation was digested with the restriction enzyme *Hind*III and cloned in plasmid pBR322 linearized with the same enzyme. Each recombinant plasmid was tested for the presence of MLO-DNA inserts by differential hybridization with DNA extracted from healthy or infected periwinkle plants. Nineteen recombinant plasmids giving no hybridization with DNA extracted from healthy periwinkle plants, but hybridizations with DNA extracted from apple proliferation MLO-infected ones were selected. Four MLO-DNA inserts were radiolabeled with ^{32}P-dCTP and used as probes for the detection of apple proliferation-MLO by dot-DNA hybridization (Bonnet et al., 1990). The best DNA probes could detect the MLO in as little as 7 ng of total DNA from infected periwinkle plants and 30 ng of total DNA from infected apple trees. The sensitivity of detection can be increased by preparing RNA probes. This was achieved by recloning the MLO-DNA inserts in pGEM-1 plasmid which contains the promotors for RNA polymerase of phages SP6 and T7. When such RNA probes are used for the detection of apple proliferation MLO in apple trees by dot hybridization, a positive reaction is ob-served in 4 ng of total DNA in comparison with 30 ng in the case of DNA probes.

Witches' Broom Disease MLO

DNA probes have also been produced with cloned WBDL-MLO-DNA following the same protocol (Garnier et al., 1991). They have been used to detect WBDL-MLO in lime trees and to identify the insect vector of the disease in conjunction with MAs. As previously described for the stolbur MLO, leafhoppers were captured on various plants in WBDL-affected areas, separated into species and tested by DAS-ELISA with WBDL-specific MAs and dot hybridization with the DNA probes. For the later technique, individual insects were

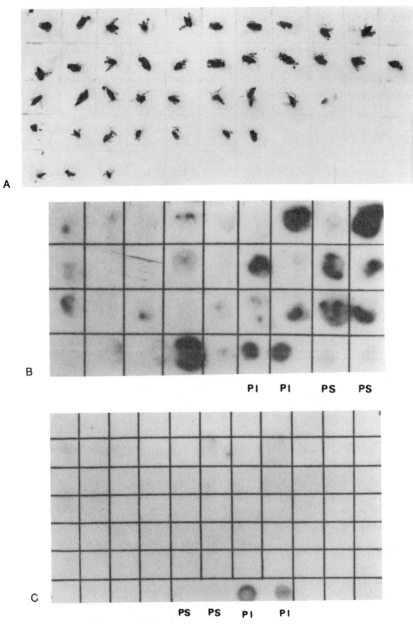

PI   PI   PS   PS

PS   PS   PI   PI

Figure 1. Dot blotting of individual leafhoppers

A - Insects crushed onto a nitrocellulose sheet.
B, C - DNA-DNA hybridization on individual
leafhoppers with a WBDL-specific probe.

All leafhoppers are *Hishimonus phycitis* (B).
All insects are different species of leafhoppers
(*Hishimonus phycitis* is not present (C)).

PS: DNA from healthy periwinkle plants.
PI: DNA from WBDL infected periwinkle plants

crushed directly onto a nylon membrane (Figure 1A), the DNA bound to the membrane was denatured and hybridized with the radiolabeled probes. Only one insect species, *Hishimonus phycitis* (Figures 1B and C), gave positive reactions in both DAS- ELISA and dot hybridization. Experimental transmission of the WBDL-MLO to healthy lime seedling with *Hishimonus phycitis* has not been obtained so far.

DETECTION OF *SPIROPLASMA CITRI* BY *IN SITU* HYBRIDIZATION

As pure cultures of *Spiroplasma citri* are available, it was easy to purify total *S. citri* DNA and to use it as a probe, after nonradioactive labeling with digoxigenin-UTP, to detect the spiroplasmas directly on sections from infected plants. The digoxigenin-labeled probe was detected using antidigoxigenin anti--bodies labeled with alkaline phosphatase (AP), followed by addition of the AP substrate (5- bromo-4-chloro-3-indolyl phosphate) in the presence of nitroblue tetrazolium. Using this procedure, a purple-blue coloration resulting from the action of AP on its substrate could be observed and, as expected, only in the phloem from infected periwinkle midrib sections, but not in that from healthy midrib sections.

DETECTION OF *SPIROPLASMA CITRI* BY POLYMERASE CHAIN REACTION (PCR)

PCR was developed very recently (Saiki *et al.*, 1988) and allows detection of very little amounts (fentograms) of a target DNA sequence. To use this technique it is necessary to know at least part of the nucleotide sequence of the fragment to be amplified. The gene coding for spiralin, the major membrane protein of *S. citri*, has been cloned and entirely sequenced. It was therefore easy to determine, from this sequence, primers to be used in the PCR reaction. Several primer pairs were chosen and used in PCR with *S. citri* purified DNA. Amplification of fragments of the spiralin gene were obtained. The size of the amplified fragment was determined after electrophoresis on polyacrylamide gels, and possessed the expected size. The specificity of the reaction was further verified by digestions of the amplified DNA by restriction enzymes corresponding to internal restriction sites. PCR was then used to detect *S. citri* in plants. For this, leaf midribs from healthy or infected plants were chopped with a razor blade in 3 ml of 0.3 M sodium chloride for one gram of plant material. The liquid phase was pipetted and either used directly for PCR (undiluted or after a ten fold dilution) or the liquid phase was first centrifuged at 12,000 g for 5 minutes and the pellet resuspended in 50 µl of sterile water. Both the pellets and the supernatants were used for PCR. Each assay was performed with 50 µl of the various samples. No amplification was obtained with extracts from healthy plants (periwinkle or citrus plants) nor with the undiluted liquid phase or with the centrifugation supernatant. Amplified fragment of the expected size were obtained with the 10 fold diluted liquid phase and with the resuspended pellet. A positive amplification was still observed when the initial liquid phase was diluted up to 1000 fold. These results indicate that inhibitors of the PCR reactions are present in plant extracts, but that they can be eliminated by dilution or centrifugation of the extract. When compared for sensitivity with the culture assay, PCR gave identical results, but within a few hours, while culture requires at least a week.

CONCLUSION

Many methods are becoming available for the detection of mollicutes. In the case of *Spiroplasma citri*, culture and serological assays were available as early as 1971. Culture is still the best assay to be used for the detection of *Spiroplasma citri*. However, DNA hybridization and PCR, which are in the course of development, are high potential techniques, since they are very sensitive and more rapid than the culture assay. In the case of MLOs, the lack of a culture has made the development of specific reagents more difficult. Monoclonals, antibodies and DNA probes have become available only recently, but have already proven very powerful in the detection and study of these prokaryotes. As of today, MAs and DNA probes are available for only a few MLOs (about 10) and, therefore, detection of other MLOs relies only on electron microscopy observations, a time consuming technique, giving no information on the nature of the MLO observed. Specific conserved sequences in the mollicutes rDNA genes of mollicutes have now been identified, it is therefore likely that in the near future, amplification of these genes by PCR will allow the detection of most mollicutes.

REFERENCES

Bonnet, F., Saillard, C., Kollar, A., Seemuller, E. and Bové, J. M. (1990) Detection and differentiation of the mycoplasma-like organism associated with apple proliferation disease using cloned DNA probes. Mol. Plant-Microbe Interact. 3:438-443.

Bové, J. M. (1986) Witches' broom disease of lime. FAO Plant Prot. Bull. 34:217-218.

Doi, Y., Teranaka, M., Yora, K. and Asuyama, H. (1967) Mycoplasma or PLT group-like microorganism found in the phloem elements of plants infected with mulberry dwarf, potato witches' broom, aster yellows or paulownia witches' broom. Ann. Phytopathol. Soc. Jpn. 33:259-266.

Garnier, M., Martin-Gros, G., Iskra, M. L., Zreik, L., Gandar, J., Fos, A. and Bové, J.M. (1990) Monoclonal antibodies against the MLOs associated with tomato stolbur and clover phyllody, in: "Recent Advances in Mycoplasmology", Proc. 7th Cong. IOM, Baden near Vienna, 1988. (Stanek, G., Cassell, G. H., Tully, J. G. and Whitcomb, R. F., Eds.), pp. 263-269. Zbl. Bakt., suppl. 20, Gustav Fischer Verlag, Stuttgart, New York.

Garnier, M., Zreik, L. and Bové, J. M. (1991) Witches' broom, a lethal mycoplasmal disease of lime trees in the Sultanate of Oman and the United Arab Emirates. Plant Disease 75:546-551.

Kirkpatrick, B. C., Stenger, D. C., Morris, T. and Purcell, A. H. (1987) Cloning and detection of DNA from a non-culturable plant pathogenic mycoplasma-like organism. Science 238:197-200.

Kollar, A., Seemuller, E., Bonnet, F., Saillard, C. and Bové, J. M. (1990) Isolation of the DNA of various plant pathogenic mycoplasma-like organisms from infected plants. Phytopathol. 80, 233-237.

Lim, P. O. and Sears, B. B. (1989) 16S rRNA sequence indicates that plant-pathogenic mycoplasma-like organisms are evolutionarily distinct from animal mycoplasmas. J. Bacteriol. 171:5901-5906.

Lim, P. O. and Sears, B. B. (1991) The genome size of a plant-pathogenic mycoplasma-like organism resembles those of animal mycoplasmas. J. Bacteriol. 173:2128-2130.

Lin, C.P. and Chen, T.A. (1985) Monoclonal antibodies against the aster yellows agent. Science 227:1235-1236.

Martin-Gros, G., Garnier, M., Iskra, M. L., Gandar, J. and Bové, J. M. (1987) Production of monoclonal antibodies against phloem limited prokaryotes of plants: a general procedure using extracts from infected perwinkles as immunogen. Ann. Microbiol. (Inst. Pasteur) 138:625-637.

Renaudin, J., Pascarel, M. C., Saillard, C., Chevalier, C. and Bové, J. M. (1986) Chez les spiroplasmes le codon UGA n'est pas non sens et semble coder pour le tryptophane. C. R. Acad. Sc. Paris 303, serie III, no 13: 539-540.

Saglio, P., Lafleche, D., Bonissol, C. and Bové, J. M. (1971) Isolement, culture et observation au microscope electronique des structures de type mycoplasme associées à la maladie du stubborn des agrumes et leur comparaison avec les structures observées dans le cas de la maladie du greening des agrumes. Physiol. Vég. 9:569-582.

Saglio, P., L'Hospital, M., Lafleche, D., Dupont, G., Bové, J. M., Tully, J. G. and Freundt, E. A. (1973) *Spiroplasma citri* gen. and sp. nov.: a mycoplasma-like organism associated with stubborn disease of citrus. Int. J. Syst. Bact. 23:191-204.

Saiki, R. K., Gelfand, D. H., Stoffel, S., Scharff, S. J., Higuchi, R., Horn, G. T., Mullis, K. B. and Erlich, H. A. (1988) Primer-directed enzymatic amplification of DNA with a thermostable DNA polymerase. Science 239:487-492.

Saillard, C., Vignault, J. C., Bové, J. M., Tully, J. G., Williamson, D. L., Fos, A., Garnier, M., Gadeau, A., Carle, P. and Whitcomb, R. F. (1987) *Spiroplasma phoeniceum*, sp. nov., a new plant pathogenic species from Syria. Intern. J. Syst. Bacteriol. 37:106-115.

Whitcomb, R. F., Chen, T. A., Williamson, D. L., Liao, C., Tully, J. G., Bové, J. M., Mouches, C., Rose, D. L., Coan, M. E. and Clark, T. B. (1986) *Spiroplasma kunkelii* sp. nov.: characterization of the etiological agent of corn stunt disease. Int. J. Syst. Bacteriol. 36:170-178.

Yamao, F., Muto, A., Kawauchi, Y., Iwami, M., Iwagami, S., Aumi, Y. and Osawa, S. (1985) UGA is read as tryptophan in *Mycoplasma capricolum*. Proc. Natl. Acad. Sci. USA 82:2306-2309.

DETECTION AND IDENTIFICATION OF MYCOPLASMAS WITH
DIAGNOSTIC DNA PROBES COMPLEMENTARY TO RIBOSOMAL RNA

Karl-Erik Johansson

The National Veterinary Institute
P.O.Box 7073
S-750 07 Uppsala, Sweden

INTRODUCTION

Hybridization is the reaction by which two single stranded and comple-mentary nucleic acid molecules can form a duplex molecule by base pairing through hydrogen bonds. This reaction has been known for more than 30 years (Hall and Spiegelman, 1961) and proved very useful in research but has, not until recently, been utilized in diagnostic microbiology (for a review, see Tenover, 1988). Nucleic acid molecules used in the hybridization reaction for a diagnostic or a detective purpose are referred to as nucleic acid (DNA or RNA) probes, gene probes or simply probes. The first generation of probes was com-posed of labeled pieces of whole genomic DNA and these probes gave a compar-atively low specificity, but have been extensively used to study phylogenetic re-latedness of bacteria in so-called DNA hybridization experiments. The second generation of probes are those which are composed of labeled restriction endo-nuclease fragments and produced by molecular cloning. These probes represent a more well-defined system and give, in general, a higher specificity. The third generation of probes consists of short oligonucleotides (15-50 nucleotides in length) and they are produced by chemical oligonucleotide synthesis from avail-able sequence information. Oligonucleotide probes give the highest possible spe-cificity and diagnostic methods based on oligonucleotide probes represent ex-tremely well-defined and reproducible systems. As an example, if the target molecule for an oligonucleotide probe of 15-20 nucleotides in length has one single mismatched base pair of the unstable type (Ikuta *et al.*, 1987) close to the middle of the duplex molecule, the stringency can be selected to avoid cross-hy-bridization with this particular target.

A special group of probes which can be used for detection and identifica-tion of microorganisms (except viruses) are those which are complementary to ribosomal RNA (rRNA) and rRNA genes. Such probes are referred to as rDNA

Rapid Diagnosis of Mycoplasmas, Edited by I. Kahane
and A. Adoni, Plenum Press, New York, 1993

probes and the application of rDNA probes for detection and identification of mycoplasmas is the topic of this chapter. The term RNA probe should be avoided in this context, since that in general refers to a probe composed of ribo-nucleotides, irrespectively of the target molecule.

RIBOSOMAL RNA

Ribosomes are present in all life forms (except viruses) and they con-stitute the essential part of the protein synthesizing machinery of the cell. The molecular mechanisms for protein biosynthesis have been fairly conserved throughout the evolution, but the different components show varying degrees of evolutionary variability. The ribosome is built up of a small and a large sub-unit which, in prokaryotes, are referred to as the 30S and the 50S subunit. The Svedberg (S) unit is proportional to the sedimentation velocity in the ultracen-trifuge and reflects the size of the molecule. The subunits are composed of pro-teins and rRNA and in prokaryotes the large subunit contains 5S and 23S rRNA. The small subunit contains the 16S rRNA molecule which in prokary-otes is about 1500 nucleotides in length. The rRNA molecules originating from the small subunit of the ribosome are sometimes referred to as the small ribosomal subunit RNA or srRNA and this term can be used for both pro-karyotic and eukaryotic RNA. The genetic information for rRNA is organized on the chromosome in so-called rRNA operons with the following organi-zation in prokaryotes:

5' - 16S rRNA - Spacer tRNA - 23S rRNA - 5S rRNA - Trailer tRNA - 3'

The number of spacer and trailer tRNAs varies with species. *Mycoplas-mas* have 1-2 rRNA operons (Razin, 1985) while *Escherichia coli*, for instance, has 7 rRNA operons. Some mycoplasmas, however, have been shown to have an unusual organization of the rRNA genes (Taschke *et al.*, 1986; Chen and Finch, 1989). So far, *Acholeplasma laidlawii* is the only mycoplasma which has been shown to have spacer tRNA genes in the rRNA operon (Nakagawa *et al.*, 1992). The discussion below will be focused on 16S rRNA, since that molec-ule contains more useful sequence information for design of diagnostic probes than the 5S rRNA molecule. Furthermore, the 16S rRNA species has been more extensively studied than the 23S rRNA molecule and, so far, more se-quence information is available. The principles, however, are general and can be applied on the other rRNAs as well.

rRNA as a Molecular Chronometer

A general misunderstanding is that the rRNA molecules are extremely conserved and, therefore, not useful as targets for diagnostic probes. The sec-ondary structure of rRNA is very conserved, but it is important to keep in mind that it is the sequence information in the primary structure which is utilized for diagnostic purposes. In the primary structure of, for instance, the 16S rRNA molecule, there are regions of both extremely low and extremely high evolutionary variability and these regions have been accurately localized (see Fig. 1). Conserved regions of very low evolutionary variability are termed

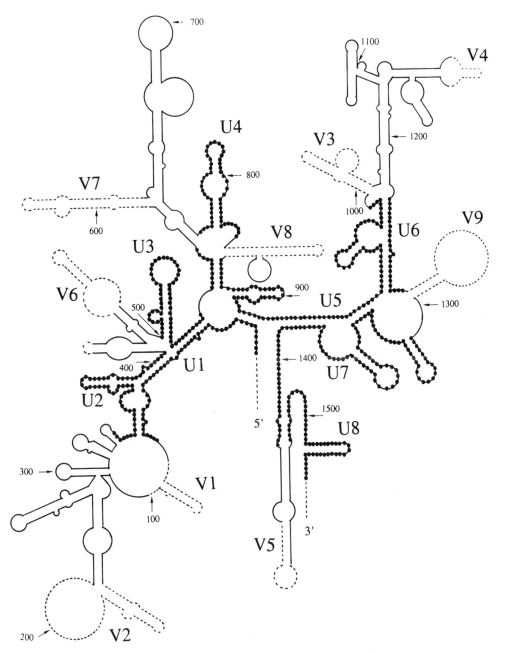

Figure 1. Secondary structure of 16S rRNA from *E. coli* based on the model published by Woese *et al.* (1983) and adapted from Gray *et al.* (1984) where more details are shown. Variable (V) regions are denoted by ----, semi-conserved regions by ___ and universal (U) regions by -•-•-. The position of each 100th nucleotide is indicated with an arrow.

universal (U-) regions and regions of very high evolutionary variability are termed variable (V-) regions (Gray *et al.*, 1984). There are 8 variable regions in prokaryotic 16S rRNA and they are 20-80 nucleotides in length. In this review, the nomenclature of Gray *et al.* (1984) will be used to define the different variable regions. Compare, however, de Rijk *et al.* (1992). Interspersed between U- and V-regions are also regions of intermediate variability, which are termed semi-conserved (S-) regions.

The fact that there exist defined regions of different evolutionary variability makes the rRNA molecules particularly useful for phylogenetic studies, since both long- and short-range relations can be investigated with the same molecular species (Woese, 1987). This, in combination with the fact that ribosomes are ubiquitous in all life forms and have the same function, makes the rRNAs ideal molecules for phylogenetic investigations. Molecules having the same function in different cells are also subjected to the same evolutionary pressure which is very important for drawing the correct phylogenetic inferences (Olsen and Woese, 1993). The phylogeny of mycoplasmas was first studied by comparing short 16S rRNA oligonucleotide sequences and the mycoplasmas were found to form a coherent group of organisms related to clostridia, but with an elevated mutation rate (Woese *et al.*, 1985). Phylogenetic trees based on almost complete 16S rRNA sequences have recently been constructed for about 50 mycoplasmas (Weisburg *et al.*, 1989). The phylogeny of mycoplasmas is discussed in two reviews (Razin, 1989; Maniloff, 1992) and today it is generally believed that mycoplasmas evolved from gram-positive bacteria with low G+C content.

rRNA as the Target Molecule for Probes

There are five factors that are important for the utility of rRNA as the target molecule for diagnostic probes. First, the fact that in a population of rapidly dividing bacteria there is a large number of ribosomes (about 10^4/cell) and consequently a corresponding high copy number of the target molecules (rRNA). Diagnostic systems based on probes complementary to rRNA will, therefore, be very sensitive as compared to probes complementary to single copy genes. Second, the presence of regions of different evolutionary variability which makes it possible to predetermine the specificity of the probe according to the need. Probes complementary to V-regions can be designed to be species- or even subspecies-specific and probes complementary to S regions can be designed to be group-specific. Third, a large number of 16S rRNA sequences have been reported in the literature, because of the usefulness of rRNA as a tool for phylogenetic studies. Sequences of small ribosomal subunit RNA are also regularly compiled in a supplement to the journal *Nucleic Acids Research* (de Rijk *et al.*, 1992). A great number of srRNA sequences have been deposited in data bases like the EMBL (European Molecular Biology Laboratory, Heidelberg, Germany) data bank for nucleotide sequences or GenBank® (c/o Intelligenetics, Mountain View, CA, USA). Fourth, standard methods are available for sequencing of rRNA. The modified dideoxy-nucleotide chain termination method with reverse transcriptase and primers complementary to U-regions upstream of the V-region to be sequenced can be used for rapid sequencing of variable regions, (Lane *et al.*, 1985). However, due to the high degree of secondary structure in an rRNA molecule, it is difficult (or impossible) to completely determine the primary structure by direct RNA sequencing with reverse transcriptase. For complete sequencing of the whole rRNA molecule, it is, therefore, better to clone and sequence the rRNA gene or to sequence the product of *in vitro* amplified rRNA or the rRNA gene by standard methods for DNA sequencing (Sogin, 1990; Weisburg *et al.*, 1991) or direct automated solid phase sequencing (Pettersson *et al.*, 1993). Finally, the fifth factor which is important to consider is the fact that the evolution of the ribosome and its constituents has been comparatively slow. The stability of a diagnostic system, based on rRNA sequences, will therefore be high, which means that a probe or a PCR system which is used to identify one species will most probably also identify all other subspecies of that particular species. On the other hand, it is difficult to design systems based on rRNA sequences which can be used to differentiate between closely related subspecies, although it has proved possible in some instances. Thus, the slow evolution of the ribosome can be an advantage in certain applications, but a drawback in others.

Stanbridge (1976) was the first to suggest that rRNA genes should be useful as the target for diagnostic probes. This idea originated from the observation that rRNA genes of mycoplasmas have conserved regions which might be possible to utilize as the target for a group-specific probe. Such a probe would be useful for detection of mycoplasma contamination in cell cultures. This idea was later proved to be correct (see below).

16S rRNA Sequences of Mycoplasmas

A number of complete or nearly complete 16S rRNA sequences from mycoplasmas have been determined and deposited in the above data bases. The first 16S rRNA sequence from a mycoplasma to be determined was that of *Mycoplasma capricolum* (Iwami *et al.*, 1984) followed by the mycoplasma strain PG50 (Frydenberg and Christiansen, 1985) and *M. hyopneumoniae* (Taschke *et al.*, 1987). These three sequences were determined on DNA level after cloning of rRNA genes and they are complete. Weisburg *et al.*, (1989) reported 45 different 16S rRNA sequences which are all available from the EMBL data bank or GenBank. The 16S rRNA sequences of *Acholeplasma laidlawii* and *M. gallisepticum* were determined by cloning of the rRNA genes and sequencing on DNA-level and they are, therefore, complete. The other sequences were determined by direct RNA sequencing using reverse transcriptase and they are only 70 to 97% complete. The sequence information obtained in that work was used for a phylogenetic grouping of the mycoplasmas and they were found to cluster into 5 distinct groups (the pneumoniae, the hominis, the spiroplasma, the anaeroplasma and the asteroleplasma group). The sequence of 16S rRNA from *M. synoviae* was deposited in 1992 by Dr. Morrow *et al.* in the EMBL data bank under the accession number L7757. Several other 16S rRNA sequences have recently been reported, for instance those of *M. iowae*, strain PPAV (Grau *et al.*, 1991), *M. flocculare* (Stemke *et al.*, 1992) and two biovars of *Ureaplasma urealyticum* (Robertson *et al.*, 1993). The complete sequence of the 16S rRNA gene of the *rrnB* operon and the partial sequence of the *rrnA* operon from *Mycoplasma* sp. strain F38 have been deposited in GenBank by Dr. Ros Bascuñana *et al.* under the accession numbers M94728 and L14607, respectively.

The following partial sequences have also been reported: *M. collis* (van Kuppeveld *et al.*, 1992), *A. axanthum, M. canadense, M. meleagridis, M. mycoides* subsp. *capri.* and *M. ovipneumoniae* (Pettersson *et al.*, 1993). All these sequences are indispensable for design of species- or group-specific rDNA probes for mycoplasmas.

The Sequence Analysis Software Package from the Genetics Computer Group (GCG) at the University of Wisconsin (Devereux *et al.*, 1984), implemented on a VAX computer, is often used in concert with the databases for analysis of nucleotide sequences. The sequences of interest can be retrieved from the database and sequence analysis can then be performed by using different programs in the software package. However, even if the computer does not have nucleotide sequence files or any software for nucleotide sequence analysis, it can still be used to download sequences from the databases to the host computer, provided that this computer is connected to an academic network with a gateway to international networks and that the "MAIL" system has been implemented on the host computer. Sequences can be retrieved and sequence similarity searching can be done in the databases for nucleotide sequences administered by the National Center for Biotechnology Information (National Library of Medicine, USA). Information on how to use the servers can be obtained by sending an electronic mail (E-mail) with the word **help** only, in the body of the message to the following E-mail (Internet) addresses:

retrieve@ncbi.nlm.nih.gov (for sequence retrieval) or
blast@ncbi.nlm.nih.gov (for sequence similarity searching).

The subject field should be left empty and the requested information will be received after a few minutes as an E-mail text file at no cost, if the computers and the lines are not too busy. A nucleotide sequence database with special facilities for rRNA has been created (Olsen *et al.*, 1992). The data in this ribosomal database are available via anonymous ftp (file transfer protocol) or by automated E-mail access.

STRATEGIES FOR DESIGN AND CONSTRUCTION OF rRNA PROBES

The different steps in design and construction of a species-specific rDNA probe are outlined in Fig. 2. First, the data base and/or the literature has to be searched for the sequence of interest. If the sequence has not earlier been determined, it is necessary to do it by any of the above procedures. The next step will be to compare the sequence of interest with the corresponding sequences of related organisms and microorganisms that are likely to be found in the same ecological niche. A suitable target region can then be selected and a complementary probe can be synthesized and tested in, for instance, direct filter hybridization experiments (Mattsson *et al.*, 1991). Direct filter hybridization can conveniently be used for mycoplasmas, since they lack the cell wall and the hybridization target can, therefore, easily be made accessible for the probe (Johansson *et al.*, 1990). The length of the oligonucleotide probe should be 25±10 nucleotides and the G+C content should not be too low (preferably about 40-60%). There should be as many mismatched base pairs as possible with the corresponding regions of rRNA from species to which cross-hybridization must be avoided and the mismatched base pairs should preferably be of the unstable

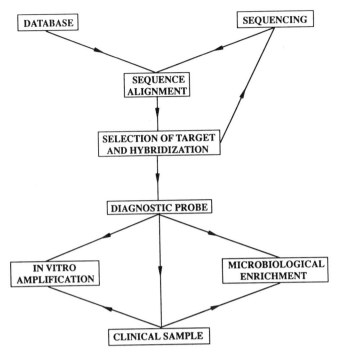

Figure 2. Strategies for design and construction of rDNA probe.

type (Ikuta *et al.*, 1987). If cross-hybridization occurs with species with unknown 16S rRNA sequences, these have to be determined as well. Finally, a new alignment and a new selection of target sequence has to be done and, hopefully, this will result in a useful diagnostic probe of the desired specificity. The sensitivity must also be determined and if the clinical material is likely to contain fewer organisms than the sensitivity threshold, the target molecules have to be enriched by microbiological culture or by *in vitro* amplification of the target molecule (Mullis and Faloona, 1987).

APPLICATIONS

Cell Culture Mycoplasmas

Göbel and Stanbridge (1984) and Razin *et al.* (1984) showed that it was possible to utilize rRNA as the target sequence for diagnostic probes for cell culture mycoplasmas, as predicted by Stanbridge (1976). The H900 probe developed by the first authors is a *Hind*III restriction fragment derived from the 23S rRNA gene of *M. hyorhinis* and it is approximately 900 nucleotides in length. The H900 probe was labeled with ^{32}P by nick-translation and tested in filter hybridization experiments. It was found to cross-hybridize with all mycoplasmas tested (including all mycoplasmas usually found as cell culture contaminants). The H900 probe can cross-hybridize with closely related gram-positive bacteria, but not with eukaryotic nucleic acids which is essential for cell culture screening. This probe has been shown to be extremely useful for screening of cell culture samples for mycoplasmas by using a modified direct filter hybridization procedure (Johansson *et al.*, 1990). A typical result from our diagnostic mycoplasma laboratory is shown in Fig. 3. Razin *et al.* (1984) used the entire plasmid pMC5 containing the main part of one of the two rRNA operons of *M. capricolum* for detection of mycoplasma contamination in cell cultures. The pMC5 probe cross-hybridized with *E. coli* and will probably also cross-hybridize with other prokaryotes, but not with eukaryotes.

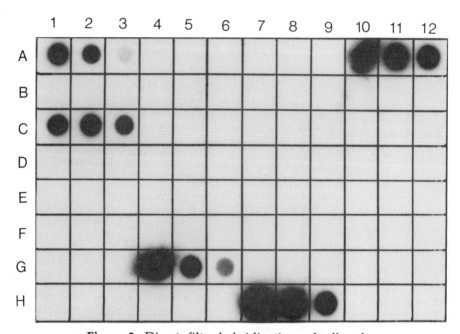

Figure 3. Direct filter hybridization of cell culture samples with the H900 probe. Every sample was applied in 10-fold dilutions in three positions. The following samples were applied. A1-3, positive control, HeLa cells infected with *M. arginini*; B1-3, negative control, mycoplasma-free Sp2/0 cells; C1-3, positive control, promyelotic leukemia cells infected with *M. fermentans*; in the other positions, 24 authentic cell culture samples were applied. Three of these samples were positive, all others were negative.

To overcome the specificity problem with the probes based on restriction fragments, two oligonucleotide probes (MYC14 and MYC25) were designed for group specific detection of mycoplasmas by Göbel *et al.* (1987a). The authors took advantage of the fact that the S-regions often are identical or very similar for related organisms and the MYC25 probe was designed to be complementary to the semi-conserved region S1a of *M. capricolum, Mycoplasma* species (strain PG50) and *M. pneumoniae*. The probe MYC25 was found to cross-hybridize with all mycoplasmas tested in filter hybridization experiments, except *Ureaplasma urealyticum*, but not with other bacteria. However, due to lack of sequence information at that time, the specificities of the MYC14 and the MYC25 probes were not optimal. A set of oligonucleotides Mcc1-3 complementary to 16S rRNA of mycoplasmas from the different phylogenetic groups as defined by Weisburg *et al.* (1989) were therefore designed for detection of mycoplasmas in cell cultures (Mattsson and Johansson, 1993). All mycoplasmas so far isolated from cell cultures can be detected with these probes and they do not cross-hybridize with bacteria. Furthermore, when labeled with 32P, the sensitivity of the filter hybridization system based on Mcc1-3 was shown to be adequate for detection of mycoplasma contamination in cell cultures.

Gen-Probe® (San Diego, CA, USA) is a company developing diagnostic kits with rDNA probes to be used in solution hybridization experiments. In 1985 Gen-Probe released their first version of a screening system for mycoplasma contamination in cell cultures based on an rDNA probe. The probe solution contains tritiated restriction fragments of cDNA cloned rRNA from *A. laidlawii* and *M. hominis*. The probe cross-hybridizes with all mycoplasmas tested and with some Gram-positive bacteria. After hybridization, the probe-rRNA duplex is bound to hydroxy apatite, the excess of probe is washed away and the degree of hybridization is determined in a scintillation counter. Several versions of the mycoplasma detection kit with improved performance have been released since 1985 and some of them have been evaluated (McGarrity and Kotani, 1986; Johansson and Bölske, 1989).

Human Mycoplasma

Two rDNA probes were constructed by Göbel *et al.* (1987 b) for detection of *M. pneumoniae*, the etiological agent of atypical pneumonia in man. The probes were termed MP20 and MP30 and they are complementary to the V6- and the V3- region, respectively, of 16S rRNA from *M. pneumoniae*. The probes were used in filter hybridization experiments with different mycoplasmas and MP20 was found to be specific, while MP30 cross-hybridized with *M. genitalium* which is a closely related species. It proved possible to detect about 10^3 mycoplasmas with 32P-labeled MP30 which means that the MP30 probe is about 100 times more sensitive than a DNA probe directed against a single copy gene would be.

Gen-Probe has developed a diagnostic system for *M. pneumoniae*, based on an rDNA probe produced by cDNA cloning and labeled with 125I. This probe was found to cross-hybridize with *M. genitalium* (Shaw, 1989).

Mycoplasmas of Veterinary Interest

M. bovis can cause mastitis, arthritis and respiratory disease in cattle. An rDNA probe termed Mbo29 has been constructed for the detection of *M.*

bovis in cattle (Mattsson *et al.*, 1991). The probe Mbo29 is complementary to the V6-region of 16S rRNA from *M. bovis* and it did not cross-hybridize with any other bovine mycoplasma. However, a weak cross-hybridization was obtained with the closely related species *M. agalactiae*. This species causes contagious agalactia in goats, but has never been isolated from cattle and Mbo29 should, therefore, be a useful diagnostic tool.

Another probe, Mag30, was developed for detection of *M. agalactiae* in goats (Mattsson *et al.*, 1991). This probe is complementary to the V8-region of 16S rRNA from *M. agalactiae* and it cross-hybridized with some bovine mycoplasma species. However, no cross-hybridization was observed with species commonly isolated from goats or sheep and it should, therefore, be useful for a diagnostic purpose. The sensitivity of the two above probes should, for instance, be adequate for detection of the organisms in milk from diseased animals.

Enzootic porcine pneumonia which is caused by *M. hyopneumoniae* is a disease of great concern in many swine producing countries. An rDNA probe (Mhp6/30) complementary to the V6-region (Fig. 4) of 16S rRNA from *M. hyopneumoniae* has been shown to be specific for *M. hyopneumoniae* and does not give cross-hybridization with the closely related species *M. flocculare* or any other mycoplasma regularly isolated from swine (Johansson *et al.*, 1992). The probe was used in direct filter hybridization experiments of lung tissue and *M. hyopneumoniae* was detected in experimentally infected animals which were in the acute phase of the disease. Three other rDNA probes (MHP1-3) were constructed for detection of *M. hyopneumoniae* by Futo *et al.* (1992). MHP1, which is complementary to the V2-region, was found to be species-specific for *M. hyopneumoniae*, whereas the other probes cross-hybridized with *M. flocculare*

M. hyorhinis can cause polyserositis and may cause pneumonia in piglets and an rDNA probe (Mhy2/27) complementary to the V2-region was, therefore, constructed (Johansson *et al.*, 1992). The Mhy2/27 probe gave almost no cross-hybridization with other porcine mycoplasmas, but was not further tested on clinical material.

Oligonucleotide probes complementary to the V8-regions of 16S rRNA from the avian mycoplasmas *M. gallisepticum* and *M. synoviae* have recently been designed and shown to be species-specific (Fernández *et al.*, 1993). *M. gallisepticum* and *M. synoviae* cause severe respiratory diseases in chickens and turkeys. The probes were used in direct filter hybridization experiments to characterize a number of field isolates and laboratory strains.

Plant Pathogens

The pMC5 probe was used to analyze plant and insect material for the presence of spiroplasmas and mycoplasma-like organisms (Nur *et al.*, 1986). This probe was, however, found to be less useful for that purpose, since it cross-hybridized with plant chloroplasts.

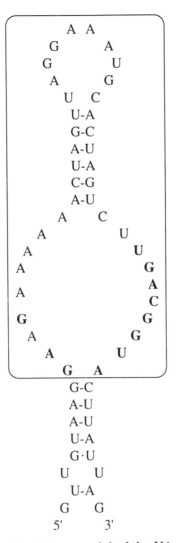

Figure 4. Tentative model of the V6-region of 16S rRNA from *M. hyopneumoniae* with surrounding nucleotide (outside the box). The sequence information was obtained from Taschke *et al.* (1987) and the program StemLoop in the Sequence Analysis Software Package from the GCG (Devereux *et al.,* 1984) was used to find the stem. Ordinary base pairs are denoted with a bar (-), while non-Watson-Crick base pairs of the stable-type (Ikuta *et al.,* 1987) are denoted with a dot (•). The signature positions for gram-positive bacteria in the V6-region (Weisburg *et al.,*1989) are shown in boldface.

FUTURE PROSPECTS

23S rRNA

Since the length of the 23S rRNA molecule is about 2900 nucleotides, it contains more phylogenetic information than the 16S rRNA molecule which will increase the chance to find species-specific regions also for very closely related species or subspecies. However, it is more cumbersome to sequence the whole 23S rRNA molecule and, therefore, less sequence information is available in the literature. When more sequence data of this molecule will be available in the future, it will probably also be more commonly used as the target molecule for diagnostic probes and for *in vitro* amplification by PCR.

In the future, when sequencing of rRNA or rRNA genes becomes fully automatic and when more sequences have been deposited in the data bases, sequencing of 16S or 23S rRNA should be a standard procedure for species determination or for grouping of new isolates. A semi-automated system for PCR with biotinylated primers and solid phase sequencing of the PCR product has been described (Wahlberg *et al.*, 1992). The potential of this system for sequencing of mycoplasmal 16S rRNA has been demonstrated (Pettersson *et al.*, 1993).

Non-Radioactive Labeling

For a diagnostic laboratory it is essential in the long run to be able to avoid radiolabeled probes. There are, unfortunately, still a number of problems associated with nonradioactive labeling which has not always been satisfactorily solved, such as lower sensitivity and unspecific binding unless nucleic acid is prepared from the sample. A system based on modification of the target molecule by sulfonation and detection by using a biotinylated primary antibody against sulfonated nucleic acid and secondary antibodies conjugated with alkaline phosphatase has been developed (Nur *et al.*, 1989). This system was used for detection of mycoplasma contamination in cell cultures by utilizing the pMC5 probe.

In vitro Amplification

In vitro amplification of DNA (or RNA) is treated elsewhere in this volume and will only be very briefly discussed here. *In vitro* amplification (by, for instance, PCR, the polymerase chain reaction) can be used to amplify the target and thereby increase the sensitivity (Mullis and Faloona, 1987) to make it possible to use probes which are not radiolabeled. Another interesting possibility is to use PCR for incorporation of suitable markers in the final product by decorating the primers with these markers (Wahlberg *et al.*, 1990), which can be very useful for diagnostic microbiology in the future. *In vitro* amplification can also be used for sequencing of rRNA from noncultivable microorganisms, since the primers can be selected to be complementary to U-regions. *In vitro* amplification can sometimes be very useful to regulate the specificity, since certain mismatches (particularly A#G and C#C) at the 3'-end of the primer will strongly reduce amplification while internal mismatches are of much less importance (Kwok *et al.*, 1990).

A pair of primers for amplification of regions of the 16S rRNA gene of species belonging to the genus *Mycoplasma* has been constructed (Blanchard *et al.*, 1991). Species determination was done either by using a species-specific probe for the amplified region (*M. pirum*) or by sequencing of the amplified region and comparing the result with known 16S rRNA sequences (*M. fermentans*).

Sets of PCR-primers were recently described to amplify different segments of the 16S rRNA gene (or 16S rRNA) from mycoplasmas (van Kuppeveld *et al.*, 1992). Specific amplification was obtained for *M. pneumoniae*, *M. hominis*, *M. fermentans*, *U. urealytium*, *M. pulmonis*, *M. arthritidis*, *M. neurolyticum*, *M. muris* and *M. collis* with the different primer sets. A primer set for group-specific amplification of a segment of the 16S rRNA gene of all mycoplasmas was also reported. This primer set can be used for detection of mycoplasma contamination of cell cultures.

In vitro amplification of rRNA or rRNA genes is a very useful tool for detection and identification of mycoplasmas and will probably be a standard method in many diagnostic laboratories in the future. The difficulties should, however, not be neglected and if PCR is to be used in a diagnostic laboratory for detection of, for instance, mycoplasma contamination in cell cultures, one has to be careful to avoid the contamination problems.

ACKNOWLEDGMENTS

I thank Dr. Ulf Göbel for generous help and many invaluable discussions, Professor Göran Hugoson for valuable support and Jens Mattsson for constructive criticism of the manuscript. Research leading to this review has been financially supported from the Swedish Council for Forestry and Agricultural Research, SAREC and Swedish Farmers' Foundation for Agricultural Research.

REFERENCES

Blanchard, A., Gautier, M. and Mayau, V. (1991) Detection and identification of mycoplasmas by amplification of rDNA. FEMS Microbiol. Lett. 81:37-42.

Chen, X. and Finch, L. R. (1989) Novel arrangement of rRNA genes in *Mycoplasma gallisepticum*: Separation of the 16S rRNA gene of one set from the 23S and 5S genes. J. Bacteriol. 171:2876-2878.

De Rijk, P., Neefs, J.-M., Van de Peer, Y. and De Wachter, R. (1992) Compilation of small subunit RNA sequences. Nucleic Acids Res. Suppl. 20:2075-2089.

Devereux, J., Haeberli, P. and Smithies, O. (1984) A comprehensive set of sequence analysis programs for the VAX. Nucleic Acids Res. 12:387-395.

Fernández, C., Mattsson, J. G., Bölske, G., Levisohn, S. and Johansson, K.-E. (1993) Species-specific oligonucleotide probes complementary to 16S-rRNA of *Mycoplasma gallisepticum* and *Mycoplasma synoviae*. Res. Vet. Sci. (in press).

Frydenberg, J. and Christiansen, C. (1985) The sequence of 16S rRNA from mycoplasma strain PG50. DNA 4:127-137.

Futo, S., Soto, Y., Mitsuse, S. and Mori, Y. (1992) Detection of *Mycoplasma hyopneumoniae* by using rRNA-oligonucleotide hybridization. J. Clin. Microbiol. 30:1509-1513.

Göbel, U.B. and Stanbridge, E. J. (1984) Cloned mycoplasma ribosomal RNA genes for the detection of mycoplasma contamination in tissue cultures. Science 226:1211-1213.

Göbel, U., Maas, R., Haun, G., Vinga-Martins, C. and Stanbridge, E. J. (1987a) Synthetic oligonucleotide probes complementary to rRNA for group- and species-specific detection of mycoplasmas. Israel J. Med. Sci. 23:742-746.

Göbel, U.B., Geiser, A. and Stanbridge, E. J. (1987 b) Oligonucleotide probes complementary to variable regions of ribosomal RNA discriminate between *Mycoplasma* species. J. Gen. Microbiol. 133:1969-1974.

Grau, O., Laigret, F., Carle, P., Tully, J. G., Rose, D. and Bové, J. M. (1991) Identification of a plant-derived *Mollicute* as a strain of an avian pathogen, *Mycoplasma iowae*, and its implications for *Mollicute* taxonomy. Int. J. Syst. Bacteriol. 41:473-478.

Gray, M. W., Sankoff, D. and Cedergren, R. J. (1984) On the evolutionary descent of organisms and organelles: a global phylogeny based on a highly conserved structural core in small subunit ribosomal RNA. Nucleic Acids Res. 12:5837-5852.

Hall, B. D. and Spiegelman, S. (1961) Sequence complementarity of T2-DNA and T2- specific RNA. Proc. Natl. Acad. Sci. 47:137-146.

Ikuta, S., Takagi, K., Wallace, R. B. and Itakura, K. (1987) Dissociation kinetics of 19 base paired oligonucleotide-DNA duplexes containing different single mismatched base pairs. Nucleic Acids Res. 15:797-811.

Iwami, M., Muto, A., Yamao, F. and Osawa, S. (1984) Nucleotide sequence of the rrnB 16S ribosomal RNA gene from *Mycoplasma capricolum*. Mol. Gen. Genet. 196, 317-322.

Johansson, K.-E. and Bölske, G. (1989) Evaluation and practical aspects of the use of a commercial DNA probe for detection of mycoplasma infections in cell cultures. J. Biochem. Biophys. Methods 19:185-200.

Johansson, K.-E., Johansson, I. and Göbel, U. B. (1990) Evaluation of different hybridization procedures for the detection of mycoplasma contamination in cell cultures. Mol. Cell. Probes 4: 33-42.

Johansson, K.-E., Mattsson, J.G., Jacobsson, K., Fernández, C., Bergström, K., Bölske, G., Wallgren, P. and Göbel, U. B. (1992) Specificity of oligonucleotide probes complementary to evolutionarily variable regions of 16S rRNA from *Mycoplasma hyopneumoniae* and *Mycoplasma hyorhinis*. Res. Vet. Sci. 52:195-204.

Kwok, S., Kellogg, D. E., McKinney, N., Spasic, D., Goda, L., Levenson, C. and Sninsky, J. J. (1990) Effects of primer-template mismatches on the polymerase chain reaction: human immunodeficiency virus type 1 model studies. Nucleic Acids Res. 18:999-1005.

Lane, D. J., Pace, B., Olsen, G. J., Stahl, D. A., Sogin, M. L. and Pace, N.R. (1985) Rapid determination of 16S ribosomal RNA sequences for phylogenetic analysis. Proc. Natl. Acad. Sci. USA 82:6955-6959.

Maniloff, J. (1992) Phylogeny of Mycoplasmas, in "Mycoplasmas: Molecular Biology and Pathogenesis" (Maniloff, J., McElhaney, R. N., Finch, L. R. and Baseman, J. B., Eds.), pp. 549-559, ASM Press, Washington.

Mattsson, J. G. and Johannsson, K.-E. (1993) Oligonucleotide probes complementary to 16S rRNA for rapid detection of mycoplasma contamination in cell cultures. FEMS Microbiol. Lett. 107:139-144.

Mattsson, J. G., Gersdorf, H., Göbel, U.B. and Johansson, K.-E. (1991) Detection of *Mycoplasma bovis* and *Mycoplasma agalactiae* by oligonucleotide probes complementary to 16S rRNA. Mol. Cell. Probes 5:27-35.

Mullis, K. B. and Faloona, F. A. (1987) Specific synthesis of DNA *in vitro*: a polymerase-catalyzed chain reaction. Methods Enzymol. 155:335-350.

McGarrity, G. J. and Kotani, H. (1986) Detection of cell culture mycoplasmas by a genetic probe. Exp. Cell Res. 163:273-278.

Nakagawa, T., Uemori, T., Asada, K., Kato, I. and Harasawa, R. (1992) *Acholeplasma laidlawii* has tRNA genes in the 16S-23S spacer of the rRNA operon. J. Bacteriol. 174:8163-8165.

Nur, I., Bové, J. M., Saillard, C., Rottem, S., Whitcomb, R. M. and Razin, S. (1986) DNA probes in detection of spiroplasmas and mycoplasma-like organisms in plants and insects. FEMS Microbiol. Lett. 35:157-162.

Nur, I., Reinhartz, A., Hyman, H. C., Razin, S., Herzberg, M. (1989) Chemi-probe™, a nonradioactive system for labeling nucleic acid. Principles and applications. Ann. Biol. Clin. 47:601-606.

Olsen, G. J. and Woese, C.R. (1993) Ribosomal RNA: a key to phylogeny. FASEB J. 7:113-123.

Olsen, G. J., Overbeek, R., Larsen, N., Marsh, T. L., McCaughey, M. J., Maciukenas, M. A., Kuan, W.-M., Macke, T. J., Xing, Y. and Woese, C. R. (1992) The ribosomal database project. Nucleic Acids Res. Suppl. 20:2199-2120.

Pettersson, B., Johansson, K.-E. and Uhlén, M. (1993) Direct automated solid phase sequencing in an *in vitro* amplified segment of 16S rDNA from bacteria, in: "Proceedings of the 6th European Congress on Biotechnology" (Alberghina, L., Frontali, L. and Sensi, P., Eds.). Elsevier, Amsterdam (in press).

Razin, S. (1985) Molecular biology and genetics of mycoplasmas (*Mollicutes*). Microbiol. Rev. 49:419-455.

Razin, S. (1989) Molecular approach to mycoplasma phylogeny, in: "The Mycoplasmas, Vol. V. *Spiroplasmas, Acholeplasmas* and *Mycoplasmas* of Plants and Arthropods" (Whitcomb, R. F. and Tully, J. G. Eds.), pp. 33-69. Academic Press, New York.

Razin, S., Gross, M., Wormser, M., Pollack, Y. and Glaser, G. (1984) Detection of mycoplasmas infecting cell cultures by DNA hybridization. In Vitro 20:404-408.

Robertson, J. A., Vekris, A., Bébéar, C. and Stemke, G. W. (1993) Polymerase chain reaction using 16S rRNA gene sequences distinguishes the two biovars of *Ureaplasma urealyticum*. J. Clin. Microbiol. 31:824-830.

Shaw, S. B. (1989) DNA probes for the detection of *Legionella* species, *Mycoplasma pneumoniae*, and members of the *Mycobacterium tuberculosis* complex, in: "DNA Probes for Infectious Diseases" (Tenover, F. C., Ed.), pp. 101-117. CRC Press, Boca Raton.

Sogin, M. L. (1990) Amplification of ribosomal RNA genes for molecular evolution studies, in: "PCR Protocols, a Guide to Methods and Applications" (Innis, M. A., Gelfund, D. H., Sninsky, J. J. and White, T. J., Eds.), pp. 307-317. Academic Press, New York.

Stanbridge, E. J. (1976) A reevaluation of the role of mycoplasmas in human disease. Annu. Rev. Microbiol. 30:169-187.

Stemke, G.W., Laigret, F., Grau, O. and Bové, J. M. (1992) Phylogenetic relationships of three porcine mycoplasmas, *Mycoplasma hyopneumoniae, Mycoplasma flocculare,* and *Mycoplasma hyorhinis,* and complete 16S rRNA sequences of *M. flocculare.* Int. J. Syst. Bacteriol. 42:220-225.

Taschke, C., Klinkert, M.-Q., Wolters, J. and Herrmann, R. (1986) Organization of the ribosomal RNA genes in *Mycoplasma hyopneumoniae:* the 5S rRNA gene is separated from the 16S and 23S rRNA genes. Mol. Gen. Genet. 205:428-433.

Taschke, C., Ruland, K. and Herrmann, R. (1987) Nucleotide sequence of the 16S rRNA of *Mycoplasma hyopneumoniae.* Nucleic Acids Res. 15:3918.

Tenover, F. C. (1988) Diagnostic deoxyribonucleic acid probes for infectious diseases. Clin. Microbiol. Rev. 1: 82-101.

Van Kuppeveld, F. J. M., van der Logt, J. T. M., Angulo, A. F., van Zoest, M. J., Quint, W. G.V., Niesters, H. G. M., Galama, J.M.D. and Melchers, W.J.G. (1992) Genus- and species-specific identification of mycoplasmas by 16S rRNA amplification. Appl. Environ. Microbiol. 58:2606-2615.

Wahlberg, J., Lundeberg, J., Hultman, T. and Uhlén, M. (1990) General colorimetric method for DNA diagnostics allowing direct solid-phase genomic sequencing of the positive samples. Proc. Natl. Acad. Sci. USA 87:6569-6573.

Wahlberg, J., Holmberg, A., Berg, S., Hultman, T. and Uhlén, M. (1992) Automated magnetic preparation of DNA templates for solid phase sequencing. Electrophoresis 13:547-551.

Weisburg, W. G., Tully, J. G., Rose, D. L., Petzel, J. P., Oyaizu, H., Yang, D., Mandelco, L., Sechrest, J., Lawrence, T. G., Van Etten, J., Maniloff, J. and Woese, C.R. (1989) A phylogenetic analysis of the mycoplasmas: Basis for their classification. J. Bacteriol. 171:6455-6467.

Weisburg, W. G., Barns, S. M., Pelletier, D. A. and Lane, D. J. (1991) 16S ribosomal amplification for phylogenetic studies. J. Bacteriol. 173:697-703.

Woese, C. R. (1987) Bacterial evolution. Microbiol. Rev. 51:221-271.

Woese, C. R., Gutell, R., Gupta, R. and Noller, H. F. (1983) Detailed analysis of the higher-order structure of 16S-like ribosomal ribonucleic acids. Microbiol. Rev. 47:621-669.

Woese, C. R., Stackebrandt, E. and Ludwig, W. (1985) What are mycoplasmas: The relationship of tempo and mode in bacterial evolution. J. Mol. Evol. 21:305-316.

MYCOPLASMAS IN CELL CULTURE

Michael F. Barile[1] and Shlomo Rottem[2]

[1]Laboratory of Mycoplasma
Office of Biologics Research, FDA, Bethesda, MD, USA
[2]Hebrew University-Hadassah Medical School
Jerusalem, Israel

INTRODUCTION

This report will briefly review our current knowledge of: 1) the incidence, prevalence and sources of mycoplasma contamination in cell cultures; 2) the procedures for isolation, detection and identification of mycoplasmas, including procedures recommended for testing biological products produced for human use; 3) the effects of mycoplasma contamination and/or infection on the function and activities of various infected cell cultures; and 4) the recommended procedures for prevention and elimination of mycoplasma contamination. Extensive reviews on mycoplasma contamination in cell culture have been reported earlier (Barile, 1979; DelGiudice and Hopps, 1978; McGarrity and Kotani, 1985).

MYCOPLASMA CONTAMINATION OF CELL CULTURES.

Historical Aspects

Robinson *et al.* (1956) first isolated a mycoplasma from a contaminated cell culture. They were investigating the effect of a mycoplasma infection on cell cultures and found that their uninoculated, negative control cell cultures were contaminated. At that time, one of us (MFB) was stationed in Japan, developing research programs on improving the existing procedures for the isolation and detection of mycoplasmas (Barile *et al.*, 1958). Within weeks of Robinson's report, it was found that the four cell lines used routinely in the laboratory were contaminated with mycoplasmas. These contaminants were subsequently identified as *M. hominis*.

On returning home in 1958 to the National Institutes of Health, polio virus vaccine was being produced in primary cell cultures. Because many of

Rapid Diagnosis of Mycoplasmas, Edited by I. Kahane
and A. Adoni, Plenum Press, New York, 1993

the cell cultures used in the United States were found to be contaminated with mycoplasmas, concerns were raised regarding the safety of vaccines produced in cell cultures. Consequently, in 1962, the United States Public Health Service established a mycoplasma test requirement for viral vaccines produced in cell cultures. This test requirement will be discussed later.

Epidemiology: Continuous Cell Cultures

It is now well-established that stable, continuous cell lines are frequently contaminated. In our studies, over 20,000 cell cultures were examined during the past 30 years and over 3,000 mycoplasma contaminants (15%) were isolated, detected and speciated. Similar findings have been reported by others (DelGiudice and Hopps, 1978; McGarrity and Kotani, 1985). Higher incidences of contamination have been reported in other countries. Three different surveys in Japan showed an incidence of mycoplasma contamination of 80% (Koshimizu and Kotani, 1981) and an incidence of 65% was reported in Argentina (Coronado and Coto, 1987), and more recently, about 32% of the cell cultures examined during recent years (1984-1991) in Israel were found to be contaminated (Rottem and Wormser, unpublished data). In spite of numerous reports on the high incidence and the diverse, adverse effects on cell functions and activities, contamination continues to be a frequent and troublesome problem today (Barile, 1979; Barile and Grabowski, 1977; Barile et al.. 1973; 1977; McGarrity and Kotani, 1985).

Bovine Mycoplasma Species. In our studies, the bovine species were the most common contaminants (Barile, 1979). Of 2,800 mycoplasmas isolated, 1,262 (45%) were bovine species and the most frequent isolated species were *Mycoplasma arginini* (26%), *Acholeplasma laidlawii* (8.5%), and *M. pirum* (7%). The other species isolated include *M. bovis*, *M. bovoculi*, *A. axanthum*, and a number of other unspeciated *Acholeplasma* species.

Human Mycoplasma Species. Of the 2,800 isolated, 929 (33%) were human species, the second most frequent recovered.*Mycoplasma orale* accounted for 29.5% of these, but strains of *M. hominis*, *M. fermentans*, and *M. salivarium* were also isolated.

Swine Mycoplasma Species. The swine species were the next most frequent contaminants; 591 (21%) of the 592 swine strains isolated were *Mycoplasma hyorhinis*. One strain of *A. oculi* was also isolated.

Murine, Avian, and Canine Mycoplasma Species. Seventeen (less than 1%) were either murine, avian or canine species. These include: *M. arthritidis* *M. pulmonis*, *M. canis* and the canine serogroup 689 strains. Most of these were isolated from primary, rather than continuous, cell cultures.

Epidemiology: Primary Cell Cultures:

The first viral vaccines were produced in primary cell cultures. Thus, our primary interest initially was to examine these types of cell cultures. From 1958 to 1972, over 3,200 primary cell culture lots were examined. Forty two lots were contaminated and 51 strains, representing 12 different *Mycoplasma* species, were isolated and identified. A primary cell culture lot is derived from one chick or duck embryo, or one or two, rarely more, sets of monkey or rabbit kidneys. Five primary monkey and four rabbit kidney cell culture lots were contaminated with two different *Mycoplasma* species. Only five rodent strains of *M. arthritidis* were isolated during these studies, and each was recovered from a primary rabbit kidney cell culture. None were isolated from continuous cell lines. The only two strains of *M. buccali* isolated were recovered from primary monkey kidney cell cultures. We showed earlier that *M. buccali* is a common oral isolate of normal monkeys (DelGiudice *et al.*, 1969). The only two strains of canine serogroup HRC 689 (Barile *et al.*, 1970) isolated were from primary canine kidney cells. The only four rodent strains of *M. pulmonis* were recovered from primary rat embryo cells. One of the three avian strains of *M. gallisepticum* isolated was recovered from a primary chick embryo cell culture. Thus, the probable source of most, or all, of the canine, murine and avian mycoplasma contaminants was the original tissues used to develop the primary cell culture lot. Only 1% of the total contaminants isolated came from the original tissues, leading to the conclusion that the original tissues were not a major source of contamination. The frequency of contamination depended on the primary organ tissue used. For example, the foreskin, lower female urogenital tract or tumor tissues, which are subject to mycoplasma colonization, generally had a slightly higher rate of contamination.

Summation: Cell Culture Contamination

Continuous, stable cell cultures are frequently contaminated. About 15% of the cell lines examined in the U.S.A. were contaminated (Barile, 1979; DelGiudice and Hopps, 1978; McGarrity and Kotani, 1985). Contamination occurs during cell propagation and comes from exogenous sources. Primary cell cultures account for about 1% of the contaminations. At least 20 distinct *Mycoplasma* or *Acholeplasma* species have been isolated from contaminated cell cultures. Ninety five percent of the contaminants were identified as either *M. orale, M. arginini, M. hyorhinis, M. fermentans,* or *Acholeplasma laidlawii*. The frequency of isolations for each species varies with the particular study. For example, McGarrity and Kotani (1985) isolated many more strains of *M. hyorhinis, A. laidlawii* and *M. salivarium*, but far less isolates of *M. pirum* or *M. arginini* than found by us (Barile, 1979). DelGiudice and Hopps (1978) isolated many more strains of *M. fermentans* than either of us. In fact, during the period 1985 to 1988, almost 30% of their isolates were *M. fermentans* (Del Giudice, unpublished data). Nine percent of our cell cultures were contaminated with two or more *Mycoplasma* species. Some cell lines were infected with as many as four different *Mycoplasma* species. All cell types were subject to contamination. These include normal, virus-infected, transformed or neoplastic cell cultures grown in monolayers and/or in suspension and derived from all hosts examined. The mammalian and avian derived cell lines were the most commonly contaminated. Occasionally, cell cultures derived from reptilian, fish, insect or plant origin were also contaminated. In addition to mycoplasmas, about 8% of our cell cultures were contaminated with low orders, less than 10^5 CCU/ml of bacteria. Because of growth suppression by antibiotic, most of these low order bacterial contaminations went undetected. They did not produce turbid growth, destroy the cell cultures, or grow on standard culture media. Contamination was detected by the DNA staining procedure to be described later. Occasionally, the DNA staining procedure detected yeast infections before the cultures were completely destroyed.

Most studies have examined fibroblastic cells, but epithelial, endothelial, lymphocytic and hybridoma cell culture lines have also been found to be contaminated. The available information on differentiated cell culture lines is limited and more data are needed before a proper assessment can be made. Mycoplasmas have been isolated from or detected in circulating blood lymphocyte preparations. *M. orale* was isolated from "buffy coats" of patients with leukemia (Anderson and Barile, 1966). *M. fermentans, M. pirum* and unspeciated species were recovered from lymphocyte cultures of patients with AIDS (Lo *et al.*, 1985; 1989; 1991; Montagnier *et al.*, 1990; Saillard *et al.*, 1989). Many of the lyphocyte cultures examined by R.A. DelGiudice (unpublished data) were infected with *M. fermentans*. Thus, the mycoplasmas isolated from infected differentiated cell cultures, such as lymphocyte cultures, may differ from the mycoplasmas isolated from fibroblastic cell lines.

Sources of Contamination

Because mycoplasma contamination of vaccines would present a potential health hazard, the sources of contamination have been of major concern to us. We had already established that the continuous cell cultures were the most frequently contaminated substrates and that contamination came from exogenous sources.

Bovine Sera Contamination. Because bovine mycoplasma species were common contaminants, bovine serum was considered a probable source of contamination for years. Prior to 1970, all attempts to recover mycoplasmas from sera failed. At that time, a standard amount of the serum specimen was inoculated onto the standard agar (0.1 ml) or into broth media (1.0 ml). Successful isolations were made when a large volume of the test serum specimen was examined (Barile and Kern, 1972). Initially, a 100 ml volume of several "suspect" bovine serum products distributed by the manufacturer were examined. Each was found contaminated with mycoplasmas. The standard broth medium was supplemented with yeast extract and phenol red as a pH indicator. The bovine serum specimen replaced the horse serum component of this medium. In an extensive study, 104 bottles of final-processed serum representing 395 separate lots produced by 5 commercial suppliers were contaminated (Barile and Kern, 1972; Barile, 1979). The number of organisms in the final processed sera was quite small. Frequently there were only one to ten viable mycoplasmas per ml of sera. Thus, the standard inoculum using agar or broth media was an inadequate volume for successful isolation. The use of larger serum specimen volumes increased the sensitivity of the test. We subsequently showed that cell cultures were exquisitely sensitive for the isolation of mycoplasmas. Only one mycoplasma cell could grow to 10^6 CCU/ml within 3 to 5 days in an infected cell culture. The unprocessed sera examined were heavily contaminated. Of 438 lots of "raw" fetal bovine serum obtained from eight different abattoirs, 159 lots were contaminated. Of 55 lots of unprocessed calf serum tested, 22 were contaminated. Many of the unprocessed serum lots were heavily contaminated with mixed cultures of mycoplasmas, bacteria and yeast. Most contained 10^4 or more mycoplasma/ml. In fact, if we had examined "raw" unprocessed bovine serum earlier, contamination would have been detected much sooner.

The Large Specimen Volume Broth Culture Procedure. Presently, the large volume serum specimen procedure is used routinely as a standard test for bovine sera. As a result, the incidence of contamination in commercially-prepared sera has decreased over the past 20 years and, presently, it is relatively low. However, even today, the incidence among commercially prepared sera varies with the supplier. Before each serum lot is accepted, it must be tested by the investigator and found mycoplasma-free.

Bovine Serum Contaminants. The bovine serum contaminants were primarily bovine *Mycoplasma* species with one exception; a swine strain of *M. hyorhinis* was also isolated from one lot of bovine serum. Because swine and cattle are processed through the same abbatoirs, the probably source of the swine isolate was of swine origin. Of the 285 strains isolated from the contaminated sera, 193 were identified representing at least eight distinct bovine species (Barile and Kern, 1972; Barile, 1979). The bovine species isolated from bovine sera were identical to those isolated from contaminated cell cultures. The two most frequently isolated bovine species in both contaminated bovine sera and contaminated cell cultures were *Acholeplasma laidlawii* and *Mycoplasma arginini*. The other species isolated include *M. alkalescens*, *M. bovis*, *M. pirum* (strain HRC 70-159) and *A. axanthum*.

Infected Cell Cultures. Since the decline of bovine serum contamination, the major sources of contamination today are contaminated cell cultures maintained and processed in the same laboratory. Contamination is spread to other cell culture by contaminated vessels, equipment, media, reagents and/or pipets used earlier to process the mycoplasma-infected cell cultures. New cell culture acquisitions must be quarantined, tested, and found mycoplasma-free before they enter the work area of the laboratory. Occasionally, commonly-used laboratory reagents, such as virus pool or a monoclonal antibody can be the primary source of contamination. Recommended procedures for prevention and quality control will be discussed later.

ISOLATION AND DETECTION

We have used four approaches for isolation and detection of mycoplasmas. These include: i) agar and broth culture media for examination of routine specimens, including cell cultures; ii) a semi-solid agar broth culture medium for screening cell cultures for microbial contamination, iii) the large specimen volume-broth culture medium, described earlier, for examination of bovine sera or other fluids; and iv) various virological-types of *in vitro* cell culture procedures with special emphasis on the indicator cell system for isolation and detection of fastidious pathogens or cryptic "non-cultivable" strains of *M. hyohrinis*. (Hopps *et al.*, 1973; DelGiudice and Hopps, 1978).

Standard Agar and Broth Culture Procedure

Our standardized medium (Barile, 1974) is a modification of the Edward-Hayflick medium formulation. It consists of a rich basal medium, 10% pretested select horse serum, and 10% freshly prepared yeast extract. The medium is supplemented with either arginine (0.1%) or dextrose (0.5%) as energy and carbon sources, thymic DNA, vitamins as used in tissue culture medium

(RPMI medium 1640) and phenol red as an indicator. Penicillin (500 U/ml) is added to medium used for examining specimens subject to bacterial contamination. Other investigators have used the SP-4 medium formulation (Tully *et al.*, 1977). Herderschee (1963) reported that the addition of 10% sucrose improved the growth-promoting properties of medium. These findings were confirmed by Vogelzang and Van Klingeren (1974). Mycoplasma colonies are identified and speciated by the agar immunofluorescent procedure (Barile and DelGiudice,1972). In brief, 0.1 ml of cell culture suspension is inoculated onto agar media, in duplicate. The culture is incubated at 36±1ºC in a 5% carbon dioxide and 95% nitrogen atmosphere either by replacing the environment or by using the commercial Gaspak jars (Baltimore Biological Laboratories, Baltimore. Agar plates are observed weekly for at least 3 weeks before being considered negative.

We first demonstrated that a 5% carbon dioxide and 95% nitrogen atmosphere was superior to air for primary isolation and growth of various mycoplasmas (Barile *et al.*, 1958; 1962; 1966a; 1973; Barile and Schimke, 1963). It has been effective for isolation of mycoplasmas from contaminated cell cultures and from normal or infected tissues of humans and animals. These findings have been confirmed by many other investigators (see Barile, 1979).

This medium has also been used for examining other tissues. Throat culture specimens are obtained by firmly scraping the infected area with a sterile cotton-tipped applicator. The specimen is then rolled gently across the surface of the agar medium. The preparation of the specimen can influence successful isolation and growth of mycoplasmas. For example, solid tissues release inhibitory substances, such as specific antibodies and complement. Accordingly, tissues were not homogenized in studies to establish the mycoplasma flora of dogs (Barile *et al.*, 1970) or monkeys (DelGiudice *et al.*, 1969; Barile, 1973). One of the inhibitory substances released from tissues is lysolecithin (Kaklamanis *et al.*, 1969). Mardh and Taylor-Robinson (1973) found that cholesterol-requiring *Mycoplasma* species were four times more susceptible to lysolecithin than noncholesterol-requiring *Acholeplasma* species.

Most mycoplasmas produce microscopic (100-400 mm) colonies with a fried egg appearance and grow embedded beneath the surface of the agar. Freshly isolated cultures of certain mycoplasma pathogens, such as *Mycoplasma pneumoniae*, may produce a more diffuse, granular type of colony. Some, such as *Mycoplasma pulmonis*, may not grow completely embedded. In addition, the gel strength of agar can affect colony growth and morphology. Each lot of agar must be pretested for optimal concentration (see section on Standardization of Media). Because mycoplasmas grow embedded, they maintain their morphologic shape. Consequently, they are easily distinguishable from bacterial colonies. Most microcolonies of bacteria are a collection of surface grown cells that can be readily scraped away. Mycoplasma colonies can not.

Semisolid Broth Medium

To prepare this medium, a small amount of purified agar (0.05%) is added to broth medium dispersed in screw-cap tubes. The specimen is delivered at the bottom of the broth tube and is released throughout the medium as the pipet is withdrawn. The agar in the broth provides an oxygen gradient.

It also permits mycoplasmas to produce turbid growth and microcolony formation. Arginine utilizers release ammonia, causing an alkaline shift. The fermenters cause an acid shift. The shift in pH causes a color change that, along with turbid colony formation, facilitates the detection of growth by visual examination. Semisolid broth medium is more sensitive than broth for isolating small numbers of arginine utilizing mycoplasmas. The mycoplasma fermenters prefer broth to semisolid broth.

Large Specimen-Volume-Broth Culture Procedure

This procedure was successful for isolating small numbers of mycoplasma from contaminated bovine sera (Barile and Kern, 1971) and has been discussed earlier.

Standardization of Culture Procedures

Numerous media formulations and various culture procedures have been used successfully for the isolation of mycoplasmas by various laboratories throughout the world (see Barile, 1974; Razin and Tully, 1983; Tully and Razin, 1983). Medium formulations are very important, but standardization of the procedures is equally important. Each formulation must be standardized and each prepared medium must be pretested for growth promoting efficacy. It must be emphasized that medium components vary with the batch and with the manufacturer. Each lot of component must be tested for growth promoting properties and toxicity and found satisfactory before use. Routinely, each newly-purchased component is pretested separately, including the basal broth or agar medium, serum and all other supplements. Whereas 10% yeast extract of a particular lot or manufacturer may be toxic, 2% can stimulate growth. Thus, the optimal concentration must be predetermined. The arginine supplement can also be toxic. Whereas 0.1% of arginine stimulates the growth of most arginine-utilizing mycoplasma species, 0.5% can be toxic for certain strains, (Leach, 1976; Washburn and Somerson, 1977). Certain types of agar preparations can be very toxic. Only purified agar products should be used, such as Ion agar #2 (Oxoid), Noble agar (Difco), Agarose, or an equivalent purified product. The optimal gel strength of the purified agar varies and must be determined experimentally. We prefer not to purchase complete basal agar media. The agar component of the medium should be purchased and tested separately. In practice, the new lot of any component replaces the working lot of the component in a complete medium. The growth-promoting properties of the newly formulated medium is compared to the existing working medium. If the newly-purchased component is equal to or better than the existing, working component, a large, adequate amount should be purchased for future use. In summary, each culture procedure must be standardized. A standardized, good quality control broth or agar culture procedure must be used to compare the efficacy of the new formulated media. We have used a limiting dilution titer in broth (CCU/ml) with subcultures to agar. Several positive control, fastidious species and strains should be used to test efficacy. Other equivalent test methods have also been used successfully, such as using a small, standardized inoculum (10^{-1}-10^2 CFU for agar or CCU for broth) of a frozen stock suspensions of selected fastidious mycoplasma strains, *e.g.*, *M. hyorhinis*, *M. hyopneumoniae* or *M. pneumoniae*. The cell culture medium components and cell culture isolation and detection procedures described below should also be standardized.

CELL CULTURE PROCEDURES FOR ISOLATION, DETECTION AND SPECIATION

Nonspecific Procedures

Hopps *et al.* (1973) first showed that "non-cultivable" strains of M. *hyorhinis* could not be grown readily on standardized agar or broth culture medium. Virological-type cell culture procedures were required for their isolation, detection and speciation. The significance of these findings is very important. It showed, for the first time, that cell culture procedures are an absolute requirement for inclusion in any protocol used for the isolation of mycoplasmas. Various nonspecific cell culture procedures have been developed. Most are based on exploitation of a basic biological, biochemical, enzymatic, antigenic and/or genomic property of mycoplasmas that distinguishes them from tissue cell cultures. These procedures are especially effective for detecting cytadsorbing mycoplasma strains. These procedures use the cells with their attached mycoplasmas, rather than the medium fluids, as the specimens. The cytadsorbing mycoplasmas also produce a characteristic pattern of infection and a typical cytopathic effect (CPE). Nonspecific staining procedures permit the visualization of the mycoplasmas attached to the infected cell membranes.

Historical Aspects.

Hopps *et al.* (1973) first reported the existence of "noncultivable" mycoplasma contaminants. These mycoplasmas grow poorly or not at all on well-standardized broth and agar media. This "noncultivable" agent was first considered to be an unidentified virus. It was called the "fuzzy agent" because infected cell cultures had a "fuzzy" appearance. The agent was filterable and produced a virus-like CPE, including plaque formation, but a virus could not be isolated or identified. We suspected that it might be a mycoplasma because small dark bodies could be visualized along the infected tissue cell membrane on Giemsa staining. In addition, the unstained cell cultures had a granular appearance. They looked "dirty", and had an abnormal "sick" appearance, similar to known mycoplasma-infected cells. Nonetheless, we were unable to grow mycoplasmas using our best standardized broth or agar culture procedures. When agar cultures were examined by the Dienes stain, minute, granular colony growth was observed surrounding the infected cell culture specimen. When the colonies were examined by epi-immunofluorescence, the infected cell culture specimen and the surrounding areas produced positive reactions with fluoroscein conjugated antisera specific for *Mycoplasma hyorhinis*. When the infected cell cultures themselves were examined, they also produced a positive immunofluorescence reaction and the "noncultivable", "fuzzy agent" was identified as *Mycoplasma hyorhinis* Subsequently, Del Giudice and Hopps (1978) showed that about 70% of the *Mycoplasma hyorhinis* strains isolated from contaminated cell cultures were shown to be for the "noncultivable" mycoplasmas. Live viral vaccines were found contaminated with a "noncultivable" strain of *Mycoplasma hyorhinis* (Woods, 1983; Barile, unpublished data).

Table 1. Detection of mycoplasmas in experimentally infected VERO cel cultures using specific immunofluorescence and non-specific DNA-fluorochrome staining procedures

Mycoplasma & Acholeplasma species & strains		Natural host	Immunofluorescence		DNA-Fluorochrome		Degree of cytadsorption
			Cells infected (%)	No. mycoplasmas Infected cell	Cells infected (%)	No. mycoplasmas Infected cell	
M. hyorhinis,	DBS1050	Swine	100	200-500	100	300-1000	###
M. pulmonis,	Ash	Rodent	100	50-150	100	200-400	###
M. fermentans,	PG18	Human	100	400-500	95	2-20	##
M. arginini,	G230	Bovine, etc.	100	20-40	90	50-100	##
M. hominis,	PG21	Human	90	50-100	100	50-150	##
A. axanthum,	S743	Bovine, etc.	75	4-10	100	20-100	# - ##
A. laidlawii,	PG8	Bovine, etc.	100	10-50	75	5-30	# - ##
A. granularum,	BTS39	Bovine, etc.	100	20-50	10	1-2	#
M. arthritidis,	PG27	Rat	80	50-100	50	10-20	#
M. gallinarum,	PG16	Avian	75	5-50	50	4-6	#
M. orale,	CH19299	Human	60	20-50	50	10-30	#
M. gallisepticum,	PG31	Avian	40	10-20	55	10-15	+ - #
M. salivarium,	PG20	Human	60	20-50	20	5-10	+ - #
M. faucium,	DC333	Human	60	20-50	10	1-2	+
M. pneumoniae,	FH	Human	80	1-2	30	2-4	+
M. buccale,	CH20247	Human	30	10-20	10	1-2	+
A. modicum,	PG49	Bovine, etc.	N.T.	-	45	20-500	#

The DNA-fluorochrome stain is Hoechst Chem. Co. No. 33258. Two or more tests done; All tests were examined blind by 3 investigators. Inoculum varied from 10^2 to 10^6 cfu. Similar results obtained using 3T6 mouse fibroblast cell culture.

163

The Indicator Cell Culture Procedure. Because cell culture systems are a valuable ancillary tool for the isolation and detection of mycoplasmas, we developed an indicator cell culture procedure. Either VERO (African green monkey kidney) or the NIH 3T3 cell cultures were used with equal success. In brief, a series of cell cultures preparations in dishes or equivalent containers is prepared. One, or more, cell culture dish is inoculated with one or more mycoplasma strains. These serve as positive mycoplasma controls to test the sensitivity of the indicator test system. Additional cell culture dishes are not inoculated and serve as negative controls. These also serve to monitor the sterility of the indicator cell culture passage. Still other cell dishes are inoculated with the test specimens. One of the advantages of an indicator system is that it has positive and negative controls to monitor the validity of the test system. The indicator system has been used for species-specific tests, such as immunofluorescence for speciation, or for nonspecific tests, such as the DNA-binding staining procedures, for detection of mycoplasmas. Spierenburg *et al.* (1988) adapted the indicator cell culture system for use in the nonspecific adenosine phosphorylase screening test. Any nonspecific or specific test procedure would benefit from using the indicator cell culture system. Details of the procedure are presented in Appendices A and B, and elsewhere (McGarrity and Barile, 1983).

Nonspecific Staining Procedures. The procedures reported include the DNA-binding fluorochrome stains; histologic stains; autoradiographic procedures (Studzinski *et al.*, 1973; Keprtova *et al.*, 1981); electron microscopy and luminol-dependent chemiluminescence (Bertoni *et al.*, 1985). A detailed review of these procedures was reported earlier (Barile, 1979; McGarrity and Kotani, 1985).

DNA-bisbenzimidazole Stain: Historical Aspects. While using the chromosome banding procedures to characterize cell cultures, Dr. T.R. Chen observed extrachromosomal bodies in his preparations. These slides were sent to Dr. R. Kirchstein at NIH, Bethesda, who first suggested that these small extra chromosomal DNA staining bodies might be due to mycoplasmas. Dr. Kirschstein suggested that the cell cultures be sent to us for examination. When examined, the cell cultures containing these abnormalities were contaminated with mycoplasmas. Subsequently, ten mycoplasma-infected and five noninfected cell cultures were sent to Dr. Chen in a randomized, blind manner for examination. When the code was broken, the results indicated that Dr. Chen was able to distinguish mycoplasma contaminated from non contaminated cell cultures. This led to the development of his bisbenzimidazole (Hoechst #33258 stain) staining procedure (Chen, 1977).

The sensitivity of the bisbenzimidazole staining procedure was examined. VERO cell cultures were experimentally infected with a series of 17 different *Mycoplasma* species. Following infection, duplicate specimens were examined by both the nonspecific DNA-binding and by specific immunofluorescence. The two staining procedures were compared by estimating the percent of cultured cells infected and the number of mycoplasmas per infected cell. A series of ten-fold dilutions of each of the 17 mycoplasmas was made and each dilution of each mycoplasma was inoculated into a series of indicator cell culture dishes. Following incubation, duplicate preparations of the infected cell cultures were examined daily for five days by both staining procedures. The indicator cell fluids were also monitored for infection by CCU/ml titers in

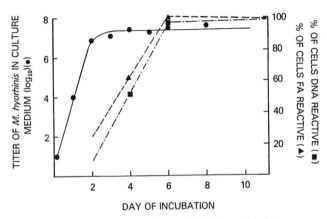

Figure 1. Detection of *M. hyorhinis* in cell culture by fluorescent antibody and DNA fluorochrome staining procedures.

broth (Table 1). When only 10 CCU inoculum of strain PG-29 of *Mycoplasma hyorhinis* was used, the infected cell culture fluids reached peak titers of 10^6 to 10^7 CCU/ml within three days post-inoculation. At four days, mycoplasmas were attached to 50-60% of the individual cultured cells as determined by both staining procedures (Figure 1). An important advantage of the indicator cell system is that small populations of mycoplasmas growth are amplified rapidly from 10^1 to 10^6 CCUs within days in infected cell cultures. This increases the sensitivity of the test system and results in expeditious detection of mycoplasmas by the DNA-binding staining procedures.

The time and extent of the infection and the severity of the CPE produced in the indicator cells was directly proportional to the mycoplasma strain and inoculum used. The larger the inoculum, the more extensive the infection. The same inoculum of a given mycoplasma gave the same results with either staining procedure. When the DNA staining results were compared to specific immunofluorescence, there was 100% agreement between the two procedures. Thus, the specific immunofluorescence findings confirmed the ability of the bisbenzimidazole stain to effectively detect mycoplasmas in infected cell cultures.

All 17 mycoplasmas were readily detected by either staining procedure, but there were considerable variations in the extent and patterns of cytadsorption among different species and strains (Table 1). In fact, the staining procedures provided a qualitative measurement of a strain to cytadsorb. In general, the DNA staining procedure was most effective in detecting the cytadsorbing strains and the poor cytadsorbing stains were best detected by growth on agar or broth media. These findings indicate the agar, broth and DNA bisbenzimidazole staining procedure are each required to detect and isolate all mycoplasma contaminants.

The other DNA-binding stains used include the 4'-6-diamidino-2-phenylindole (DAPI) stain (Russell *et al.*, 1975), the olivomycin fluorescent dye (Polster, 1986) and a conjugated benzoxazinone kanamycin fluorescent probe (Monsigny *et al.*, 1991). The protocol for the bisbenzimidazole staining procedure is given in Appendix A.

Histological Stains. Most of the classic histologic staining procedures have been used to detect mycoplasmas in infected cell cultures. These include the hematoxylin and eosin, intensified Giemsa, May-Grunwald-Giemsa, hypotonic orcein (see Barile, 1979, for references) and acridine orange fluorescent stains (Ebke and Kuwert, 1972). Occasionally, these staining procedures have provided the initial evidence to indicate that a cell culture was contaminated; *e.g.*, see section on historical aspects. In stained preparations, the mycoplasmas appear as small, microscopic dots lining the infected cell membrane. These staining procedures are especially effective for detecting cytadsorbing mycoplasmas, such as *Mycoplasma hyorhinis* They are least effective in detecting non cytadsorbing mycoplasmas. However, chronically infected cell culture provides selective pressures to retain the cytadsorbing mycoplasmas. The spent medium fluids containing the noncytadsorbing mycoplasmas are discarded on passage. The cell cultures infected with the cytadsorbing mycoplasmas are propagated on passage.

Electron Microscopy and Cell Morphology. Occasionally, transmission or scanning electron microscopy has provided the initial evidence to suggest that a cell culture is contaminated (see Barile, 1979 for references). Electron microscopy has been especially useful in examining mycoplasma-cell interactions. In collaboration with Douglas Anderson (1964), we provided some of the earliest evidence to show that certain mycoplasmas, such as *Mycoplasma pulmonis*, initiated infection by attachment to the tissue cell membrane. The thin-section micrographs suggested that attachment was mediated by a terminal tip and that some of the attached mycoplasmas were being engulfed by endocytosis (Barile and Anderson, 1965). Following attachment, the mycoplasma multiplied along the membrane, colonizing the entire monolayer causing cell damage and, eventually, death. A similar course also develops during a mycoplasma infection in man and animals.

The mycoplasma cell consists of a membrane, ribosomes, and a network of nuclear strands. Unlike other prokaryotes, it has no cell wall (Anderson, 1965). Because the membranes of the mycoplasma and the tissue cell are morphologically, structurally, and functionally similar (Razin and Rottem, 1982; Rottem and Kahane, 1992; Razin, 1992), they have been a model of choice to study membrane structure and function. The autoimmune abnormalities that develop during mycoplasma infections may be due, in part, to antigenically similar, cross-reaction membrane components among these two cells Biberfeld, 1985).

Summation: Staining Procedures. Of the nonspecific staining procedures reported, we recommend the use of the Hoechst #33258, bisbenzimidazole DNA-fluorochrome staining procedure. It is simple, inexpensive, and sensitive. The results obtained with the nonspecific DNA stain were comparable to those obtained by specific immunofluorescence. One of the most extensive studies using the DNA-binding procedures for testing cell culture specimens routinely submitted for examination have been published by Del Giudice and Hopps (1978).

Chemical and Enzymatic Methods and Nucleic Acid Probes

Extensive reviews on the use of these procedures have been reported earlier (Barile, 1979; McGarrity and Kotani, 1985). These approaches are based on the detection of an enzymatic activity present in mycoplasmas, but minimal or absent in tissue cells. The enzymic activities exploited include the arginine deiminase; thymidine, uridine, adenosine or pyrimidine nucleoside phosphorylase; or hypoxanthine or uracil phosphoribosyl transferase activities (see Levine and Müller, 1983). Of these procedures, the adenosine phosphorylase assay is probably the best, but each method has shortcomings. Two-dimensional electrophoresis was also suggested as a means of detecting mycoplasmas in infected human fibroblasts (Yang *et al.*, 1990). The other procedures used are based on the isolation and identification of mycoplasmal RNA or on the comparative utilization of uridine versus uracil in contaminated versus mycoplasma-free cell cultures. McGarrity *et al.* (1985) developed a rather novel procedure using the substrate 6-methyl purine deoxyriboside (6-MPDR). Mycoplasma adenosine phosphorylase converts 6- MPDR into a toxic metabolite that destroys the cell culture.

DNA probes have also been used. These include the use of mycoplasma ribosomal RNA genes (Göbel and Stanbridge, 1984), synthetic oligonucleotide probes complementary to rRNA for group- and species-specific mycoplasmas (Göbel *et al.*, 1987), as well as other genetic probes (McGarrity and Kotani, 1986; Johansson and Bölske, 1989; Johansson *et al.*, 1990). DNA hybridization procedures have been also used (Razin *et al.*, 1984; Borchsenius *et al.*, 1987).

The enzymatic and chemical procedures are especially effective for detecting cytadsorbing mycoplasmas. The infected cells cultures themselves, rather than the fluids, are used as the specimen. These procedures have several disadvantages. Not all mycoplasma contaminants are good cytadsorbing agents or possess higher distinguishing levels of enzymic activity. Negative and positive mycoplasma controls are not used. Positive reactions are based on arbitrary values making low orders of mycoplasma activity difficult to detect. These procedures can be useful to screen cell culture specimens if these technologies are available in the laboratory, but their shortcomings must be appreciated. Each of these procedures would benefit from the use of the indicator cell culture system approach using positive and negative controls. Studies are needed to validate the sensitivity of these methods by comparing them to the bisbenzimidazole DNA-fluorochrome test that has become the "gold standard".

Species-Specific Stains: Immunofluorescence

Barile *et al.* (1962) first reported the use of immunofluorescence to detect and identify mycoplasmas in contaminated cell cultures. A cell culture strain of *Mycoplasma hominis* was isolated and grown in broth. Antisera were prepared, conjugated with fluorescein and used to test cell cultures for the presence of mycoplasma. At that time, most of the early contaminants in our studies were due to *Mycoplasma hominis*.

A number of other excellent immunofluorescence procedures have also been reported using species-specific polyclonal antisera (DelGiudice and Barile,

1974; Barile and Grabowski, 1983) or monoclonal antisera conjugated with fluorescein or peroxidase. Buck *et al.* (1982) first used monoclonal antibodies to detect cell culture mycoplasmas and others followed (Radka *et al.*, 1984; Blazek *et al.*, 1990). Rose *et al.* (1983) used monoclonal antibodies as probes to detect antigens of *Mycoplasma pulmonis*. Gabridge *et al.* (1986) detected and speciated common cell culture mycoplasmas using an enzyme linked immunosorbent assay with biotin-avidin amplification on solid phase microporous membranes. Other investigators used immunobinding onto nitrocellulose paper (Kotani *et al.*, 1987) or combinations of specific and nonspecific staining procedures (Freiberg and Masover, 1990). Of these, we recommend the immunofluorescence procedure using the indicator cell culture system. Details are presented in Appendix B and reported elsewhere (Barile *et al.*, 1974; Barile and Grabowski, 1983; Olson and Barile, 1988).

Specific immunofluorescence is used primarily for mycoplasma speciation. Because numerous mycoplasma species contaminate cells, numerous specific conjugated antisera must be prepared. The specific conjugates can be used alone or in combination. Immunofluorescence is especially effective for speciation of cytadsorbing mycoplasmas. These contaminants colonize the tissue cell membrane and are readily visualized attached to the infected cells. In practice, contamination is detected by the nonspecific DNA staining procedure and the mycoplasmas are speciated by specific immunofluorescence.

Cell Cultures for Isolation and Propagation

Because primary atypical pneumonia was first considered to be a viral disease, the "Eaton agent" was first grown in cell cultures and developing chick embryos. Using fluorescein-labeled antibody procedures, the agent was visualized on epithelial cells lining the bronchioles and in the air sacs of the developing chick embryo and attached to the surface of monkey kidney cell cultures. These findings suggested that the agent was probably not a virus (see Clyde, 1979, for early references). Subsequently, the causative agent was grown on artificial medium producing typical colonies and was identified as a mycoplasma (Chanock *et al.*, 1962).

Cell cultures were also used effectively to isolate other mycoplasma agents that were thought initially to be viral diseases. These include the causative agents of chronic respiratory disease of mice (Nelson, 1960) caused by *M. pulmonis,* and enzootic pneumonia of swine caused by *Mycoplasma pneumoniae* (Goodwin and Whittlestone, 1963). Presently, cell culture procedures are used routinely for isolation, detection and speciation of mycoplasmas.

Test Requirements for Human Biologics

The current recommended test requirements for biologics in the U.S.A. are as follow: The master cell and working cell seed banks must be free of mycoplasmas. The product harvest concentrates must be free of mycoplasmas. The test is required for all products produced in cell substrates, a generic term used for all tissue cells grown *in vitro*. This includes viral vaccines (polio virus, adenovirus, measles, rubella, mumps, rabies, *etc.*), monoclonal antibodies, immunologic modifiers and cell culture derived blood products, such as tissue plasminogen activator, erythropoitein, *etc.*

In brief, the harvest concentrate is inoculated onto agar medium and into broth that is subcultured periodically onto agar media. The indicator cell culture system is also included in each test. An equivalent procedure is acceptable when detailed data presented to the FDA demonstrates that it is equal to, or better than, the recommended procedures. The current test requirements and the "points to consider" for biologics marketed in the U.S.A. can be obtained from the Office of Biologics Research, FDA, Bethesda, MD 20892, U.S.A.

MYCOPLASMA EFFECTS ON CELL CULTURES

For additional information and reference citations, see the extensive reviews by Barile (1979) and McGarrity and Kotani (1985).

Effects on Cell Function and Metabolism

From the very beginning, mycoplasmas have been established as common troublesome contaminants. They are capable of altering the function and activities of cultured cells and affecting the results of study. The nature of the infection depends on the contaminating species and strain of mycoplasma and on the type of cell infected. Many mycoplasma species produce severe cytopathic effects. Others produce very little overt cytopathology, and covert contamination may go undetected for months. The biological, biochemical and enzymatic activities of the mycoplasma determine the effect on cells and the degree of CPE. Arginine is an energy source for certain mycoplasmas (Schimke and Barile,1963a, b; Barile *et al.*, 1966b). The arginine utilizing mycoplasmas rapidly deplete arginine, frequently overnight, depriving the cell culture of an essential amino acid. Arginine depletion can cause alterations of protein synthesis and affect cell division and growth. They can also inhibit or stimulate lymphocyte blast formation or viral growth. A mycoplasma infection results in profound effects on cell functions and activities, metabolism, virus propagation and karyology. It may also cause chromosomal aberrations (see Barile, 1979 for references).

Fermenting mycoplasmas rapidly degrade sample sugars to acid. They generate copious amounts of acid metabolites that alter cell functions and/or produce severe CPE. All mycoplasmas require nucleic acid precursors (free bases, nucleosides, or oligonucleotides), amino acids and energy sources (either arginine or dextrose, seldom both) for growth (Razin, 1985a). Several genera, *e.g.*, *Mycoplasma* and *Ureaplasma* species) have an absolute requirement for sterols (such as cholesterol). All species require fatty acids for growth (Razin and Rottem, 1982; Razin 1992; Rottem and Kahane, 1993). Because the chemical composition and function of the mycoplasma and tissue cell membranes are similar, their nutritional needs are similar. Attachment can alter and disrupt the integrity of the host cell membrane causing leakage of membrane components. These components, their enzymatic activities or by-products may then be assimilated by the cytadsorbing pathogen (O'Brien *et al.*, 1981; 1983). Frequently there are from 100 to 1000 mycoplasmas attached to each infected cell. Thus, there are far more mycoplasmas than tissue cells in an infected cell culture. Those overwhelming numbers permit the mycoplasmas to compete effectively for medium nutrients. Mycoplasma infections deprive the infected cell culture of essential nutrients and this results in profound effects on cell metabolism and function (see Barile, 1979).

Perez *et al*. (1972) observed an altered incorporation of nucleic acid precursors in mycoplasma-infected mammalian cell cultures. Hellung-Larsen and Fredriksen (1976) reported that mycoplasmas can alter the incorporation of different precursors into the RNA components of infected culture cells. As a consequence, the precursors are incorporated into mycoplasmal RNA rather than host cell RNA. Mycoplasmas can also affect pyruvate dehydrogenase activity in cultured fibroblasts (see Razin, 1985). Kouri *et al*. (1983) reported that *Mycoplasma pulmonis* can affect protein and glycosaminoglycan synthesis in infected connective tissue cells. Koch and Bigalow (1983) showed that the insensitivity of cells to cyanide respiration was an artifact resulting from mycoplasmal contamination.

Kluve and colleagues (1983) reported that *Mycoplasma orale* induces the secretion of murine type I and III collagenase production in infected 3T3 cell cultures. They discussed the possible implications of these findings in the induction of arthritis. Crowell *et al*. (1989) suggested that mycoplasma attachment to infected cell membrane can interfere with membrane receptors or alter signal transduction inhibiting the cellular autocrine response. Almagor *et al*. (1983) showed that *Mycoplasma pneumoniae* inhibited catalase activity and suggested that this was a possible mechanism for cell injury (Almagor *et al*., 1984). Hatcher (1983) reported that mycoplasma infected cells secrete larger amounts of plasminogen activator factor. They suggested that this activity may play a role in tissue destruction in mycoplasma disease states.

Effects on Morphology

Covert Infection. Contamination may go undetected because mycoplasma infections do not produce overt turbid growth commonly associated with bacterial and fungal contamination. The morphological cellular changes can be minimal or unapparent. Frequently, the cellular changes are similar to those caused by nutritional effects, such as the depletion of amino acids, sugars, or nucleic acid precursors. These morphological effects can be reversed by changing the medium or by replenishing the medium with fresh nutrients. Thus, mycoplasma contamination may go undetected.

Overt Effects. Collier (1957) was one of the first investigators to report that mycoplasmas produced CPE in contaminated cell cultures. The CPE was characterized by stunted, abnormal growth and rounded, degenerated cells. The cells had a macroscopic, "moth-eaten" appearance at the edge of the culture. O'Malley *et al*. (1961) isolated a "cytolytic viral agent" that produced a generalized, destructive CPE. It also produced plaque formation in agar overlay of primary rabbit kidney cell cultures. The agent was subsequently identified as *M. gallisepticum*. Certain strains of *Mycoplasma arginini* cause the lysis of cells in some, but not all, human lymphoblastoid cell cultures. The addition of arginine to the medium prevented the lytic activity. Most toxic, cytolytic agents are mycoplasma fermenters that produce large amounts of acid metabolites from glycolysis. This causes destructive damage to the cell culture. The large amounts of acids drastically reduce the pH causing the monolayer of cells to detach from the glass. A V-shaped destruction of the cell culture is produced in monolayers grown in test tubes (see Barile, 1973, for illustrations).

Attachment permits the mycoplasma contaminant to release noxious, enzymatic and cytolytic metabolites directly onto the tissue cell membrane. Some mycoplasmas selectively colonize defined areas of the cell culture. This results in microcolony formation producing microlesions and small foci of necrosis, *e.g.*, *M. pulmonis*, or form plaques, *e.g.*, *M. gallisepticum*, in an agar overlay system (O'Malley *et al.*, 1966). Microcolonization suggests that mycoplasma-specific receptors are localized in defined areas of the cell monolayer. However, other fermenting mycoplasmas, *e.g.*, *M. hyorhinis*, attach to every cell, and it produces a generalized CPE and destroys the entire monolayer.

Effects on Chromosomal Aberration

Arginine-utilizing and fermenting mycoplasmas, ureaplasmas and acheloplasmas induce chromosomal aberrations *in vitro.* Mycoplasma infections cause disturbances in chromosomal patterns. They were observed in: i) human amnion cell cultures infected with an unspeciated mycoplasma; ii) in human diploid W1-38 cells with either *Mycoplasma orale, A. laidlawii, M. hyorhinis* and *M. pulmonis*; iii) in hamster fibroblasts infected with *M. salivarium*; and iv) in human lymphocyte cultures infected with either *M. salivarium, M. fermentans, M. arthritidis,* or ureaplasmas (see Barile, 1979; McGarrity and Kotani, 1985). The most commonly induced aberrations were chromosomal breakage, multiple translocation, reduction in chromosome number and the appearance of new and/or additional chromosome varieties. Histones, the protein portion of nucleoproteins, are rich in arginine. One postulation was that mycoplasmas inhibit histone synthesis by depleting arginine. Because fermenting mycoplasmas and ureaplasmas, neither of which utilize arginine for energy, also induce chromosomal aberrations, other mechanisms are involved. These include competition for nucleic acid precursors or degradation of host cell DNA by mycoplasma nucleases.   Mycoplasmas endonucleases and mycoplasma DNAs have been isolated from contaminated cell cultures (Schaeffer *et al.*, 1991).

Although mycoplasmas can induce chromosomal aberrations *in vitro,* attempts to induce tumor formation in animals have been uniformly unsuccessful. The newborn hamsters or the cheek pouch of cortisonized weanling hamsters procedures failed to induce tumors.

Mycoplasmas can inhibit viral transformation of cell cultures by known oncogenic viruses. *M. orale* can inhibit the effects of Rous sarcoma and Rous-associated viruses in chick embryo fibroblasts. Other mycoplasma contaminants reduce the number of foci in simian SV40 and polyoma-infected cell cultures. Arginine-utilizing mycoplasmas inhibit the growth of certain oncogenic DNA viruses, such as adenoviruses (see Barile, 1979 and McGarrity and Kotani, 1985, for references).

Effects on Virus Propagation

Some mycoplasmas have no detectable effect on viral growth. Others can either increase or decrease virus yields in infected cell culture. Some alter viral infections in animals (Barile, 1979; McGarrity and Kotani, 1985). The effect depends on the strain or species of mycoplasma, the virus, and the cell culture substrate used. *M. hyorhinis* can inhibit reverse transcriptase activity and replication of a retrovirus (Lipp *et al.*, 1979). They reported that a mycoplasma infection can interfere with the detection of these agents.

Decreased Virus Yields. At least two mechanisms have been established for decreasing viral yields *in vitro* The cytolytic, fermenting mycoplasmas suppress metabolism and growth. This results in severe CPE, causing a decrease in viral yields. Arginine-utilizing mycoplasmas decrease titers of arginine-requiring DNA viruses by depleting arginine from the medium. This includes various DNA viruses, such as: i) Herpes simplex virus (Manischewitz *et al.*, 1975); ii) vaccinia virus (Singer *et al.*, 1970); iii) simian SV40 virus; iv) adeno-virus types 1, 2, and 5; v) polyoma virus; and vi) human and simian cytomegaloviruses (see Barile, 1979; McGarrity and Kotani, 1985). Changing the medium or replenishing arginine reversed the effect. Measles virus titers were decreased by either *M. hyorhinis,* a cytolytic fermenter, or by various nonfermenting, arginine-utilizing mycoplasmas. Thus, reduction in titer can be caused by more than one mechanism. The immunoreactivity of varicella zoster virus was also reduced in mycoplasma-infected cell cultures (Harper *et al.*, 1988). Scott *et al.* (1989) showed the previously reported immunosuppressive effects by cytomegalovirus were due to mycoplasma contamination and not the virus.

Increased Virus Yields. Effect on Interferon. Mycoplasmas can also increase virus yields by inhibiting interferon induction and interferon activity (Barile 1973a, 1977; Singer *et al.*, 1973). Singer *et al.* (1969a, b) showed that *M. arginine* or *M. hyorhinis* inhibited interferon production, interferon activity, and cell resistance. This resulted in increased yields of Semiliki Forest virus. Mycoplasmas inhibited interferon activity induced by either viruses, *e.g.,* vesicular stomatitis virus, or synthetic RNA copolymers, *e.g.,* polyinosinic and polycytidylic acids. Mycoplasmas can render cell cultures less sensitive to exogenously supplied interferon. Consequently, mycoplasma infections can affect the results of titers obtained by the standard cell culture interferon assay (Singer *et al.*, 1969a, b; 1973). The same species can affect cell cultures in several ways. *M. hyorhinis* can produce CPE and reduce virus yields. If the CPE is suppressed by changing the medium, it can inhibit interferon production and increase virus yields. A mycoplasma infection can be used to advantage. Decreased interferon induction and activity by a mycoplasma infection could be exploited to increase titers of latent, interferon sensitive viruses.

Induction of Intrerferon Activity. Various mycoplasmas induced interferon expression in ovine leukocyte cultures or in animals (Cole *et al.* 1974a, b; 1978). Beck *et al.* (1982) induced interferon by infecting mouse spleen cell cultures with mycoplasmas. Mice inoculated with a strain of *Acholeplasma* were protected against infection with Semliki Forest virus, and resistance to infection was mediated by the induction of interferon. Most *Acholeplasma* species lipoglycans have endotoxin-like activities that induce interferon activity in mice. Some species induced an earlier response in mice (6 h after inoculation) while other species produced a delayed response. Conversely, viable or nonviable sonicated preparations of various mycoplasmas and acheloplasmas suppressed the interferon response in mice to Newcastle disease virus. Prior exposure to mycoplasmas can either suppress or enhance a virus infection in mice (Cole *et al.*, 1985).

Effect on Viral Infections.   Mycoplasmas can also alter viral infections in organ cultures or in animals. Dual infections produced greater destruction of the ciliated epithelium in swine tracheas than either *M. hyorhinis* or swine influenza alone. *M. gallisepticum* infection of pullets reduced symptoms in Marek's disease, but increased the severity of Newcastle disease. Influenza A infections were enhanced in: i) ducks infected with *M. anatis;* ii) in chickens infected with *M. gallisepticum;* and iii) in mice experimentally infected with *M. pneumoniae.* Swine adenovirus infections were more severe in gnotobiotic pigs infected with *M. hyopneumoniae* (see Barile, 1979).

Mistaken Identity

Because mycoplasmas produce destructive virus-like CPE, a surprising number of investigators have mistaken cytolytic mycoplasmas for viruses (see Barile, 1979, for earlier reports. Mycoplasmas share various properties with viruses. They are: i) filterable; ii) hemadsorbant; iii) hemagglutinate; iv) resistant to certain antibiotics; v) inhibited by antisera; vi) able to induce chromosomal aberrations; and vii) sensitive to detergents, ether, and chloroform. O'Malley *et al.* (1964) reported that the reputed "human hepatitis agent" was a *M. gallisepticum* contaminant. Kapikian *et al.* (1979) showed that the reputed "Crohn's disease agent" was a *M. hyorhinis* contaminant. In fact, the first established mycoplasma pathogen of humans *(M. pneumoniae)*, or of animals *(M. mycoides* subsp. *mycoides)*, or of plants was each believed initially to be a virus. Sydiskis *et al.* (1981) reported that a mycoplasma contaminant cosedimented with the mouse mammary tumor virus in sucrose density gradients affecting the results of study. Thus, the virologist must be cognizant of mycoplasmas and their properties to avoid misinterpretation of data.

Effects on Lymphocytes.

Biberfeld and Gronowicz (1976) reported that *M. pneumoniae* can activate a polyclonal population of mouse B lymphocytes. Because the mitogenic component was heat-stable, it was postulated that it might be an endotoxin-like substance. Some mycoplasmas and acholeplasmas have lipoglycans with endotoxin-like activity (Seid *et al.*, 1980). Others induce interferon expression (Cole *et al.*, 1985). Ruuth and Lundgren (1986) reported the enhancement of immunoglobulin secretion by the lymphokine-like activity of a *Mycoplasma arginini* strain. Proust *et al.* (1985) examined a soluble "lymphokine-like" product in the serum-free supernatant of a T-cell hybridoma. They showed that it induced proliferation and maturation of B cells as a consequence of mycoplasmal contamination. Other mycoplasmas were shown to alter the Fc receptors of rat basophilic leukemia cells for IgE (Chan *et al.*, 1986).

Ruckdeschel *et al.* (1975) reported that mycoplasma contamination inhibited the ability of membrane-associated measles antigens to induce *in vitro* responsiveness of lymphocytes obtained from measles patients. Makhoul *et al.* (1987) induced production of both interleukin-2 and colony stimulating activity in mycoplasma infected cell cultures. Levin *et al.* (1985) reported that *My-*

coplasma pulmonis membranes could stimulate the production of interleuk-in- 2 by rat lymph node cells.

Mycoplasma hyorhinis can attach to and acquire differential alloanti-gen from the mouse lymphocyte surface (Wise *et al.,* 1982). This results in mycoplasma capping on the immune cell in culture (Stanbridge and Weiss, 1975; Stanbridge *et al.,* 1981). Carrington *et al.* (1988) observed the conversion of a mycoplasma-infected melanoma cell line from an HL-A class II positive to a negative phenotype following treatment with antimycoplasma drugs. The effect of mycoplasmas on the expression of HL-A antigens in cultured human fibroblasts was reported by Brautbar *et al.* (1973). Mycoplasmas also induce cyto-toxic responses in normal mouse lymphocytes against allogeneic and syngene-ic target cells.

Franzoso *et al.* (1992) reported that the AIDS-associated *M. fermentans,* strain incognitus, can fuse with either CD4+ (Molt 3 lymphocyte cell culture) or the CD4- CEM cell variant lacking CF4 cells. The amount of fusion was rela-tively low and ranged from 5-10% of the cells with either cell culture. They sug-gested that the intracellular delivery of mycoplasma components into the lymphocyte cells as a result of fusion could affect the normal functions of the cell. If the mycoplasma membrane components were inserted into the lym-phocyte membranes, this could alter receptor recognition sites or the express-ion of lymphokines. It would affect communication between the cellular ele-ments of the immune system. It might also influence binding, integration, in-sertion or expression of HIV. This could decrease host resistance to infection. However, the effect, if any, remains to be determined.

Vasudevachari *et al.* (1990) reported that mycoplasma contamination in-terfered with the viral reverse transcriptase assay of HIV-1 infected cultures and obscured virus detection. Coinfection with the AIDS-associated *Mycoplas-ma fermentans,* strain incognitus, (Lo *et al.,* 1985; 1989) enhanced the ability of human immunodeficiency virus to induce cytopathic effects on human T-lymphocytes *in vitro* (Lo *et al.,* 1991). Chowdhury *et al.* (1990) reported that my-coplasmas can enhance HIV replication *in vitro* They suggested that this might be a possible cofactor responsible for the progression of AIDS. Alym-baeva *et al.* (1985) showed that mycoplasma infections of cell cultures in-creased production and synctial formation of HTLV by facilitating virion bud-ding. Mycoplasma infection can also immunosuppress the humoral antibody response of animals to various antigens (Kaklamanis and Pavlotos, 1972; Berquist *et al.,* 1974).

Specific Mitogenic Activity.

Leventhal *et al.* (1986) first demonstrated that *M. pneumoniae* stimu-lated transformation (blast formation) and mitosis of lymphocyte cultures from patients with primary atypical pneumonia. These findings were con-firmed by others (Biberfeld, 1977, 1985; Cole *et al.,* 1985). *In vitro* lymphocyte stimulation procedures are sensitive methods for demonstrating cell-medi-ated immunity to *M. pneumoniae.* These procedures were used to obtain useful information in establishing the possible role of cellular immunity in resistance to mycoplasma disease (Fernald, 1979). Exposure of lymphocytes to both *M. pneumoniae* and PHA stimulated erythrophagocytosis. PHA or mycoplasmas given alone did not (Leventhal *et al.*, 1968). The mechanism of erythrophagocytosis is not well understood, but it could play an important role in the pathogenesis of mycoplasma disease.

Nonspecific Mitogenic Activity. The nonspecific mitogenic properties of mycoplasmas were first observed by Ginsburg and Nicolet (1973). These findings were confirmed by many others (see Cole *et al.*, 1985). Various mycoplasmas can stimulate nonspecific blast formation *in vitro* (Aldridge *et al.*, 1977a, b). Murine mycoplasma species were strong mitogens for human lymphocytes. Mouse lymphocytes were stimulated by nonmurine mycoplasmas (Naot, 1982; Gideoni and Naot, 1984). Soluble cytotoxic factor (lymphotoxins) were liberated during mycoplasma-induced blastogenesis of normal unsensitized lymphocytes. The mitogenic activity against normal lymphocytes may provide an explanation for mycoplasma induced lymphocytotoxicity (Cole *et al.*, 1985). Mitogenicity may be a general property and provide mycoplasma pathogens a potential mechanism for damaging tissue cells (Cole *et al.*, 1985). Cole and colleagues (1982) reported that the Ir gene control of lymphocyte transformation correlates with binding of the *Mycoplasma arthritidis* mitogen to specific Ia-bearing cells. Murine T-hybridoma cells exhibited differential accessory cell requirements for activation by the *M. arthritidis* T-cell mitogen (Cole *et al.*, 1986). The cross-reactive recognition by the antigen-specific, major histocompatibility complex-restricted T cells of the *Mycoplasma arthritidis* mitogen is clonally expressed and I-E restricted (Lynch *et al.*, 1986) The mechanism of *Mycoplasma arthritidis* mitogen stimulation of T-cells and the possible role of class II IE molecules were postulated by Bekoff *et al.* (1987).

Inhibition of Mitogenic Activity by Arginine Depletion. Copperman and Morton (1966) first showed that PHA stimulation of a lymphocyte culture was inhibited by viable or nonviable cultures of *M. hominis*. The inhibitory effect was reversible. Barile and Leventhal (1968) extended these studies and demonstrated that the inhibitory effect was due to arginine depletion by the arginine-utilizing mycoplasmas. The lymphocytes were not killed. Changing the culture medium or replenishing it with arginine reversed the effect. These findings were confirmed by others using *M. arthritidis,* another arginine-utilizing species (Spitler *et al.*, 1968; Cochrum *et al.*, 1969). The fermenting mycoplasmas examined either had no effect or they stimulated blast formation. Certain *Mycoplasma* species utilize arginine for energy (Schimke and Barile, 1963a, b). They rapidly deplete and deprive cells of an essential amino acid and cause lymphocyte dysfunction. Simberkoff *et al.* (1969) showed that the purified arginine-splitting enzyme (arginine deiminase) produced the same inhibitory effect. The effect was reversed by enzyme specific antisera. The antisera reversed the inhibitory effect of all arginine-utilizing mycoplasma species tested, and they concluded that all arginine deiminase enzymes were closely related or identical. Subsequently, at least three antigenically distinct arginine deiminase moieties have been reported (Weikmann and Fahrney, 1977). The purified enzyme of Simberkoff *et al.* (1969) also blocked the response of sensitized lymphocytes to tuberculin, to homograph antigens, and to secondary production of antibody to diphtheria toxoid *in vitro.*

Summation: Effects on Cell Cultures. Mycoplasma infections have numerous deleterious effects on lymphocytes in culture. Mycoplasmas are nonspecific mitogens and polyclonal B-cell activators (see review by Cole *et al.*, 1985).

Effect on Macrophages

Jones *et al.* (1972) were the first to investigate attachment, ingestion and phagocytosis of *Mycoplasma pulmonis* by mouse peritoneal macrophages. Subsequently, mycoplasma infections were shown to affect the functions and activities of macrophage cultures. Stuart and colleagues (1989; 1990) reported that some, but not all, mycoplasma membrane preparations cause the differential induction of bone marrow macrophage proliferation and that it involved granulocyte macrophage stimulating factor. The deliberate infection of a myelomonocytic cell line with at least five different mycoplasmas caused significant induction of class II MHC surface expression. Makhoul *et al.* (1987) showed that *Mycoplasma pneumoniae* caused the induction of interleukin-2 and colony stimulating activity by human peripheral blood mononuclear cells. Lowenstein *et al.* (1983) reported that mycoplasmas induced macrophage-mediated cytolysis of neoplastic cells. They suggested that undetected mycoplasma infections were responsible for some reports of lysis of neoplastic cells by nonactivated macrophages. Gallily *et al.* (1989) showed that either viable or heat-killed *Mycoplasma orale* induces a cytolytic effect on murine macrophages. The activity was mediated by tumor necrosis factor (TNF) because the effect was neutralized by specific antiserum against murine cloned recombinant TNF. Extensive studies by Sher *et al.* (1990a, b, 1991) revealed that *Mycoplasma capricolum* and *Spiroplasma* sp. strain MQ1 are very efficient TNF-inducing agents, activating bone marrow macrophages to secrete very high levels of TNFα and to mediate tumor cytolysis. The capacity to induce TNFα secretion by macrophages was found to reside exclusively in the cell membrane. It was also found that *M. capricolum* or *Spiroplasma* sp. strain MQ1 membranes and lipopolysaccharide synergize to augment TNFα secre-tion by C57BL/6-derived macrophages. Moreover, lipopolysaccharide unresponsive C3H/HeJ-derived macrophages were pronouncedly activated by my-coplasma membranes which do not contain lipopolysaccharide. These findings suggest that the mechanism by which mycoplasma membranes activate macrophages differs from that of lipopolysaccharide. Further studies showed that human monocytes also secrete TNFα following activation by mycoplasma membranes. Hommel-Berrey and Brahmi (1987) detected soluble cytotoxic factors generated by mycoplasma contaminated target cells. They discussed the significance and relevance of infection on natural killer cell-mediated killing. Arai and colleagues (1990) showed that the supernatants of mycoplasma-infected macrophage cultures contained a potent cytotoxic activity to TNFα-sensitive L-cells, but not to insensitive L-cells (Furukawa *et al.*, 1989). They suggested that the mycoplasma induced TNFa activity might be responsible for the enhanced cytotoxic activity of macrophages. It could also induce resistance to mycoplasma infections in the host (Arai *et al.*, 1990). Lai *et al.* (1990) reported that infection of mice with *Mycoplasma pulmonis* enhanced natural killer cell function both *in vitro* and *in vivo*.

ELIMINATION OF MYCOPLASMA CONTAMINATION

Ever since mycoplasma contamination of cell cultures was first reported, attempts to develop methods for elimination of the mycoplasma have been made. A variety of procedures were utilized, including the use of antibiotics such as tetracyclines, kanamycin, novobiocin, tylosin, gentamycin, doxycycline, thiayline, and quinolones (reviewed by Barile, 1979; Rottem and Barile, 1992); surface active agents (Mardh, 1975); and the use of antimycoplasma antisera (Barile, 1979; McGarrity and Kotani, 1985). Many of the methods were shown to be unreliable. Some techniques may apply to some, but not all, mycoplasma species; some of them are laborious and/or time consuming. Therefore, it was suggested that, whenever possible, the infected cell culture should be discarded and replaced with a mycoplasma-free culture (McGarrity and Kotani, 1985). When the cell culture is irreplaceable, the use of antibiotic mixtures, detergents, prolonged heating treatments (40-42°C), treatment with specific antisera or the combined use of high titer specific neutralizing antisera and a high concentration of a pretested antibiotic (Barile, 1973, 1979; McGarrity and Kotani, 1985) are the most common approaches. One also has to keep in mind that cell culture contaminants that have been continuously exposed to antibiotics develop resistance to the drug. Antibiotic-resistant strains have been isolated for most mycoplasma species tested. Treatment may also induce the selection of a cell population and the treated cell culture may not retain all its initial properties.

Elimination of mycoplasmas from contaminated cell cultures by passage through nude mice has been successful for some, but not all, mycoplasmas and by some, but not all, investigators. Animals have a rich oral and/or urogenital mycoplasma flora. Consequently, mycoplasmas are frequently isolated from infected or neoplastic tissues. They have also been recovered from exudates or ascites, and especially from immunosuppressed humans or animals. Passage through animals could conceivably contaminate the test cell culture with the indigenous mycoplasma flora. Pristine, trauma and other stressful conditions permit mycoplasmas and other agents to gain entry and infect the peritoneal cavity.

Twelve years ago, we described the selective killing of mycoplasmas from contaminated cell culture (Marcus et al., 1980). The method is based on the selective incorporation of 5-bromouracil (5-BrUra) into mycoplasmas and the induction of breaks by light in the 5-BrUra containing DNA. This photosensitivity was greatly increased by the binding of the fluorochrome 33258-Hoechst to the DNA. The unusually high content of A+T makes the mycoplasma DNA an excellent candidate for the induction of breakage by the combined action of 5-BrUra, 33258 Hoechst and visible light. Thus, treating cell culture in this way was shown to provide an efficient method for the selective killing of mycoplasmas. Throughout the years, a number of laboratories have reported the successful elimination of mycoplasmas from cell cultures using this technique (McGarrity and Kotani, 1985; Machatkova et al., 1986; Calozini and Ruggieri, 1989). Nevertheless, the method was not widely accepted, apparently since the procedure is laborious and time consuming (four sequential treatments and subsequent cloning of 50-100 cells in microtiter plates). Mycoplasmas can be readily eliminated from solvent-resistant virus pools by treatment with 2:1 parts ether and chloroform overnight in the cold. Treatment with detergents such as Triton-X has been effective. Filtration through a 100 or 220 nm (depending on virus size) filter twice has worked. Treatment with high concentrations of a pretested, effective antibiotic, *e.g.*, 10,000 µg/ml kanamycin or tetracycline, or combinations of these treatments has also been effective.

CELL CULTURE MODELS AS *IN VITRO* MODELS

We have already shown that cell cultures are an exquisitely sensitive procedure for isolation and detection of fastidious mycoplasma pathogens and the noncultivable strains of *M. hyorhinis* (see Section IV. C.). Cell cultures are also invaluable tools for investigating pathogenic properties of mycoplasmas. It is important to emphasize, however, that the cell culture systems used must be free of mycoplasmas. We have successfully used the indicator cell culture procedure for the propagation, detection, identification and speciation of mycoplasmas. The system is effective because it has built in positive and negative controls.

Cell culture systems have been used successfully to examine and characterize various virulence properties of pathogenic mycoplasma, such as adhesins (see Razin, 1985; Razin and Jacobs, 1992). They have been used to identify and characterize tissue cell receptor sites (Chandler *et al.*, 1982b; Kriven *et al.*, 1989; Roberts *et al.*, 1989). We have used the WIDR cell line to examine and compare the attachment activities of five strains of *Mycoplasma pneumoniae* (Chandler *et al.*, 1982a). These *in vitro* activities were compared with the ability of the strain to colonize and produce lung pathology and disease in hamsters. The attachment activity of the five strains to cell cultures correlated directly with colonization of lungs in inoculated animals. The strains with good cytadsorption activity produced disease. The noncytadsorbing strain did not produce disease. Thus, attachment is an important virulence factor for this pathogen. The Mac strain produced the same *in vivo* attachment activity, and the same amount of lung colonization as the pathogenic strains M-129, 1428 and FH, but it did not produce lung lesions nor disease. These findings indicate that whereas attachment is important, other factors are required to produce disease. These may include the factors responsible for ciliotoxic and leukocyte recruitment activities (Barile *et al.*, 1988a, b).

We showed that strain 1620 of *M. hominis* isolated from a patient with septic arthritis had very good attachment activity to cell cultures, but the reference type strain PG-21 had very poor attachment activity (Izumikawa *et al.*, 1987). The cytadsorbing strain induced septic arthritis in experimentally injected chimpanzees, but the noncytadsorbing type strain did not. These findings indicate that attachment is probably an important virulence factor for *Mycoplasma hominis* as well (Barile *et al.*, 1987). Therefore, *in vitro* culture studies have provided useful information on the attachment and these findings correlated directly with colonization in inoculated animals.

CONCLUSIONS

We have presented a broad, sweeping overview of mycoplasma-cell interactions. We have discussed mycoplasma infection and contamination of cell cultures; the effects of infection on cell function and activities; the proced- ure for isolation, identification and speciation of mycoplasmas; and the use of cell cultures as *in vitro* models to examine virulence properties of mycoplas- mas. It is especially important to emphasize that mycoplasma contamination can affect virtually every parameter and every function and activity of a cul- tured cell. The prudent investigators must be aware of this. They must main- tain constant vigilance for the presence of contamination in order to properly interpret the results of study.

REFERENCES

Aldridge, K. E., Cole, B. C. and Ward, J.R. (1977a) Mycoplasma-dependent act- ivation of normal lymphocytes: role of arginine and nonviable myco- plasma antigen in the induction of lymphocyte-mediated cytotoxicity for syngeneic mouse target cells. Infect. Immun. 18:386-392.

Aldridge, K. E. and Cole, B. C. (1977b) Mycoplasma-dependent activation of normal lymphocytes: induction of a lymphocyte-mediated cytotoxicity for allogeneic and syngeneic mouse target cells. Infect. Immun. 18:377-385.

Almagor, M., Yatziv, S. and Kahane, I. (1983) Inhibition of host catalase by *My- coplasma pneumoniae*: a possible mechanism for cell injury. Infect. Im- mun. 41:251- 256.

Almagor, M., Kahane, I. and Yatziv. S. (1984) Role of super-oxide anion in host cell injury induced by *Mycoplasma pneumoniae* infection. A study in normal and trisomy 21 cells. J. Clin. Invest. 73:842-847.

Alymbaeva, D. B., Miller, G. G., Rakovskaia, I. V. and Bykovskii, A. F. (1985) In- fluence of mycoplasma on the production of the onocogenic leukemia virus HTLV by HUT-102 T-lymphoblastoid cells. Vopr. Virusol. 30:75-78.

Anderson, D. R. (1965) Subcellular particle associated with human leukemia as seen with the electron microscope. In: " Methodological Approaches to the Study of Leukemias" (V. Defendi, Ed.) Wistar Institute Press, Philadelphia, pp. 113-146.

Anderson, D. R. and Barile, M. F. (1966) Ultrastructure of *Mycoplasma orale* isolated from patients with leukemia. J. Natl. Cancer. Inst. 36:161-167.

Arai, S., Furukawa, M., Munakata, T., Kuwano, K., Inoue, H. and Miyazaki, T. (1990) Enhancement of cytotoxicity of active macrophages by mycoplas- ma: role of mycoplasma-associated induction of tumor necrosis factor α (TNFα) in macrophages. Microbiol. Immunol. 34:231-243.

Barile, M. F. (1962) Discussion: Detection and Elimination of Contaminating Organisms. Bethesda, J. Natl. Cancer Inst., Monograph Series #7, pp. 50-53.

Barile, M. F. (1965) Mycoplasma (PPLO), leukemia and auto-immune disease. In: "Methodological Approaches to the Study of Leukemias" (V. Defendi, Ed.). Wistar Institute Press, Philadelphia, pp. 171-181.

Barile, M. F. (1973) Mycoplasma Contamination of Cell Cultures: Mycoplasma- Virus Cell Culture Interactions. In: "Tissue Culture" (J. Fogh, Ed.) Academic Press, New York, pp. 131-172.

Barile, M. F. (1974) General principles of isolation and detection of mycoplas- mas. In: "Les Mycoplasmes" (J. M. Bové and J. F. Duplan, Eds.) Colloques INSERM 33:135- 142.

Barile, M. F. (1976) Mycoplasma Contamination of Cell Cultures. Proc. Workshop on Cell Substrates for Vaccine Production, Bowers Reporting Co., pp. 82-88.

Barile, M. F. (1977) Mycoplasma contamination of cell cultures: A status report. In: "Cell Culture and Its Applications" (R. Acton, Ed.) Academic Press, New York, pp. 291-334.

Barile, M. F. (1979) Mycoplasma Contamination of Cell Cultures. In: "Handbook Series in Clinical Laboratory Science: Virology and Rickettsiology", Section H, Vol. I, Part II. (G.D. Hsuing and R. Green, Eds.) CRC Press, Inc., West Palm Beach, FL, pp. 381-406.

Barile, M. F. (1979) Mycoplasma-tissue cell interactions. In: "The Mycoplasmas", Vol. II (J. G. Tully and R. F. Whitcomb, Eds.) Academic Press, New York, pp. 425-474.

Barile, M. F. (1981) Mycoplasma infection of cell cultures. Isr. J. Med. Sci. 17:555-562.

Barile, M. F. and DelGiudice, R. A. (1972) Isolations of mycoplasmas and their rapid identification by plate epi-immunofluorescence. In: "Pathogenic Mycoplasmas". Ciba Foundation Symposium, Elsevier and North-Holland, Amsterdam, pp. 165-185.

Barile, M. F. and Grabowski, M. W. (1977) Mycoplasma-cell culture-virus interactions: A brief review. In: "Mycoplasma Infection of Cell Cultures" (G. J. McGarrity, D. G. Murphy, and W. W. Nichols, Eds.) Plenum Press, New York, pp. 135-150.

Barile, M. F. and Grabowski, M. W. (1983) Detection and identification of mycoplasmas in infected cell cultures by direct immunofluorescence staining. In: "Methods in Mycoplasmology", Vol. II, (J. G. Tully and S. Razin, Eds.) Academic Press, New York, pp. 173-182.

Barile, M. F. and Kern, J. (1971) Isolation of *Mycoplasma arginini* from commercial bovine sera and its implication in contaminated cell cultures. Proc. Soc. Exp. Biol. Med. 138:432-437.

Barile, M. F. and Leventhal, B. G. (1968) Possible mechanism for mycoplasma inhibition of lymphocyte transformation induced by phytohemagglutinin. Nature 219:751-752.

Barile, M. F. and McGarrity, G. J. (1983a) Special techniques for isolation and identification of mycoplasmas from cell cultures. In: "Methods in Mycoplasmology", Vol. II (J. G. Tully and S. Razin, Eds.). Academic Press, New York, pp. 155-190.

Barile, M. F. and McGarrity, G. J. (1983b) Isolation of mycoplasmas from cell cultures by agar and broth techniques. In: "Methods in Mycoplasmology", Vol. II (J. G. Tully and S. Razin, Eds.) Academic Press, New York, pp. 159-165.

Barile, M. F. and Schimke, R. T. (1963) A rapid chemical method for detecting PPLO contamination of tissue cell cultures. Proc. Soc. Exptl. Biol. Med. 114:676-679.

Barile, M. F., Yaguchi, R. and Eveland, W. C. (1958) A simplified medium for the cultivation of pleuropneumonia-like organisms and the L-forms of bacteria. Am. J. Clin. Path. 30:171-176.

Barile, M. F., Malizia, W. F. and Riggs, D. B. (1982) Incidence and detection of pleuropneumonia-like organisms in cell cultures by fluorescent antibody and cultural procedures. J. Bacteriol. 84:130-136.

Barile, M. F., DelGiudice, R. A., Carski, T. R., Yamashiroya, H. M. and Verna, J. A. (1970) Isolation and rapid identification of *Mycoplasma* species from canine tissues by plate immunofluorescence. Proc. Soc. Exp. Biol. & Med. 134:146-148.

Barile, M. F., Hopps, H. E., Grabowski, M. W., Riggs, D. B., and DelGiudice, R. A. (1973) The identification and sources of mycoplasmas isolated from contaminated tissue cultures. Ann. NY Acad. Sci. 225:251-264.

Barile, M. F., DelGiudice, R. A., Grabowski, M. W. and Hopps, H. E. (1974) Media for the isolation of mycoplasmas from biologic materials. Develop. Biol. Standard 23:128-133.

Barile, M. F., Hopps, H. E., and Grabowski, M. W. (1977) Incidence and sources of mycoplasma contamination: A brief review. In: "Mycoplasma Infection of Cell Cultures" (G. J. McGarrity, D. G. Murphy and W. W. Nichols, Eds.). Plenum Press, New York, pp. 35-45.

Barile, M. F., Grabowski, M. W., Snoy, P. J., and Chandler, D. K. F. (1987) The superiority of the chimpanzee animal model to study the pathogenicity of known (*M. pneumoniae*) and reputed mycoplasma pathogens. Isr. J. Med. Sci. 23:556-560.

Barile, M. F., Chandler, D. K. F., Yoshida, H., Grabowski, M. W., Harasawa, R., and Razin, S. (1988a) Parameters of *Mycoplasma pneumoniae* infection in the Syrian hamster. Infect. Immun. 56:2443-2449.

Barile, M. F., Chandler, D. K. F., Yoshida, H., Grabowski, M. W. and Razin, S. (1988b) A challenge potency assay in hamsters for evaluation of *Mycoplasma pneumoniae* vaccine. Infect. Immun. 56:2450-2457.

Beck, J., Brunner, H., Marcucci, F., Kirchner, H. and Wietzerbin, J. (1982) Induction of interferon by mycoplasmas in mouse spleen cell cultures. J. Interferon Res. 2:31-36.

Beckoff, M. C., Cole, B. C. and Grey, H. M. (1987) Studies on the mechanism of stimulation of T cells by the *Mycoplasma arthritidis*-derived mitogen. Role of class II IE molecules. J. Immunol. 139:3189-3194.

Bertoni, G., Keist, R., Groscurth, P., Wyler, R., Nicolet, J. and Peterhans, E. (1985) A chemiluminescent assay for mycoplasmas in cell cultures. J. Immunol. Methods. 78:123-133.

Biberfeld, G. (1977) Activation of human lymphocyte subpopulations by *Mycoplasma pneumoniae*. Scand. J. Immunol. 6:1145-1150.

Biberfeld, G. (1985) Infection Sequelae and Autoimmune Reactions in *Mycoplasma pneumoniae* Infection. In: "The Mycoplasmas", Vol. IV. (S. Razin and M. F. Barile, Eds.) Academic Press, New York, pp. 293-311.

Biberfeld, G. and E. Gronowicz (1976) *Mycoplasma pneumoniae* is a polyclonal B-cell activator. Nature 261:238-239.

Blazek, R., Schmitt, K., Krafft, U. and Hadding, U. (1990) Fast and simple procedure for the detection of cell culture mycoplasmas using a single monoclonal antibody. J. Immunol. Methods. 131:203-212.

Borchsenius, S. N., Chernova, O. A., Merkulova, N. A. and Are, A. F. (1987) Detection and identification of Mycoplasma infections by DNA hybridization. Tsitologiia 29:934-941.

Brautbar, C., Stanbridge, E. J., Pellegrino, M. A., Ferrone, S., Reisfeld, R. A., Payne, R. and Hayflick, L. (1973) Expression of HL-A antigens on cultured human fibroblasts infected with mycoplasmas. J. Immunol. 111:1783-1789.

Buck, D. W., Kennett, R. H. and McGarrity, G. J. (1982) Monoclonal antibodies specific for cell culture mycoplasmas. In Vitro. 18:377-381.

Calorini, L. and Ruggieri, S. (1989) Eradication of mycoplasma contamination from cell lines of different origin by the 5-bromouracil-fluorochrome procedure. Cancer Letts. 46:107-112.

Carrington, M. N. and Ward, F. E. (1988) Conversion of a melanoma cell line from an HLA class II positive to negative phenotype after treatment with anti-mycoplasma drugs. Hum. Immunol. 22:275-282.

Chan, B. M., McNeill, K., Berczi, I. and Froese, A. (1986) Effects of mycoplasma infection on Fc receptors for IgE of rat basophilic leukemia cells. Eur. J. Immunol. 16:1319-1324.

Chandler, D. K. F., Razin, S., Stephens, E. B., Harasawa, R. and Barile, M. F. (1982a) Genomic and phenotypic analysis of *Mycoplasma pneumoniae* strains. Infect. Immun. 38:607-609.

Chandler, D. K. F., Grabowski, M. W. and Barile, M. F. (1982b) *Mycoplasma pneumoniae* attachment: competitive inhibition by mycoplasmal binding component and by sialic acid-containing glycoconjugates. Infect. Immun. 38:598-603.

Chanock, R. M., Hayflick, L. and Barile, M. F. (1962) Growth on artificial medium of an agent associated with atypical pneumonia and its identification as a PPLO. Proc. Natl. Acad. Sci. 48:41-49.

Chen, T. R. (1977) *In situ* detection of mycoplasma contamination in cell cultures by fluorescent Hoechst 33258 stain. Exp. Cell Res. 104:255-262.

Chowdhury, I. H., Munakata, T., Koyanagi, Y., Kobayashi, S., Arai, S. and Yamamoto, N. (1990) Mycoplasma can enhance HIV replication *in vitro*: a possible cofactor responsible for the progression of AIDS. Biochim. Biophys. Res. Commun. 170:1365-1370.

Clyde, W. A., Jr. (1979) *Mycoplasma pneumoniae* Infections of Man. In: "The Mycoplasmas", Vol. II (J. G. Tully and R. F. Whitcomb, Eds.) Academic Press, New York, pp. 275-306.

Cochrum, K. C., Dykman, L., Najarian, J. S. and Fudenberg, H.H. (1969) A new source of large numbers of lymphocytes and studies on their culture. Proc. 3rd Ann. Leucocyte Cult. Conf. 169-176

Cole, B. C., Araneo, B. A. and Sullivan, G. J. (1986) Stimulation of mouse lymphocytes by a mitogen derived from *Mycoplasma arthritidis*. IV. Murine T-hybridoma cells exhibit differential accessory cell requirements for activation by *M. arthritidis* T-cell mitogen, concanavalin A., or hen egg-white lysozyme. J. Immunol. 136:3572-3578.

Cole, B. C., Daynes, R. A. and Ward, J .R. (1982) Stimulation of mouse lymphocytes by a mitogen derived from *Mycoplasma arthritidis*. III. Ir gene control of lymphocyte transformation correlates with binding of the mitogen to specific Ia-bearing cells. J. Immunol. 129:1352-1359.

Cole, B. C., Lombardi, P. S., Overall, J. C., Jr. and Glasgow, L. A. (1978) Inhibition of interferon induction in mice by mycoplasmas and mycoplasmal fractions. Proc. Soc. Exp. Biol. Med. 157:83-88.

Cole, B. C., Naot, Y., Stanbridge, E. J., and Wise, K. S. (1985) Pathogenesis of mycoplasma diseases. In: "The Mycoplasmas", Vol. IV. (S. Razin and M. F. Barile, Eds.) Academic Press, New York, pp. 204-258.

Cole, B. C., Overall, J. C., Jr. and Glasgow, L. A. (1974a) Induction of interferon in mice by mycoplasmas. Infect. Immun. 10:1296-1301.

Cole, B. C., Overall, J. C., Jr., Ward, J. R. and Glasgow, L. A. (1974b) Induction of interferon in ovine leukocytes by species of mycoplasma and acheleoplasma, Proc. Soc. Exp. Biol. Med. 146:613-618.

Collier, L. H. (1957) Contamination of stock lines of human carcinoma cells by pleuropneumonia-like organisms. Nature. 180:757.

Coronato, S. and Coto, C. (1987) Mycoplasmas contaminating tissue cultures. Rev. Argent. Microbiol. 4:165-172.

Crowell, S. L., Burgess, H. S. and Davis, T. P. (1989) The effect of mycoplasma on the autocrine stimulation of human small cell lung cancer *in vitro* by bombesin and β-endorphin. Life Sci. 45:2471-2476.

DelGiudice, R. A. and Barile, M. F. (1974) Immunofluorescent procedures for mycoplasma identification. Develop. Biol. Standard 23:134-137.

DelGiudice, R. A. and Hopps, H. E. (1978) Microbiological methods and fluorescent microscopy for the direct demonstration of mycoplasma infection of cell cultures In: "Mycoplasma Infection of Cell Cultures" (G. J. McGarrity, D. Murphy and W. W. Nichols, Eds.) Plenum Press, New York, pp. 57-69.

DelGiudice, R. A., Carski, T. R., Barile, M .F., Yamashiroya, H. M. and Verna, J. E. (1969) Recovery of human mycoplasmas from simian tissues. Nature 222:1088-1089.

Ebke, J. and Kuwert, E. (1972) Detection of *Mycoplasma orale* type I in tissue cultures by means of the acridine orange stain. Zentralbl. Bakteriol. 221:87-93.

Franzoso, G., Dimitrov, D. S., Blumenthal, R., Barile, M .F. and Rottem, S. (1992) Fusion of *Mycoplasma fermentans*, strain incognitus, with T-lymphocytes. FEBS Letts. 303:251-254.

Fernald, G. W. (1979) Humoral and cellular immune responses to mycoplasmas In: "The Mycoplasmas", Vol. II (J. G. Tully and R. F. Whitcomb, Eds.) Academic Press, New York, pp. 399-423.

Freiberg, E. F. and Masover, G. K. (1990) Mycoplasma detection in cell culture by concomitant use of bisbenzamide and fluoresceinated antibody. In Vitro Cell Dev. Biol. 26:585-588.

Gabridge, M. G., Lundin, D. J. and Gladd, M. F. (1986) Detection and speciation of common cell culture mycoplasmas by an enzyme-linked immunosorbent assay with biotin-avidin amplification and microporous membrane solid phase. In Vitro Cell Dev. Biol. 22:491-498.

Gallily, R., Sher, T., Ben-Av, P. and Lowenstein, J. (1989) Tumor necrosis factor as a mediator of *Mycoplasma orale* induced tumor cell lysis by macrophages. Cell Immunol. 121:146-153.

Gardella, R. S. and DelGuidice, R. A. (1984) Antibiotic sensitivities and elimination of mycoplasmas from infected cell cultures. Isr. J. Med. Sci. 20:931-934.

Gideoni, O. and Naot, Y. (1984) Interactions of mycoplasmas with lymphocytes and macrophages. Ann. Microbiol. (Paris) 135A:55-62.

Ginsburg, H. and Nicolet, J. (1973) Extensive transformation of lymphocytes by a mycoplasma organism. Nature New Biol. 246:143-146.

Göbel, U. B. and Stanbridge, E. J. (1984) Cloned mycoplasma ribosomal RNA genes for the detection of mycoplasma contamination in tissue cultures. Science 226:1211-1213.

Göbel, U., Maasm, R., Haun, G., Vinga-Martins, C. and Stanbridge, E. J. (1987) Synthetic oligonucleotide probes complementary to rRNA for group- and species-specific detection of mycoplasmas. Isr. J. Med. Sci. 23:742-746.

Goodwin, R. F. W. and Whittlestone, P. (1963) Production of enzootic pneumonia in pigs with an agent grown tissue culture from the natural disease. Brit. J. Exp. Path. 44:291-299.

Harper. D. R., Kangro, H. O., Argent, S. and Heath, R. B. (1988) Reduction in immunoreactivity of varicella-zoster virus proteins induced by mycoplasma contamination. J. Virol. Methods. 20:65-72.

Hatcher, V. B. (1983) Modulation of plasminogen activator activity in human skin fibroblasts infected with mycoplasmas. Proc. Soc. Exp. Biol. Med. 173:324-327.

Hellung-Larsen, P. and Frederiksen, S. (1976) Influence of mycoplasma infection on the incorporation of different precursors into RNA components of tissue culture cells. Exp. Cell Res. 99:295-300.

Herderschee, D. (1963) An improved medium for the cultivation of Eaton agent (cause of primary atypical pneumonia in man is a PPLO). Anton van Lowen J. Microbiol. Serol. 29:154-166.

Hommel-Berrey, G. A. and Brahmi, Z. (1987) Relevance of soluble cytotoxic factors generated by mycoplasma-contaminated targets to natural killer cell-mediated killing. Hum. Immunol. 20:33-46.

Hopps, H. E., Meyer, B. C., Barile, M. F., and DelGiudice, R. A. (1973) Problems concerning "noncultivable" mycoplasma contaminants in tissue cultures. Ann. N.Y. Acad. Sci. 225:265-276.

Izumikawa, K., Chandler, D. K. F., Grabowski, M. W., and Barile, M.F. (1987) Attachment of *Mycoplasma hominis* to human cell cultures. Isr. J. Med. Sci. 23:603-607.

Johansson, K. E. and Bölske, G. (1989) Evaluation and practical aspects of the use of a commercial DNA probe for detection of mycoplasma infections in cell cultures. J. Biochem. Biophys. Methods. 19:185-199.

Johansson, K. E. , Johansson, I. and Gobel. (1990) Evaluation of different hybridization procedures for the detection of mycoplasma contamination in cell cultures. Mol. Cell Probes. 4:33-42.

Jones, T. C., Yeh, S. and J. G. Hirsch, J. G. (1972) Studies on Attachment and Ingestion Phases of Phagocytosis of *Mycoplasma pulmonis* by Mouse Peritoneal Macrophages. Proc. Soc. Exp. Biol. Med. 139:464-470.

Kaklamanis, E. and Pavlatos, M. (1972) The immunosuppressive effect of mycoplasma infection. I. Effect on the humoral and cellular response. Immunol. 22:695-702.

Kaklamanis, E., Thomas, L., Stavropoulos, K., Borman, I. and Boshivitz, C. (1969) Mycoplasmacidal action of normal tissue extracts. Nature 221:860-862.

Kapikian, A. Z., Barile, M. F., Wyatt, R. G., Yolken, R. H., Tully, J. G., Greenburg, H. B., Kalica, A. R. and Chanock, R. M. (1979) Mycoplasma contamination in cell culture of Crohn's Disease material. Lancet II:446-467,

Keprtova, J., Jurmanova, K., Spurna, V., Minarova, E., Hofmanova, J. and Nebola, M. (1981) An autoradiographic method of detecting A. *laidlawii* and *M. hyorhinis* in cell cultures. In Vitro 17:563-569.

Kluve, B., Merrick, W. C. and Gershman, H. (1983) Mycoplasma-induced BALB/c 3T3 collagenase is a mammalian enzyme. Biochem. J. 212:641-647.

Koch, C. J. and Bigalow, J. E. (1983) Cyanide insensitive respiration in mammalian cells: an artifact of mycoplasmal contamination. Adv. Exp. Med. Biol. 159:337-345.

Koshimizu, K. and Kotani, H. (1981) In: "Procedures for the Isolation and Identification of Human, Animal and Plant Mycoplasmas" (M. Nakamura, Ed.) Saikon, Tokyo, pp. 87-102.

Kotani, H., Huang, H. and McGarrity, G. . (1987) Identification and isolation of mycoplasmas by immunobinding. Isr. J. Med. Sci. 23:752-758.

Kouri, T., Jalkanen, M. Turakainen, H. and Leach, R. H. (1983) Effect of *Mycoplasma pulmonis* infection on protein and glycosaminoglycan synthesis of cultured connective tissue cells. Exp. Cell Res. 148:1-10.

Krivan, H. C., Olson, L. D., Barile, M. F., Ginsburg, V. and Roberts, D. D. (1989) Adhesion of *Mycoplasma pneumoniae* to sulfated glycolipids and inhibition by dextran sulfate. J. Biol. Chem. 264:9283-9288.

Lai, W. C., Bennett, M., Pakes, S. P., Kumar, V., Steuterman, D., Owusu, I. and Mikhael, A. (1990) Resistance to *Mycoplasma pulmonis* mediated by activated natural killer cells. J. Infect. Dis. 161:1269-1275.

Leventhal, B. G., Smith, C. B., Carbone, P. P. and Hersh, E. M. (1968) Lymphocyte transformation in response to *Mycoplasma pneumoniae* after experimental infection in man. Proc. 3rd Ann. Leucocyte Culture Conference, Appleton-Century Crofts, New York, pp. 519-532.

Levin, D., Gershon, H. and Naot, Y. (1985) Production of interleukin-2 by rat lymph node cells stimulated by *Mycoplasma pulmonis* membranes. J. Infect. Dis. 151:541-544.

Levine, E. M. and Müller, S. N. (1983) Biochemical Procedures for the Detection of Mycoplasmal Infection in Cell Cultures. In: "Methods in Mycoplasmology", Vol. II (J. G. Tully and S. Razin, Eds.) Academic Press, New York. pp. 191-208.

Lipp, M., Koch, E., Brandner, G. and Bredt, W. (1979) Stimulation and prevention of retrovirus-specific reactions by mycoplasmas. Med. Microbiol. Immunol. 167:127-136.

Lo, S.-C. and Liotta, L. A. (1985) Vascular tumors produced by NIH/3T3 cells transfected with human AIDS Kaposi's sarcoma DNA. Am. J. Pathol. 118:7-13.

Lo, S.-C., Shih, J., Newton, P. B., Wong, D. M., Hayes, M. M., Benish, J. R., Wear, D. J. and Wang, R. (1989) The virus-like infectious agent (VLIA) is a novel pathogenic mycoplasma. Am. J. Trop. Med. Hyg. 41:586-600.

Lo., S.-C., Tsai, S., Benish, J. R., Shih, J. W., Wear, D. J. and Wong, D. M. (1991) Enhancement of HIV-1 cytocidal effects in CD4+ lymphocytes by the AIDS-associated mycoplasma. Science 251:1074-1076.

Loewenstein, J., Rottem, S. and Gallily, R. (1983) Induction of macrophage-mediated cytolysis of neoplastic cells by mycoplasmas. Cell Immunol. 77:290-297.

Lynch, D. H., Cole, B. C., Bluestone, J. A. and Hodes, R. J. (1986) Cross-reactive recognition by antigen-specific major histocompatibility complex-restricted T-cells of a mitogen derived from *Mycoplasma arthritidis* is clonally expressed and I-E restricted. Eur. J. Immunol. 16:747-751.

Makhoul, N., Merchav, S. and Naot, Y. (1987) Mycoplasma-induced *in vitro* production of interleukin-2 and colony stimulating activity. Isr. J. Med. Sci. 23:480-484.

Manischewitz, J. E., Young, B. G. and Barile, M. F. (1975) The Effect of Mycoplasmas on Replication and Plaquing Ability of Herpes Simplex Virus. Proc. Soc. Exp. Biol. & Med. 148:859-863.

Mardh, P.-A. and Taylor-Robinson, D. (1973) Differential effects of lysolecithin on mycoplasmas and acholeplasmas. Med. Microbiol. Immunol. 158:259-266.

Machatkova, M., Jurmanova, K., Chlupova, L. and Snejdar, V. (1986) Decontamination of cell lines by selective elimination of mycoplasmas. Arch. Exper. Vet. Med. 8:151-156.

McGarrity, G. J. and Barile, M. F. (1983) Use of indicator cell lines for recovery and identification of cell culture mycoplasmas. In: "Methods in Mycoplasmology", Vol. II, (J. G. Tully and S. Razin, Eds.). Academic Press, New York, pp. 167-172.

McGarrity, G. J. and Kotani, H. (1985) Pathogenesis of Mycoplasma Diseases In: "The Mycoplasmas", Vol. IV (S. Razin and M. F. Barile, Eds.). Academic Press, New York, pp. 353-390.

McGarrity, G. J. and Kotani, H. (1986) Detection of cell culture mycoplasmas by a genetic probe. Exp. Cell Res. 163:273-278.

McGarrity, G., Gamon, L. and Sarama, J. (1983) Prevention and control of mycoplasmal infection of cell cultures In: "Methods in Mycoplasmology", Vol. II (J. G. Tully and S. Razin, Eds.) Academic Press, New York, pp. 203-208.

Monsigny, M., Midoux, P., Depierreaux, C., Bébéar, C., Le Bris, M.T. and Valeur, B. (1990) Benzoxazinone kanamycin A conjugate. A new fluorescent probe suitable to detect mycoplasmas in cell culture. Biol. Cell. 70:101-105.

Montagnier, L., Berneman, D., Guetard, D., Blanchard, A., Chamaret, S., Rame, V., VanRietschoten, J., Marbrouk, K. and Bahraoui, E. (1990) Infectivity inhibition of HIV prototype strains by antibodies directed against a peptide sequence of mycoplasma. CR Acad. Sci. III 311:425-430.

Naot, Y. (1982) *In vitro* studies on the mitogenic activity of mycoplasmal species toward lymphocytes. Rev. Infect. Dis. 4:S205-S209.

Nelson, J. B. (1960) The behavior of murine pleuropneumonia-like organisms in HeLa cell cultures. Ann. N.Y. Acad. Sci. 79:450-457.

O'Brien, S. J., Simonson, J. M., Grabowski, M. W. and Barile, M. F. (1981) An analysis of multiple isoenzyme expression among twenty-two species of mycoplasma and acholeplasma. J. Bacteriol. 146:222-232.

O'Brien, S. J., Simonson, J. M., Razin, S. and Barile, M. F. (1983) On the distribution and characterization of isoenzyme expression iosenzymes in *Mycoplasma, Acholeplasma and Ureaplasma* species. Yale J. Biol. Med. 56:701-708.

Olson, L. D. and Barile, M. F. (1988) Mycoplasma infection of cell cultures: isolation and detection. J. Tissue Culture Methods 11:175-179.

O'Malley, J. P., McGee, Z. A., Barile, M. F. and Barker, L. F. (1966) Identification of the A-1 agent as a *Mycoplasma gallisepticum*. Proc. Natl. Acad. Sci. 56:895-901.

Perez, A. G., Kim, J. H., Gelbard, A. S. and Djordjevic, B. (1972) Altered incorporation of nucleic acid precursors by mycoplasma-infected mammalian cells in culture. Exp. Cell Res. 70:301-310.

Polster, U. (1986) Fluorescent dye demonstration of mycoplasma in cell cultures using olivomycin. Arch. Exp. Veterinarmed. 40:142-146.

Proust, J. J., Buchholz, M. A. and Nordin, A. A. (1985) A lymphokine-like, soluble project that induces proliferation and maturation of B cell appears in the serum-free supernatant of a T cell hybridoma as a consequence of mycoplasmal contamination. J. Immunol. 134:390-396.

Radka, S. F., Hester, D. M., Polak-Vogelzang, A. A. and Bolhuis, R. L. (1984) Detection of mycoplasma contamination lymphoblastoid cell lines by monoclonal antibodies. Hum. Immunol. 9:111-116.

Razin, S. (1985a) Mycoplasma Adherence In: "The Mycoplasmas", Vol. IV, (S. Razin and M. F. Barile, Eds.) Academic Press, New York, pp. 161-203.

Razin, S. (1985b) Molecular Biology and Genetics of Mycoplasmas (*Mollicutes*). Microbiol. Rev. 49:419-455.

Razin, S. (1993) Mycoplasma membranes as models in membrane research In: "Mycoplasma Cell Membranes" (S. Rottem and I. Kahane, Eds.) Plenum Publications Co. (in press).

Razin, S. and Jacobs, E. (1992) Mycoplasma adhesion. J. Gener. Microbiol. 138:407-422

S. Razin and S. Rottem, Eds. (1982) Microbial membrane lipids. Current topics in membranes and transport pp. 1-383.

S. Razin and J. G. Tully, Eds. (1983) Methods in Mycoplasmology, Vol. I, Academic Press, New York. pp. 1-504.

Roberts, D. D., Olson, L. S., Barile, M. F., Ginsburg, V., Krivan, H. C. (1989) Sialic acid-dependent adhesion of *Mycoplasma pneumoniae* to purified glycoproteins. J. Biol. Chem. 264:9289-9293.

Robinson, L. B., Wichelhausen, R. H. and Roizman, B. (1956) Contamination of human cell cultures by pleuropneumonia-like organisms. Science 124:1147-1148.

Rose, F. V., Barile, M. F. and Cebra, J. J. (1983) Monoclonal antibodies as probes for antigens of *Mycoplasma pulmonis*. Adv. Exp. Med. Biol. 162:319-326.

Rottem, S. and Kahane, I., Eds. (1993) Mycoplasma Cell Membranes. Plenum Publications Co. (in press).

Russell, W. C., Newman, C. and Williamson, D. H. (1975) A simple cytochemical technique for demonstration of DNA in cells infected with mycoplasmas and viruses. Nature 253:461-462.

Ruuth, E. and Lundgren, E. (1986) Enhancement of immunoglobulin secretion by the lymphokine-like activity of a *Mycoplasma arginini* strain. Scand. J. Immunol. 23:575-580.

Saillard, C., Carle, P., Bové, J.M., Bébéar, C., Lo, S.-C., Shih, J. W.-K., Wang, R. Y.-H., Rose, D. L. and Tully, J. G.(1990) Genetic and serologic relatedness between *Mycoplasma fermentans* strains and a mycoplasma recently identified in tissues of AIDS and nonAIDS patients. Res. Virol. 141:385-395.

Schaeffer, W. I., Olson, L. D., Barile, M. F. and Sun, F. W. (1991) Selective labelling of *Mycoplasma hyorhinis* and mitochondrial DNA *in situ* with cultured cells. Their coisolation and their differentiation using restriction fragment length polymorphisms. J. Bacteriol. 173:1382-1387.

Schimke, R. T. and Barile, M. F. (1963a) Arginine breakdown in mammalian cell culture contaminated with pleuropneumonia-like organisms (PPLO). Exptl. Cell Res. 30:593-596.

Schimke, R. T. and Barile, M. F. (1963b) Arginine metabolism in pleuropneumonia-like organisms isolated from mammalian cell culture. J. Bacteriol. 86:195-206.

Scott, D. M., Rodgers, B. C., Freeke, C., Buiter, J. and Sissons, J. G. (1989) Human cytomegalovirus and monocytes: limited infection and negligible immunosuppression in normal mononuclear cells infected *in vitro* with mycoplasma-free virus strains. J. Gen. Virol. 70:685-694.

Seid, R. C., Jr., Smith, P. F., Guevarra, G., Hochstein, H. D., and Barile, M. F. (1980) Endotoxin-like activities of mycoplasmal lipopolysaccharides (Lipoglycans). Infect. Immun. 29:990-994

Sher, T., Rottem, R. and Gallily, R. (1990a) *Mycoplasma capricolum* membranes induce tumor necrosis factor α by a mechanism different from that of lipopolysaccharide. Cancer Immunol. Immunother. 31:86-92.

Sher, T., Yamin, A., Rottem, S. and Gallily, R. (1990b) *In vitro* induction of tumor necrosis factor-α, tumor cytolysis, and blast transformation by *Spiroplasma* membranes. Reports. 82:1142-1145.

Sher, T., Yamin, A., Stein, I., Rottem, S. and Gallily, R. (1991) TNF-α, IL-1 and PGE$_2$ secretion following macrophage activation by *Mycoplasma capricolum* membranes In: "Microbial Surface Components and Toxins in Relation to Pathogenesis" (E. Z. Ron and S. Rottem, Eds.) Plenum Press, New York and London.

Singer, S. H., Barile, M. F. and Kirschstein, R. L. (1969b) Enhanced Virus Yields and Decreased Interferon Production in Mycoplasma-Infected Hamster Cells. Proc. Soc. Exp. Biol. & Med. 131:1129-1134.

Singer, S. H., Barile, M. F. and Kirschstein, R. L. (1973) Mixed mycoplasma-virus infections in cell culture. N.Y. Acad. Sci. 225:304-310.

Singer, S. H., Fitzgerald, E. A., Barile, M. F. and Kirschstein, R. L. (1970) Effect of Mycoplasmas on Vaccinia Virus Growth: Requirement for Arginine. Proc. Soc. Exp. Biol. & Med. 133:1439-1442.

Singer, S. H., Ford, M., Barile, M. F. and Kirschstein, R. L. (1972) Effect of Mycoplasmas on Virus Replication and Plaque Formation in Mouse Cells. Proc. Soc. Exp. Biol. Med. 139:56-58.

Singer, S. H., Kirschstein, R. L. and Barile, M. F. (1969a) Increased yields of vesicular stomatitis virus from hamster cells infected with mycoplasmas. Nature 222:1087-1088.

Spierenburg, G. T., Polak-Vogelzang, A. A. and Bast, B. J. (1988) Indicator cell lines for the detection of hidden mycoplasma contamination using an adenosine phosphorylase screening test. J. Immunol. Methods. 114:115-119.

Stanbridge, E. J. and Weiss, R. L. (1978) Mycoplasma capping on lymphocytes. Nature. 276:583-587.

Stanbridge, E. J., Bretzius, K. A. and Good, R. F. (1981) Mycoplasma-lymphocyte interactions: Ir gene control of mitogenesis and a paradoxical interaction with thy-1 bearing cells. Isr. J. Med. Sci. 17:629-632.

Stuart, P. M., Cassell, G. H. and Woodward, J. G. (1986) Induction of class II MHC antigen expression in macrophages by *Mycoplasma* species. J. Immunol. 142:3392-3399.

Stuart, P. M., Cassell, G. H. and Woodward, J. G.. (1990) Differential induction of bone marrow macrophage proliferation by mycoplasmas involves granulocyte-macrophage colony-stimulating factor. Infect. Immun. 58:3558-3563.

Studzinski, G. P., Gierthy, J. F. and Cholon, J. J. (1973) An autoradiographic screening test for mycoplasmal contamination of mammalian cell cultures. In Vitro 8:466-472.

Sydiskis, R. J., Weber, P. A. and DelGiudice, R. A. (1981) Covert infection of a mouse mammary tumor cell line with *Mycoplasma hyorhinis*: cosedimentation with mouse mammary tumor virus in sucrose density gradients. In Vitro 17:997-1003.

Tully, J. G. and Razin, S. (Eds.) (1983) Methods in Mycoplasmology, Vol. II, Academic Press, New York, pp. 1-440.

Tully, J. G., Whitcomb, R. F., Clark, H. F. and Williamson, D. L. Pathogenic mycoplasmas: cultivation and vertebrate pathogenicity of a new spiroplasma. Science. 195:892-894.

Wise, K. S., Minion, F. C. and Cheung, H. C. (1982) Translocation of Thy-1 antigen and a fluorescent lipid probe during lymphoblastoid cell interaction with *Mycoplasma hyorhinis*. Rev. Infec. Dis. 4 Suppl,S-210-S-218.

Woods, S. B. (1983) The isolation of a 'noncultivable' strain of *Mycoplasma hyorhinis* from a mammalian live virus vaccine. J. Biol. Stand. 11:247-250.

Vasudevachari, M. B., Mast, T. C. and Salzman, N. P. (1990) Suppression of HIV-1 reverse transcriptase activity by mycoplasma contamination of cell cultures. AIDS Res. Hum. Retroviruses 6:411-416.

Vogelzang, A. A. and van Klingeren, B. (1974) Proceedings: Mycoplasmas in Cell Cultures. Antonie Van Leeuwenhoek. 40:316-317.

Yang, R. C., Tsuji, A. and Suzuki, Y. (1990) Abnormal protein spots revealed by two- dimensional electrophoresis in mycoplasma-infected human fibroblasts. Electrophoresis 11:344-346.

APPENDIX A   PROTOCOL FOR THE DNA STAINING PROCEDURE USING BISBENZAMIDE FLUOROCHROME STAIN

Reagents

Bisbenzamide fluorochrome stain. [Stock concentration (100 ml)] :

Add 5 mg bisbenzamide fluorochrome stain: (Hoechst #33258)* to 100 ml of Hank's balanced salt solution (BSS) without sodium bicarbonate and phenol red plus 0.01 gm Thimersol (merthiolate) (final concentration, 1:10,000). Mix thoroughly at 22-25°C with magnetic stirrer for 30 min and wrap bottle in aluminum foil and store in dark at 2-8°C. *Stain is light and heat sensitive.*

*Compound #33258 Hoechst (bisbenzimidazole) is 2-[2-(4 hydroxyphenyl)-6-benzimidazolyl]-6-(1-methyl-4-piperazyl)benzimidazoltrihydrochloride (Loewe): purchase in the U.S.A. from Hoechst Pharmaceuticals, Route 202-206 N., Sommerville,New Jersey 08876.

Bisbenzamide fluorochrome stain. [Stock working stain dilution (100 ml)]

Add 100 l (0.1 ml) of stock concentrate to 100 ml of Hank's BSS for final concentration of 0.05 µg/ml. Optimal fluorescence may range from a concentration of 0.05 to 0.5 µg/ml. Store in a dark bottle wrapped in aluminum foil at 2-8°C. Before use, mix thoroughly with magnetic stirrer at 22-25°C for 30 min. The "WORKING STAIN DILUTION" can be stored at 2-8°C for short periods, but must be tested periodically for microbial contamination. *Discard when contamination or when deterioration of fluorescence occurs.* Millipore filtration diminishes fluorescence. A large amount of Stock Working Stain Solution is prepared only when large amounts of specimens are being tested.

Otherwise, it is preferred that the working solution is prepared freshly as needed.

Citric acid-disodium phosphate buffer for mounting fluid (100 ml).

Add 22.2 ml of 0.1 $\underline{M}$ citric acid to 27.9 ml of 0.2 $\underline{M}$ disodium phosphate plus 50.0 ml of glycerol with final pH of 5.5 (Check periodically; pH is critical for optimal fluorescence). Store at 2-8°C until used.

Fixative

Mix 1:3 parts of glacial acetic acid and methanol.

PROCEDURE

Indicator cell culture: We have routinely used the 3T3 or 3T6 (mouse fibroblast) and VERO (African green monkey) cell cultures very effectively as indicator cells for growth and detection of mycoplasma contaminants. Many other primary and continuous cell cultures have been found suitable. Pretest before selecting cell culture for suitability. Generally, a fibroblastic cell is preferable to differentiated cells. Some transformed cell cultures may contain large amounts of extra nuclear fragments causing nonspecific artifacts and extensive background fluorescence, making interpretation of results difficult. The indicator cell culture is grown on glass coverslips (10.5 x 22 mm. No. 1 thickness) placed in a small (35 x 10 mm) plastic, nontoxic "tissue culture clean" dishes (Falcon, Corning) or equivalent containers. Three to four ml of the 3T6 cell culture suspension (approximately 10^5 cells/ml) in basal medium no. 2 (Eagle) containing 10% fetal bovine serum and 100 u/ml of penicillin G, ampicillin, or an equivalent β-lactam antibiotic that interferes with peptidoglycan bio-synthesis (mycoplasmas do not possess peptidoglycan) is added to each dish.

The cell culture dishes are incubated at 36±1°C in 5% CO_2 in air for 4-6 days. Cells are inoculated within 24 h with 0.2-0.3 ml of the specimen and positive mycoplasma control culture. Dishes are identified (code number) as to specimen inoculated.

Each test includes a positive control (*M. hyorhinis* or *M. arginini* infected cell culture) to establish the efficacy and validity of the test and a negative control (noninoculated cell culture). The negative control also provides a means of monitoring each passage of the indicator cell culture for mycoplasma contamination. Each passage of the indicator cell culture is also examined weekly for contamination using very sensitive agar and broth culture procedures (see Barile, 1974; 1973; 1979; Barile and McGarrity, 1983). The indicator cell culture system provides the advantages of having positive (*M. hyorhinis*- infected) controls to test efficacy of procedure and negative (non-inoculated) controls to monitor the sterility of the indicator cell and for comparison to the test specimens. Discard contaminated indicator cell culture immediately. In practice, a number of vials of the indicator cell culture are stored frozen and used when working cell line becomes contaminated.

Staining

Remove "working stain dilution" from refrigeration and mix thoroughly at 22-25°C with magnetic stirrer for 30 min. Aspirate the cell culture medium from the dish, but do not permit the specimen to dry because drying produces undesirable *artifacts*.

For fixation, add 3-4 ml of acetic acid-methanol fixative to the indicator cell culture specimen-coverslip and incubate for 5 min. Aspirate the fixative and repeat fixation procedure for an additional 10 min. Aspirate and permit the specimen to air dry.

For staining specimen in dishes, place 3-4 ml of the working stain solution on cell culture specimen-coverslip and incubate at 22-25°C for 30 min. To prevent dehydration, 8 specimen dishes are placed in a large covered petri dish (150 x 25 mm) during staining period. Aspirate. Rinse specimen-coverslip three times with *deionized or distilled water. Do not use salt solutions because they can cause artifacts and increase background fluorescence.* After the third rinse, remove excess water from specimen-coverslip with a Pasteur pipet or blotting paper.

Mount specimen-coverslips on a large microscope slide for microscopic examination. Remove with forceps and place 6 specimen-coverslips in two rows of three each on a large glass microscope slide (2" x 3") and cover with two large cover-slips (18 x 75 mm, No. 1 thickness), one coverslip for each of the two rows of three specimens. Mounting fluid is placed above and below the specimens. Identify and record the position of each of the six specimens. Specimens (positive and negative controls and unknowns) are observed by fluorescence microscopy at 500 X using No 50 barrier and BG12 exciter filters. (We have used and recom-mend a Carl Zeiss Universal microscope with an epi-illuminator). The filter systems recommended for other microscopes are given elsewhere (Barile and Grabowski, 1983).

APPENDIX B   PROTOCOL FOR DIRECT IMMUNOFLUORESCENCE STAINING PROCEDURE

Reagents

Antiserum

Use specific, sensitive, pretested, high quality fluorescein-isothiocyanide conjugated antiserum for each *Mycoplasma* species, *e.g.*, *M. hyorhinis*. Dilute conjugate in phosphate buffer saline at pH 7.2 (PBS) containing 10% fetal bovine serum and experimentally determine the optimal dilution of each conjugated antiserum for maximal fluorescence. The working stock solution of our conjugated antisera to *M. hyorhinis* strain, BTS 7 (NIAID No. M718-501471) is diluted 1:200.

Store a number of vials of the working stock dilution of conjugate in appropriate volumes (each vial for given number of specimens) frozen at minus 20°C or below. Six ml is generally an adequate volume for 10 specimens. Filter conjugate through 450 filter before use to remove nonspecific fluorescent debris as well as contaminating organisms. *Avoid repeated freeze-thawing because it will cause fluorescence to deteriorate. Discard conjugate if deterioration or contamination occurs.*

Evans Blue counterstain: To prepare Stock solution, add 0.1 g/100 ml in PBS and store at 4∘C. To prepared Working solution, add 1:20 parts of stock solution in PBS and store at room temperature until used.

Buffered glycerol mounting medium: Use Baltimore Biologics Laboratories lot #30825Y or equivalent.

PROCEDURE

Indicator cell culture

Pretest and select the indicator cell culture for suitability. We have routinely used the 3T6 (mouse fibroblast) and VERO (African green monkey) cell cultures very effectively as indicator cells for growth and detection of *M. hyorhinis* contaminants as well as other mycoplasma pathogens. Many other continuous cell cultures have been found acceptable for use. Generally, a fibroblastic cell is preferable to differentiated cells. Each passage of the indicator cell culture is also examined weekly for contamination using very sensitive agar and broth culture procedures (see Barile, 1974; 1973; 1979; Barile and McGarrity, 1983). The indicator cell system provides the advantage of having positive (*M. hyorhinis* infected) and negative (noninoculated) controls for comparison with inoculate specimens.

The indicator cell cultures are grown on glass coverslips (10.5 x 22 mm, No. 1 thickness) placed in small (35 x 10 mm) plastic, nontoxic tissue culture clean dishes (Falcon, Corning, etc.). We add 3 to 4 ml per dish of the 3T6 cell culture suspension (approximately 10^4 cells/ml) in Basal Medium No. 2 (Eagle) containing 10% fetal bovine serum and 100 U/ml of penicillin G. The cell cultures are incubated at 36±1∘C in 5% CO_2 in air for 5 to 7 days. Cells are inoculated within 24 h with 0.2 to 0.3 ml of the cell culture specimen or positive mycoplasma control. Dishes are identified (using a code number) as to specimen inoculated.

Each test includes a *M. hyorhinis* infected cell culture as a positive control and a noninoculated cell culture as a negative control. The negative control provides a means to monitor the indicator cell culture for contamination by *M. hyorhinis.* The indicator cell culture is also examined weekly for contamination by culture procedures (see Barile, 1974, 1973). Discard contaminated indicator cell culture immediately. In practice, a number of vials of indicator cell cultures are stored frozen and used when working cell line becomes contaminated.

Fixation

After three to five days of incubation, aspirate and remove the cell culture medium fluids from the dish, but *do not permit the specimen to dry be-*

cause drying produces undesirable artifacts. Rinse the culture coverslip-specimens in the dish twice with 5 ml of PBS with gentle agitation.

Remove the specimen-coverslip with forceps and place in a Columbia jar with the coverslip-specimen side facing forward. Properly identify and record the position of each specimen. Labels can also be used to identify each specimen in each Columbia jar. In practice, the first slot in the jar is left open for orientation and identification and the first specimen is placed in the second slot, the second specimen in the third slot, *etc.*

Fix the cell culture specimen-coverslips, while still in the Columbia jar, with 5 ml of acetone twice with gentle agitation. Aspirate and remove the acetone fixative and repeat fixation for an additional 10 min. Rinse the specimens twice with PBS. Remove the coverslip-specimen from the jar and return the specimen to its originally identified dish, specimen side up. Rinse with PBS, aspirate, and *do not permit the specimen to dry.*

Staining

Place 8 specimen dishes to each large Petri dish (150 x 25 mm). Add an adequate volume (from 0.2 to 0.8 ml) of the working dilution of filtered (through a 450 µ filter) fluorescein-conjugated antiserum onto each coverslip to completely cover the cell culture specimen and incubate at 22-25°C for 30 min. Rinse with PBS twice and aspirate fluids.

Counterstain.

Add 0.3 ml of the working dilution of Evans Blue onto each specimen in each dish and incubate at room temperature (22-25°C) for 30 min. The counter-stain reduces the amount of nonspecific background fluorescence, making specific fluorescence easier to determine. Rinse twice with PBS. Remove and place 6 coverslip specimens (in two rows of 3 each) on a large glass microscope slide (2" x 3"). Cover each row of three with two large coverslips (18 x 75 mm, No. 1 thickness) with buffered glycerol mounting fluid placed above and below the coverslip specimen.

Specimens (positive and negative controls and unknowns) are observed by fluorescence microscopy at 500 X using No. 50 barrier and BG12 exciter filters and using a Carl Zeiss Universal microscope with an epi-illuminator. The filter systems recommended for other microscopes are given elsewhere (Barile and Grabowski, 1983).

DEVELOPMENT OF A CAPTURE-ELISA FOR THE SPECIFIC DETECTION
OF *MYCOPLASMA PNEUMONIAE* IN PATIENTS' MATERIAL

B. Gerstenecker and E. Jacobs

Department for Microbiology and Hygiene
University of Freiburg
D-7800 Freiburg, Germany

INTRODUCTION

The cell wall-less prokaryote *Mycoplasma pneumoniae* causes tracheo-bronchitis and severe pneumonia, especially in children (Foy *et al.*, 1983). Out-breaks of *M. pneumoniae* infections in families, school children, or in closed populations, *i.e..* military personnel, are common (Forsyth and Channock, 1966). Approximately 15 to 40% of all community-acquired pneumonias dur-ing epidemic periods are caused by *M. pneumoniae* (Foy *et al.*, 1979). The dis-ease is self-limiting, but serious clinical complications (encephalitis, mening-itis, myocarditis) were reported (Behan *et al.*, 1986; Chen *et al.*, 1986). The rout-ine diagnostic procedures of this disease are limited to serology, mostly the complement fixation test using a glycolipid extract of *M. pneumoniae* as anti-gen (Kenny and Newton, 1973). Isolation of the pathogen by culture methods is time-consuming and mostly without success. Recently, DNA- and RNA-probes for the detection of *M. pneumoniae* in clinical specimens have been de-veloped (Harris *et al.*, 1988; Göbel *et al.*, 1987). These probes cross-hybridized with the closely related species, *Mycoplasma genitalium*, recently co-isolated with *M. pneumoniae* out of throat swabs from vaccinated volunteers (Base-man *et al.*, 1988). Approaches of enzyme immunoassays using polyclonal capture- and polyclonal peroxidase-labelled detection antibodies (Kok *et al.*, 1988) also resulted in cross-reactions with *M. genitalium*. An immunoblot assay based on a monoclonal antibody with binding to a 43,000-molecular-weight protein of *M. pneumoniae* (Madson *et al.*, 1986; Madson *et al.*, 1988) was shown to cross-react to a protein antigen of *M. genitalium* of similar size (Cimolai *et al.*, 1987).

In our study, the P1-adhesin of *M. pneumoniae* was used as a target molecule for diagnostic purposes. The P1-protein is: (i) the major adhesin of this organism (Baseman *et al.*, 1982; Feldner *et al.*, 1982); (ii) it is concentrated

Rapid Diagnosis of Mycoplasmas, Edited by I. Kahane
and A. Adoni, Plenum Press, New York, 1993

in the tip organelle (Hu *et al.*, 1982); and (iii) it comprises approximately 1.5% of the total cell protein of *M. pneumoniae* (Jacobs and Clad, 1986).

A species-specific capture-ELISA for direct *M. pneumoniae* antigen detection using anti-P1 monoclonal antibodies was developed. The sensitivity was less than 10^3 cfu *M. pneumoniae* tested with artificially infected patient sputum.

MATERIALS AND METHODS

Reagents

All reagents for the capture ELISA, *i.e.*, coating buffer, sample preparation buffer (STD), washing buffer, dilution buffers, etc., were standardized Enzygnost® reagents kindly provided by Behringwerke, Marburg.

Organisms

The mycoplasma species *M. pneumoniae* (strain FH), *M. genitalium* (strain G37), *M. hominis*, *M. salivarium*, *M. fermentans* and *M. orale* were grown in Hayflick's modified Eagles medium (Hayflick, 1965) at 37∘C. Cells were harvested by centrifugation and washed twice with sterile phosphate buffered saline (PBS). The various bacterial isolates from clinical samples (Table 1) were grown on agar plates used in diagnostic microbiology laboratories. Viral preparations and control antigens were used as antigens for complement fixation tests (Behringwerke, Marburg).

Preparation of Polyclonal Anti-*M. pneumoniae* Antibodies

Rabbits were immunized by whole *M. pneumoniae* cell antigen or purified P1-adhesin (Jacobs *et al.*, 1988). The immunization scheme consists of subcutaneous injections of antigens in Freund's complete adjuvant followed in two-week intervals by three intravenous injections of the PBS-suspended antigens. Two weeks after the final injection, the rabbits were bled and antibody titres were tested by ELISA with immobilized whole *M. pneumoniae* cell antigen and isolated P-1 protein (Jacobs *et al.*, 1986a) and by Western immunoblots as described recently (Jacobs *et al.*, 1986b). The serum IgG antibodies were purified by Protein A affinity chromatography (Behringwerke, Marburg).

Monoclonal Antibodies

Monoclonal antibodies (mAbs) were produced against viable *M. pneumoniae* cells or purified P-1 protein according to the methods of de St. Groth and Scheidegger (1980). Spleen cells were fused PEG-mediated with X63-Ag-8.653 myeloma cells (Kearney *et al.*, 1979). After selection, the hybridoma microcultures were screened for secretion of antigen-specific antibodies using the capture-ELISA method (see below). Positive cultures were further expanded and subcloned by a limiting dilution technique. Selected hybridoma clones were cultured *in vivo* in female Balb/c-mice. Monoclonal antibodies were purified from ascites fluids by Protein A affinity chromatography (Behringwerke, Marburg). Fab- and F(ab)$_2$'-fragments were enzymatically prepared and conjugated with horseradish peoxidase (Behringwerke/Marburg).

Table 1. Important human pathogens causing pneumonia tested for cross-reactivity with the monoclonal antibodies used in the capture ELISA

Gram-positive bacteria	Gram-negative bacteria
Streptococcus pneumoniae	*Klebsiella pneumoniae*
Staphylococcus aureus	*Legionella pneumophila*
	Pseudomonas aeruginosa
Viruses	*Branhamella catarrhalis*
Parainfluenza 1 and 2	*Moraxella morganii*
Respiratory Syncytial Virus	*Escherichia coli*
Adenovirus	*Neisseria meningitidis*
Herpes simplex Virus	*Acinetobacter anitratus*
Influenza A and B	*Coxiella burnetti*
	Aeromonas hydrophila
Yeasts	*Haemophilus influenzae*
Candida albicans	*Haemophilus parainfluenzae*
Candida tropicalis	*Proteus mirabilis*
Torulopsis sp.	*Serratia marcescens*
	Neisseria elongata
	Neisseria lactamica
	Citrobacter freundii
	Chlamydia psittaci

Determination of Immunoglobulin Subclasses

Subclasses of the monoclonal antibodies were determined using a capture immunoassay according to the method of McDougal *et al.* (1983).

Specificity of the Antibodies

MAbs were characterized with immobilized sonicated whole *M. pneumoniae* antigen or with isolated P1-adhesin in ELISA tests, using intact *M. pneumoniae* cells (Gerstenecker and Jacobs, 1990), and radioimmunoprecipitation technique with 125J-labelled *M. pneumoniae* cells (Morrison, 1980) solubilized with Nonidet P-40 (Müller-Lantzsch *et al* , 1979). Antibodies were further analysed for adherence inhibiting activity (Jacobs *et al.* ,1985).

Capture-ELISA

Microtiter wells (Nunc, Roskilde/DK) were coated overnight with anti-*M. pneumoniae* or anti-P1 adhesin IgG-antibodies (100 ng IgG per 100 μl). Unspecific protein binding sites were blocked with 3% bovine serum albumin in distilled water (100 μl per well, 1h, 37oC). Antigen preparations were diluted in sample preparation buffer (STD) (see above) and incubated for 1 h at 37oC under agitation. The solubilized antigen was incubated with the preblocked capture antibodies (1h, 37oC, 100 μl/well). After washing, the wells were further incubated with the various mAb preparations (1h, 37oC). Bound unlabeled antibodies were detected with peroxidase-conjugated rabbit anti-mouse antibodies (Behringwerke, Marburg). After final washing, substrate solution with tetramethyl-benzidine as a chromogen was added and incubated at room temperature for 1 h (screening with hybridoma culture supernatants) or 30 min (routine testing with purified peroxidase-labelled mAbs). Substrate react-

Table 2. Binding characteristics of different monoclonal antibodies used in the capture ELISA

mAb	Ig-suclass	Cell-ELISA[1]	Adherence inh. activity	P1-recognition in immunoblot
P1.58	IgG$_1$	+	+	+
P1.26[2]	IgG$_1$	+	+	+
M51[2]	IgG$_{2b}$	+	+	+
M46	IgG$_1$	+	+	+
P1.25	IgG$_1$	+	-	-
P1.27	IgG$_1$	-	-	-
M74	IgG$_1$	+	-	+
M75	IgG$_1$	(+)	-	-
M57	IgG$_1$	-	-	-

[1] partially fixed *M. pneumoniae* cells immobilized to a solid support were used as an antigen.
[2] mAbs are further characterized (Gerstenecker and Jacobs, 1990)

ion was stopped with 0,5 N sulfuric acid and the color development was measured photometrically at 450 nm.

Artificial Infection of Clinical Specimens

One hundred sputum samples from patients without clinical symptoms were collected and pretested in the capture ELISA. The bacterial flora was screened for Fc-receptor carrying organisms (*Staphylococcus aureus*, Streptococcus group G). Groups of 5-10 individual sputa were combined to various pools. Aliquots of each pool were inoculated with untreated *M. pneumoniae* (10 µl, 10 mg protein/ml). Inoculated aliquots from each sputum pool were solubilized in sample preparation buffer and centrifuged (10,000 g, Eppendorf). The supernatants were used for antigen detection. To determine the sensitivity of the test, *M. pneumoniae* preparations (starting with 10 µg/well) were diluted in the patient material.

RESULTS

Screening of Monoclonal Antibodies

572 hybridoma culture supernatants were screened for reactivity with solubilized *Mycoplasma pneumoniae* antigen which was captured by solid-phase bound rabbit anti-*M. pneumoniae* IgG antibodies. Antibodies from 36 supernatants showed binding to the immunofixed antigen. These monoclonal antibodies (mAbs) were further characterized with different methods: (i) ELISA with solid-phase-immobilized sonicated *M. pneumoniae* cells; (ii) ELISA with immobilized isolated P1 adhesin; (iii) ELISA using immobilized partially fixed intact *M. pneumoniae* cells; (iv) radioimmunoprecipitation with [125]J-labelled *M. pneumoniae* cells solubilized with Nonidet P-40; and (v) Western immunoblots. The specificity of the selected antibodies is shown in Table 2. All

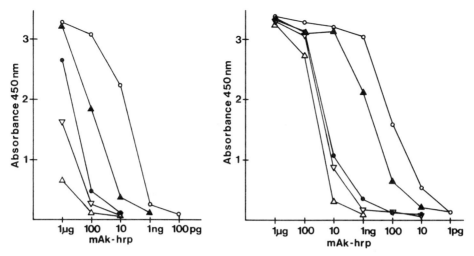

Figure 1. Avidity of peroxidase (hrp)-labelled intact mAbs P1.25 (o); P1.27 (•); M57 (Δ); M74 (▲); and M75 (▽); in capture ELISA with the catching antibodies anti-P1-IgG (left) and anti-Mp-IgG (right); capture antibodies were saturated with *M. pneumoniae* antigen (10 μg total cell protein per 100 μl).

mAbs recognized sonicated *M. pneumoniae* cells and purified P1-adhesin in ELISA. In the capture-system the mAbs were non-reactive with various bacteria, yeast and viruses found in the respiratory tract (Table 1). Furthermore, beside mAbs P1.58, P1.26, M46 and M51 which were binding to *M. salivarium* and *M. hominis*, anti-P1 mAbs P1.25, P1.27, M57, M74 and M75 proved to be species-specific.

Capture and Detection Antibodies

Two polyclonal IgG preparations with different specificities were analyzed for optimal binding and presentation of *M. pneumoniae* antigen to the mAbs: monospecific anti-P1 adhesin antibodies (anti-P1 IgG) and anti-*M. pneumoniae* antibodies directed against intact cells (anti-Mp-IgG). The avidity of the species-specific mAbs in capture assays with these two antibodies is shown in Fig. 1. All mAbs recognized the antigens bound to monospecific anti-P1-IgG with decreased avidity compared with the reactivity with anti-Mp-IgG captured antigen.

Four different *M. pneumoniae* strains isolated from patients suffering from *Mycoplasma pneumoniae* disease and four reisolates from experimentally infected guinea pigs were analyzed. As shown in Figure 2, the mAbs P1.25 and M74 recognized epitopes on all *M. pneumoniae* strains tested.

Influence of clinical specimens

One hundred sputum samples from patients with other than *M. pneumoniae*- induced pneumonia or tracheobronchitis were tested as aliquots with

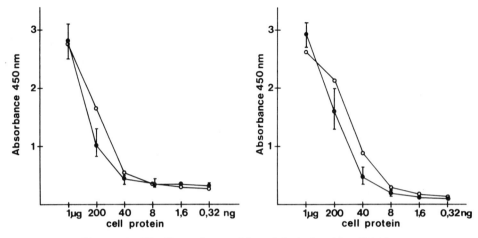

Figure 2. Binding of peroxidase-labeled mAbs P1.25 (left) and M74 (right) to epitopes on eight *M. pneumoniae* isolates (●) compared with the recognition of the reference antigen *M. pneumoniae* strain FH (o); vertical bars represent the deviations from the median.

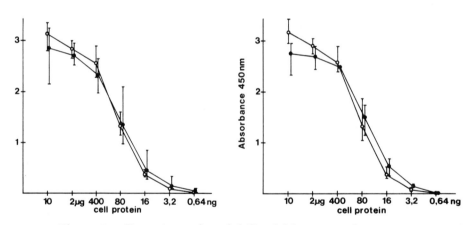

Figure 3. Detection of solubilized *M. pneumoniae* antigen in patient material (●) and in the reference system (o) (solubilization buffer only) with the species-specific mAbs P1.25 (left) and M74 (right); vertical bars indicate the deviations of individual repeats (n = 3) from the median.

Table 3. Comparison of the sensitivities resulting from capture-ELISA with anti-Mp-IgG capture antibodies and various preparations of species-specific monoclonal antibodies.

mAb	Fragment	ng mAb[1]	cut-off (ng/ml)[2]
P1.25	-	2, 5	60
	F(ab')$_2$	2	15
	Fab	2	< 7. 5
M74	-	20	< 15
	F(ab')$_2$	500	30
	Fab	5	< 15

[1] optimized concentrations of peroxidase-labeled antibodies (ng protein per 100µl).

[2] representing the *M. pneumoniae* cell protein concentration (ng/ml) which gives an absorbance at 450 nm twice of the capture ELISA performed in the absence of specific antigen.

and without experimentally added *M. pneumoniae* antigen. The recognition of the specific antigen in patient material is demonstrated for mAbs P1.25 and M74 (Figure 3). The signals (absorbance 450 nm (A_{450})) showed no difference between the detection of *M. pneumoniae* antigen in sample preparation buffer only compared to the antigen mixed in solubilized sputa. In the assay with 'uninfected' sputum samples, unspecific background was not altered (A_{450} 0.1-0.15).

Improvement of sensitivity

Purified F(ab')$_2$- and Fab-fragments of mAb P1.25 were as reactive as the intact antibody (data not shown). On the other hand, sensitivity was increased by reducing the molecular mass of the antibody P1.25 (Table 3). In contrast, reactivity of F(ab')$_2$-fragments of mAb M74 was reduced, whereas avidity of Fab fragments was comparable to the intact antibody. Sensitivity of the test with M74- Fab as detection antibody was reduced when using F(ab')$_2$ fragments (Table 3). The potential of mAb mixtures for increasing sensitivity was determined. Homogeneous monoclonal capture systems and 'additivity assays' according to the method of Friguet *et al.*, (1983) were used for epitope analysis. Fab fragments of mAbs P1.25 and M74 apparently bind independently to their epitopes on captured solubilized antigen (data not shown). Antibody concentrations of P1.25 and M74 mixtures were further optimized by chess-board titrations. Using a test with an optimal antibody mixture (100 ng protein of each mAb), it was possible to detect less than 600 pg *M. pneumoniae* protein (<6 pg P1-protein, <103 CFU). No difference in sensitivity was found when the capture-ELISA was performed either as sequential assay (two incubation steps: (i) antigen, (ii) mAbs, or as a 'one-step-assay' (one incubation step: antigen and mAbs simultaneously) (data not shown).

DISCUSSION

Main problems of antigen detection systems are specificity, sensitivity and handling. The antibodies used in the capture ELISA were tested for specificity with a wide range of microorganisms found in the human respiratory tract and the oral cavity, including pathogenic bacteria, viruses and yeasts. Additionally, several mycoplasma species including *Mycoplasma genitalium* were analyzed. Polyclonal capture anti-*M. pneumoniae*-IgG antibodies tested in a homogeneous assay did not recognize any of the various microorganisms listed in Table 1, but bound all mycoplasma species tested.

Some of the mAbs cross-reacted with *M. hominis* and *M. salivarium* antigens. About 64%, or 1% of healthy persons, carry *M. salivarium* or *M. hominis*, respectively, in the oral cavity (Watanabe *et al.*, 1983) and thus might interfere with the *M. pneumoniae* detection. Therefore, these antibodies could not be used in a specific *M. pneumoniae* antigen detection test.

A particular problem is the antigenic relationship of *M. pneumoniae* with *M. genitalium*. The latter was primarily found in the human genital tract (Tully *et al.*, 1981), but a recent report suggest a possible occurence also in the respiratory tract (Baseman *et al.*, 1988). Any diagnostic system should be able to discriminate between these two species. This is not achieved by several systems (cDNA probe (Harris *et al.*, 1988), polymerase chain reaction (Jensen *et al.*, 1989), capture-ELISA using poylclonal antibodies only (Kok *et al.*, 1988), Western immunoblots probing with mAbs (Cimolai *et al.*, 1987).

Five of our mAbs (P1.25, P1.27, M57, M74, M75) recognized only epitopes of various *M. pneumoniae* isolates, but did not cross-react with the various mycoplasma species tested, especially with *M. genitalium*.

An additional problem can occur with microorganims carrying Fc-binding proteins, *e.g.*, *Staphylococcus aureus*, streptococci group G), which could unspecifically react with intact antibodies. We therefore used Fab-fragments of the mAbs P1.25 and M74 which were as reactive as the intact antibody. The sensitivity of the assays was about 10^4 CFU in 100 µl. Using optimized antibody mixtures, the detection limit was lowered to 600 pg *M. pneumoniae* total cell protein (approximately 10^3 CFU). With this sensitivity, clinical application seems promising, because the quantities of *M. pneumoniae* cells found in patient sputum are within the range of 10^2 to 10^6 CFU/ml (Collier and Clyde, 1974). The detection limit of this capture ELISA competes with results obtained with rRNA probes ($<10^3$ CFU) (Göbel *et al.*, 1987), PCR (10^2 to 10^3 CFU (Bernet *et al.*, 1989)) and capture ELISAs based on poylclonal antibodies ($<10^3$ CFU) (Helbig and Witzleb, 1984).

The use of monoclonal antibodies as specific probes in antigen detection has further advantages as compared to oligonucleotide probes. Protein antigens as target molecles are more easily stabilized by detergents and protected against degrading activities (proteases) than RNA or DNA targets. The *M. pneumoniae* antigen can be stored by refrigerating or freezing the sample without affecting the sensitivity of the capture ELISA (data not shown). In contrast, the sensitivity of solid-phase hybridization with short DNA and rRNA probes is diminished 100-fold after freeze-thaw cycles (Göbel *et al.*, 1987).

The capture ELISA permits rapid and specific detection of M. *pneumoniae* antigen. A sample can be analyzed within 3.5 h (sequential assay) or 2.5 h (one- step assay), whereas detection methods using radiolabeled oligonucleotides need, minimally, about one day. Furthermore, an ELISA can be run automatically, without limitation of sample numbers, in automatic processors so that the test is an acceptable method for diagnostic laboratories to detect M. *pneumoniae* infections in time.

ACKNOWLEDGEMENTS

This work was supported by grants of the Bundesministerium für Forschung und Technologie (01 ZR 171). We are grateful to the Behringwerke AG (PBox 1140, D-3550 Marburg 1), especially Dr. W. Schuy for providing reagents, antibody purification, enzyme conjugation and discussion.

REFERENCES

Baseman, J. B., Dallo, S. F., Tully, J. G. and Rose, D. L. (1988) Isolation and characterization of *Mycoplasma genitalium* strains from the human respiratory tract. J. Clin. Microbiol. 26:2266-2269.

Baseman, J. B., Banai, M. and Kahane, I. (1982) Sialic acid residues mediate *Mycoplasma pneumoniae* attachment to human and sheep erythrocytes. Infect. Immun. 3:389-391.

Behan, P. O., Feldman, R. G., Segerra, J. M.and Draper, I. T. (1986) Neurological aspects of mycoplasmal infections. Acta Neurolog. Scand. 74:314-322.

Bernet, C., Garret, M., deBarbeyrac, B., Bébéar, C., and Bonnet, J. (1989) Detection of *Mycoplasma pneumoniae* by using the polymerase chain reaction. J. Clin. Microbiol. 27:2492-2496.

Chen, S.-C., Tsai, C. C., and Nouri, S. (1986) Carditis associated with *Mycoplasma pneumoniae*. Am. J. Dis. Children 140:471-472.

Cimolai, N., Bryan, L. E., Woods, D. E. (1987) Immunological cross-reactivity of a *Mycoplasma pneumoniae* membrane-associated protein antigen with *Mycoplasma genitalium* and *Acholeplasma laidlawii*. J. Clin. Microbiol. 25:2136-2139.

Collier, A. and Clyde, W. A. (1974) Appearance of *Mycoplasma pneumoniae* in lungs of experimentally infected hamsters and patients with natural disease. Am. Rev. Respir. Dis. 110:765-773.

de St.Groth, S. F. and Scheidegger, D. (1980) Production of monoclonal antibodies: strategy and tactics. J. Immun. Methods 35:1-21.

Feldner, J., Göbel, U. and Bredt, W. (1982) *Mycoplasma pneumoniae* adhesin localized to tip structure by monoclonal antibody. Nature (London) 298:765-767.

Forsyth, B. R. and Channock, R. M. (1966) *Mycoplasmae pneumoniae*, in: "Annual Review of Medicine", (A. C. DeGraff and W. P. Creger, Eds.), pp. 371-382. Annual Reviews Inc., Palo Alto.

Foy, H. M., Kenny, G. E., Cooney, M .K. and Allan, I. D. (1979) Long-term epidemiology of infections with *Mycoplasma pneumoniae*. J. Infect. Dis. 139:681-687.

Foy, H. M., Kenny, G. E., Cooney, M. K., Allan, I. D. and Van Belle, G. (1983) Naturally acquired immunity to pneumonia due to *Mycoplasma pneumoniae*. J. Infect. Dis. 147:967-973.

Friguet, B., Djavadi-Ohaniance, L., Pages, J., Bussard, A. and Goldberg, M. (1983) A convenient enzyme-linked immunosorbent assay for testing whether monoclonal antibodies recognize the same antigenic site. Application to hybridomas specific for the ß$_2$-subunit of *Escherichia coli* tryptophan synthase. J. Immunol. Meth. 60:351-358.

Gerstenecker, B. and Jacobs, E. (1990) Topological mapping of the P1-adhesin of *Mycoplasma pneumoniae* with adherence-inhibiting monoclonal antibodies. J. Gen. Microbiol. 136:471-476.

Göbel, U. B., Geiser, A. and Stanbridge, E. J. (1987) Oligonucleotide probes complementary to variable regions of ribosomal RNA discriminate between *Mycoplasma* species. J. Gen. Microbiol. 133:1969-1974.

Harris, R., Marmion, B. P., Varkanis, G., Kok, T., Lunn, B. and Martin, J. (1988) Laboratory diagnosis of *Mycoplasma pneumoniae* infection. 2. Comparison of methods for the direct detection of specific antigen or nucleic acid sequences in respiratory exudates. Epidem. Infec. 101:685-694.

Hayflick, L. (1965) Tissue cultures and mycoplasmas. Texas Reports Biol. Med. 23:285-303.

Helbig, J. H. and Witzleb, W. (1984) Enzyme-linked immunosorbent assay (ELISA) zum Antigennachweis von *Mycoplasma pneumoniae*. Zeitschrift für die Gesamte Hygiene und ihre Grenzgebiete 30:106-107.

Hu, P.-C., Cole, R. M., Huang, Y. S., Graham, J. A., Gardner, D. E., Collier, A. M. and Clyde, W. A. (1982) *Mycoplasma pneumonie* infection: role of a surface protein in attachment organelle. Science 216:313-315.

Jacobs, E., Schöpperle, K. and Bredt, W. (1985) Adherence inhibiting assay: a specific serological test for detection of antibodies to *Mycoplasma pneumoniae*. EJCM 4:113-118.

Jacobs, E. and Clad, A. (1986) Electroelution of fixed and stained membrane proteins from preparative sodium dodecylsulfate polyacrylamide gels into a mebrane trap. Analyt. Biochem. 154:583-589.

Jacobs, E., Fuchte, K. and Bredt, W. (1988) Isolation of the adherence protein of *Mycoplasma pneumoniae* by fractioned solubilization and size exclusion chromatography. Biol. Chem. Hoppe-Seyler 369:1295-1299.

Jacobs, E., Fuchte, K., and Bredt, W. (1986a) A 168 kilodalton protein of *Mycoplasma pneumoniae* used as antigen in a dot enzyme-linked immunosorbent assay. EJCM 5:435-440.

Jacobs, E., Bennewitz, A. and Bredt, W. (1986b) Reaction pattern of human anti-*Mycoplasma pneumoniae* antibodies in enzyme-linked immunosorbent assays and immunoblotting. J. Clin. Microbiol. 23:517-522.

Jensen, J. S., Sondergard-Anderson, J., Uldum, S. A. and Lind, K. (1989) Detection of *Mycoplasma pneumoniae* in simulated clinical samples by polymerase chain reaction. Acta Pathol. Microbiol. Immunol. Scand. 97:1046-1048.

Kearney, J. F., Radbruch, A., Liesegang, B. and Rajewski, K. (1979) A new mouse myeloma cell line that has lost immunoglobulin expression but permits the construction of antibody-secreting hybrid cell lines. J. Immunol. 123:1548-1550.

Kenny, G. E. and Newton, R. M. (1973) Close serological relationship between glycolipids of *Mycoplasma pneumoniae* and glycolipids of spinach. Annals of the New York Acad. Sci. 225:54-61.

Kok, T.-W., Varkanis, G. and Marmion, B.P. (1988) Laboratory diagnosis of *Mycoplasma pneumoniae* infection. 1. Direct detection of antigen in respiratory exudates by enzyme immunoassay. Epidemiology and Infection. 101:669-684.

Madsen, R. D., Weiner, L. B., McMillan, J., Saeed, F. A., North, J. A. and Coates, S. R. (1988) Direct detection of *Mycoplasma pneumoniae* antigen in clinical specimen by a monoclonal antibody immunoblot assay. Am. J. Clin. Pathol. 89:95-99.

Madsen, R. D., Saeed, F .A., Gray, O., Fendly, B. M. and Coates, S. R. (1986) Species-specific monoclonal antibody to a 43,000-molecular-weight membrane protein of *Mycoplasma pneumoniae*. J. Clin. Microbiol. 24:680-683.

McDougal, J. S., Browning, S. W., Kennedy, S. and Moore, D. D. (1983) Immunodot assay for determining the isotype and light chain type of murine monoclonal antibodies in unconcentrated hybridoma culture supernatants. J. Immunol. Meth. 63:281-290.

Morrison, M. (1980) Lactoperoxidase-catalysed iodination as a tool for investigation of proteins. Meth. Enzymol. 70:214-220.

Müller-Lantzsch, N., Yamamoto, N. and zurHausen, H. (1979) Analysis of early and late Eppstein-Barr virus associated polypeptides by immunoprecipitation. Virology 97:378-387.

Tully, J. G., Taylor-Robinson, D., Cole, R. M. and Rose, D.L. (1981) A newly discovered mycoplasma in the human urogenital tract. Lancet I., 1288-1291.

Watanabe, T., Matsuura, M. and Seto, K. (1983) Enumeration, isolation, and species identification of *Mycoplasmas* in saliva sampled from the normal and pathological human oral cavity and antibody responses to an oral *Mycoplasma* (*Mycoplasma salivarium*). J. Clin. Microbiology 23:1034-1038.

IDENTIFICATION OF MOLLICUTES BY IMMUNOBLOTTING

Shulamith Horowitz

Department of Microbiology and Immunology
Faculty of Health Sciences, Ben-Gurion
University of the Negev, Beer-Sheva, Israel

INTRODUCTION

Immunoblotting (IB) technique combines the resolution of gel electrophoresis with the specificity of immunochemical detection. It is used to detect specific antigens in a protein mixture with an antibody and to evaluate the purity or the complexity of this mixture. Since Towbin described the procedure (1979), numerous protocols evolved during the years using various gel systems, different immobilizing matrices, modified buffer systems, diversity of ligands and variety of washing and blocking conditions. There is no ideal procedure, and the technique should be examined according to one's need and the conditions be determined empirically for each specific system investigated.

The IB procedure is comprised of several steps: preparation of the antigen sample; resolution of the protein sample by gel electrophoresis; transfer of the separated polypeptides to a membrane support; blocking non-specific binding sites on the membrane; addition of the antibody; and detection of antigens. There are multiple steps and parameters, and slight modifications are frequently introduced by investigators, there are often discrepancies in results reported by various laboratories investigating the same system.

PARAMETERS THAT AFFECT BLOT ANALYSIS

Resolution of the proteins by gel electrophoresis

Sample preparation. The appropriate amount and the concentration of proteins in the sample to be used should be determined prior to IB analysis, especially when dealing with bacterial cells. To ensure that the relative amount of the antigen in the sample is above the limit of detection, one should consider either the use of µg protein (representing protein content) or growth units, *i.e.*, CFU (representing viable cells).

Introduction of proteases' inhibitors into the sample can preserve proteins from degradation and addition of DNase or RNAse is sometimes helpful, especially if staining is performed later.

Solubilization of cells and membranes is required for the extraction and the dissociation of proteins and for the optimal separation in the gel electrophoresis. This is achieved only in the presence of anionic detergents, *e.g.*, SDS, and reducing agents, *e.g.*, 2-ME. Since these reagents might be detrimental to the protein configuration, optimal conditions for solubilization of a given protein mixture should be determined prior to antigen analysis to ensure the minimal possible protein denaturation.

Protein resolution. The separation of a protein into its peptides can be performed in two types of gel systems: one-dimensional polyacrylamide-gel-electrophoresis (PAGE); and two-dimensional PAGE, which provides increased resolution of proteins due to isoelectrofocusing performed in the first dimension. In both systems, the concentration of the acrylamide and the cross-linker will affect both the migration of the proteins and their elution from the gel.

Transfer of proteins to immobilizing matrix

Electrotransfer. Immediate transfer after the PAGE is preferable, although other methods were also used. Constant voltage is usually used, but as electrolytes are eluted from the gel, the conductivity of the buffer rises and the resistance decreases. In order to maintain constant voltage, it is necessary to increase current, resulting in heating, which also reduces the resistance. The use of constant current, if a proper power supply is available, and precooling of the transfer buffer, may solve these problems.

Immobilizing matrix. The most commonly used matrix is nitrocellulose filter (NC), although it has some limitations, *i.e.*, it is negatively charged, has a moderate binding capacity for protein, and non-ionic detergents will remove bound proteins from it. The matrix density might affect the final results, as smaller pore size improves the binding of the peptides.

Other factors. The quality of the blot is affected also by: 1) the electroblot apparatus and location of the gel-NC assembly in the apparatus; 2) the buffer composition (SDS and/or methanol) which determines the buffer conductivity, the current generated, the efficiency of the elution and the binding of protein to NC. However, elution without methanol might be better, but then proteins will not adsorb well to the matrix, especially the low molecular weight ones.

Quenching

Blocking the unoccupied binding sites to prevent nonspecific binding is achieved by incubation with a buffer solution containing a quencher, most often an inert protein (BSA, gelatin, FCS, milk). Optimization of the quenching is critical in obtaining acceptable signal-to-background ratio, as overquenching may occur when detergent is used. The latter might remove proteins from the matrix, or cause non-specific binding of the probe, or interfere with association of the probe to the protein on the matrix. These points should also be considered when determining the washings conditions.

Addition of antibody

IB does not require high affinity antibodies due to both the exposure of different epitopes on denaturation and the high local concentration of antigens on the membrane. The types of antibody preparations commonly used for IB are:

Polyclonal antibodies. These are widly used, and most of them will bind to denatured epitopes, resulting in a strong signal. Due to their high concentration in serum, high dilutions of sera can be used resulting in decreased background. However, analysis of microbial antigens with polyclonal antibodies might be complicated, due to presence of antibodies against common bacterial antigens in the serum. Preadsorption of sera with antigens, non-relevant to the system investigated, is one of the ways to solve this problem

Monoclonal antibodies (mAb). The major advantage in using MAb is their high specificity to one epitope. MAb will cross-react with all polypeptides that have the same primary sequence of amino acids and, therefore, it is useful to use MAb to detect related antigens. The major disadvantage in using MAb in IB is that they may not recognize denatured epitopes (see below).

Probing

Protein blots are probed either by radiolabelled second antibody or by enzyme-conjugated second antibody. It is advisable to use large volumes of fluid at this step to avoid non-uniform background. Non-ionic detergents can be introduced if the background is high, but with caution, since excess detergent may diminish the signal.

Signal detection

The sensitivity of the IB is also determined by the detection method. Autoradigraphy is more sensitive than enzyme-conjugate detection and exposures can be repeated to obtain optimal signals; however, using enzyme conjugates is less hazardous and the resolution is superior to autoradiography.

GENERAL USES OF IMMUNOBLOTTING

Antigen detection

A major use of IB is the determination of the presence of antigens in a protein mixture, their quantity, the relative molecular weight of the polypeptide chains, and the efficiency of antigen extraction from cells and membranes. IB is useful when dealing with antigens that are insoluble, difficult to label, or easily degraded. Only the steady-state level of an antigen can be determined by IB and further analysis of its biochemical properties is not possible.

Antibody detection

Another major use of IB is assaying the presence, quantity and specificity of antibodies from different samples of polyclonal sera and monoclonal antibodies in immunized animals and in hybridomas. It can be also used to purify specific antibodies from polyclonal sera.

In conclusion, the major factor that will determine the success of an IB procedure is the nature of the epitopes recognized by the antibodies. Since most PAGE techniques involve denaturation of the antigen sample, only antibodies that recognize denaturation-resistant epitopes will bind. Most polyclonal sera contain antibodies of this type. MAbs, as highly specific probes, may not detect a determinant that is sensitive to the electrophoretic process itself.

USES OF IMMUNOBLOTTING IN MYCOPLASMOLOGY

The immunoblotting technique was applied to the field of Mycoplasmology in the last decade, and was used to identify antigens (surface and others) of animal, human and plant *Mollicutes*. Most of the work published is concerned with *Mollicutes* of pathogenic potential.

Identification of virulence factors

Once it was recognized that adherence activities of mycoplasmas are localized on the surface, and that these activities determine the virulence, membranes of these organisms were studied extensively by the use of the IB. For example, in *M. pneumoniae*, a protein of 170 kDa designated P1 was first identified by IB and characterized as the major component in the attachment and adherance of this organism to epithelial cells (Hu *et al.*, 1982). The role of this peptide in pathogenesis was demonstrated when a monoclonal antibody to P1 inhibited the attachment of this organism to its host cells (reviewed in Baseman, 1993). In other research groups, mAb anti-*M. pneumoniae* with other specificities were obtained, *e.g.*, Chandler *et al.* 1989. As expected, not every mAb that identifies antigens by IB has inhibitory biological activity. Thus, antigens that are detected by biologically active antibodies can be used for vaccine development, while antigens detected by antibodies with no biological activity can be used as a diagnostic tool, as long as they are species-specific. Along this line of thought, surface components were investigated also in other mycoplasmas, *e.g.*, *M. pulmonis*, a rodent mycoplasma which causes a pulmonary disease similar to human pneumonia in mice and rats. IB was by 1D-PAGE, or by the higher resolution 2D-PAGE, ap-peared upon staining as multiple bands or multiple spots, respectively. But, out of all these peptides of various pI and different molecular weights, the major antigens have been detected by the use of IB with sera from infected mice (Horowitz *et al.* 1987). A unique antigen with a "ladder" pattern, shown to be surface exposed, was proven by the IB to be an immunodominant antigen, as it was recognized by sera from naturally infected mice (Figure 1). This surface antigen, termed V-1, varies among the different strains of *M. pulmonis* and the heterogeneity of its structure was shown to be associated with variable degrees of virulence of these strains (Watson et al 1988; Davidson 1988).

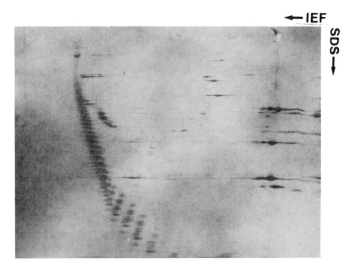

← IEF

SDS ↓

Figure 1.   Immunoblot of *M. pulmonis* membranes resolved by 2-D PAGE, and reacted with a serum from naturally infected mouse. From Horowitz *et al.*, 1987, reproduced by permission)

Other mycoplasmas were analyzed as well by this route, using IB (*e.g.* Ureaplasma urealyticum) for the purpose of characterization of antigenic determinants on the their surface. This is one of the important issues in mycoplasma research because of the direct involvment of this surface with host cells and with the host immune system (Cole *et al.*1985).

Characterization of antigens expressed in disease

Interestingly, a ladder-like antigen was also found in certain serotypes of *U. urealyticum* by IB with immune rabbit sera (Horowitz, *et al.*, 1986). Recently, we detected this antigen with sera from patients infected with ureaplasma and who had high titers of specific anti-*U. urealyticum* antibodies as measured by ELISA. In a case of chronic infection with ureaplasma that was treated and became clinically cured and culture negative, IB with the patient's convalesent serum demonstrated the disappearance of the antibodies to this "ladder" antigen. We detected this antigen in patients with pregnancy complications having an intrauterine infection with ureaplasma. Thus, it is tempting to speculate that this antigen is of pathogenic significance in humans as well.

Epitope localization and strain variability

Antigenic differences within a species is a known phenomenon, recognized in mycoplasmas long ago by antibodies possesing biological activities (Gois *et al.*, 1974). The use of IB and the availability of mAb make it possible to recognize distinct epitopes selectively expressed on the surface of some mycoplasmas, and thus differentiate among strains. Extensive work was done with *M. hyorhinis* strains. A 23 kDa membrane lipoprotein antigen, identified in one strain, bears an epitope that is shared by other strains tested, but is local-

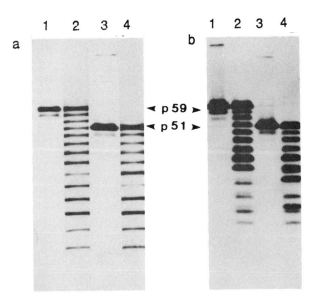

Figure 2. Immunoblots with mAb of *M. hyorhinis* size-variants (lanes 1 and 3) and of enzyme-digested variants (lanes 2 and 4), either with trypsin (A) or with carboxypeptidase Y (B). (From Rosengarten and Wise, with permission, Copyright 1990 by the AAAS)

ized on various proteins in the different strains, *e.g.*, on the 23 kDa, or 55 kDa, or 50 kDa lipoproteins (Boyer and Wise, 1989). These size-variants of one surface antigen reflects the difference among these strains. Moreover, within a given strain itself, a phenotypic instability was observed and was shown by IB with a mAb to correlate with antigenic variation of the surface lipoprotein (Rosengarten and Wise, 1990). The structural features and the orientation of the variant surface lipoproteins were characterized by immunoblotting of the enzyme-digests of these proteins (Figure 2). Thus, antigenically distinct surface proteins that contain highly repetitive structure and undergo high-frequency variation were identified.

The work described above was done with mAb, but for certain purposes, polyclonal antibodies are usful. For example, it is possible to identify differences among ureaplasmal serovars by IB with patients' sera (Horowitz *et al.*, unpublished data). Each serovar, when blotted with sera from infected humans, demonstrates a number of antigens that are either shared by all serovars of the same biotype or those that are serovar-specific. Some of these antigens were constantly expressed during the disease state. Disappearance of antibody reactivity to certain ureaplasmal antigens in convalescent sera was also reported before (Lee and Kenny, 1987). Thus, it is possible to investigate the involvement of various serotypes in the pathogenesis of disease by IB with patients' sera.

Such approach has been taken concerning *M. hominis* antigens. An antigen of 102.7 kDa was shown to be present in all strains of this mycoplasma and was detected by IB with sera from patients infected with *M. hominis* (Andersen *et al.*, 1987; Cassell *et al.*, 1988). In another research, other proteins were suggested to be indicative of a disease caused by this organism, 50 kDa and 58 kDa (Schalla and Harrison, 1987). These protein antigens were detected by IB only with sera from infected women that had pregnacy complications and were not detected in other human mycoplasmas. Therefore, by definition, the antigens identified in either of the reports described above are of diagnostic significance.

PROBLEMS IN IDENTIFICATION OF *MOLLICUTES* BY IMMUNOBLOTTING

Antigens derived from cells cultured in enriched media

Mycoplasma are cultured in broth supplemented with serum. It is possible that certain proteins detected by IB are not genuine mycoplasmal, but rather medium contaminants. This problem can be solved in several ways: a) dilution of the antibodies in broth/serum to adsorb any anti-medium cross-reactivity that might have been present; b) preadsorbtion of antisera with broth components; and c) use of purified antigens (Horowitz and Gal, 1991).

Major proteins are not necessarily major antigens

In the case of ureaplasma cells, biosynthetically labelled with ^{35}S-methionine, the major cell proteins of serovar 4 are 45 kDa and 66 kDa, while the major antigen identified by IB with patients' sera is a 50 kDa peptide (S. Horowitz, in preparation). In addition, different peptides which are detected by IB with a mAb may share the same exact epitope but they may not necessarily have the same function.

Many mycoplasmas share common epitopes

One example is the serological cross-reactivity shown between *M. genitalium* and *M. pneumoniae* (Taylor-Robinson, 1983). The crossreactive epitopes identified by IB were shown to be located on the P1 adhesin of *M. pneumonia* and the 140 kDa protein of *M. genitalium* (Morrison-Plummer *et al.*, 1987).

In *M. pulmonis,* of 250 peptides identified by 2D-PAGE, 15 were shared by other rodent mycoplasmas (Watson *et al.*, 1987). Obviously, none of these 15 peptides can serve for identification of *M. pulmonis* infection. Another example is the analysis of seven strains of caprine mycoplasmas. By 2D-PAGE combined with IB, crossreactivity among these strains was demonstrated (Olsson *et al.*, 1990).

Mycoplasmas share epitopes with eubacteria

Evidence that mycoplasma, gram-negative bacteria, and certain gram-positive bacteria share a similar protein antigen was demonstrated by IB (Sasaki, 1991). Thus, if sera from humans or from immunized animals are used in IB, cross-reactions might occur between mycoplasmal polypeptides and common epitopes derived from structurally similar non-mycoplasmal antigens.

High frequency of antigenic variation

Antigenic variation was observed in various mycoplasmas (see above) and consequently the identification of specific antigens that are relevant to pathogenesis or significant in diagnosis became more complex.

Laboratory strains might differ from the *in vivo* strains

Multiple passages of the organisms in the enriched culture media and antigenic variations described above might result in the appearance or disappearance of certain peptides in the IB analysis. Therefore, a routine examination of the laboratory strains used in repeated experiments, especially in the sensitive technique of IB, is recomended.

Highly sensitive assays are not always highly specific

The use of highly sensitive assays with a crude antigen might be misleading, since the high sensitivity results in lower specificity, demonstrating false-positive cross-reactivity. The use of purified or partially purified antigenic preparations might solve this problem.

SUMMARY

The major uses of IB in mycoplasmology have been the investigation of antigens and their role in the biology of mycoplasmas and the identification of mycoplasmal cell components that are valuable for diagnostic purposes.

It should be stressed that the interpretation of the results should be done with caution, since modifications in the conditions used in this procedure greatly affect the outcome of the IB.

In spite of the limitations described above, most of which can be overcome, IB is a powerful and important tool in the investigation of mycoplasmas. Much of the knowledge available today on structure of surface components of mycoplasmas, on variability among strains, and about homology among species would not be obtained without this technique.

PROCEDURE

SDS-PAGE

Reagents

1. Stock acrylamide:bis-acrylamide - 29.2%:0.8% (w/v) in H_2O
2. 10% SDS in water
3. 1.5 M Tris-HCL pH 8.8
4. 0.5 M Tris-HCL pH 6.8
5. TEMED (tetramethylethelenediamine)
6. 10% ammonium persulfate (APS) (fresh, in water)
7. Sample buffer (3 x concentrated):100 mM Tris-HCL pH 6.8, 20% glycerol, 4% SDS, 0.1% bromophenol-blue,2-mercapto-ethanol

8.   Running buffer: 25 mM Tris, 192 mM glycine, 0.1% SDS, pH 8.3

Equipment

1.   A pair of glass plates
2.   Spacers
3.   Comb
4.   Gel apparatus + electrical leads
5.   Power supply

Preparation of gel

1.   Clean glass plates (acetone, alcohol, water and dry by air).
2.   Assemble glass plates and spacers and secure in casting stand; mark 3.0 cm from the top.
3.   Prepare 10% polyacrylamide separating gel:mix 10 ml stock acrylamide, 7.5 ml 1.5 M Tris-HCL pH 8.8, 0.3 ml 10% SDS, add water to final volume 30 ml. Mix well, degas for 5 min, add 20 µl TEMED, mix and add 150 µl 10% APS. Mix and pour the gel up to the mark (see 2.)
4.   Overlay separating gel with iso-butanol. Allow gel to polymerize about 30-60 min.
5.   Wash interface with water and cast stacking gel:4% (1.33 ml) acrylamide:bisacrylamide in 125 mM Tris-HCL pH 6.8 (1.25 ml)/0.1% SDS (0.1 ml)/5 µl TEMED/50 µl APS (=10 ml).
6.   Insert the comb and allow to polymerize (15-30 min).
7.   Assemble gel in apparatus: Take the comb out from between the glass plates, remove bottom spacer and secure gel to the apparatus. Add electrode buffer to the lower chamber.

Preparation of samples

1.   Minimally mix protein sample 1:3 in 3 X sample buffer.
2.   Boil the sample for 2 min.
3.   Centrifuge the sample to remove insoluble material.

Resolution of proteins

1.   Load the appropriate amount of protein into the wells of the stacking gel (1-5 µg/band).
2.   Run gel at a 20-30 mA constant current for a short run (3 h) or 7 mA for overnight run. The final running conditions should be determined empirically for each gel system.
3.   End run when the tracking dye reaches the bottom of the gel, remove gel and electrotransfer it to the NC.

PROTEIN BLOTTING

The following protocol has been found to be useful in the analysis of ureaplasmal antigens. Modifications in incubation times and temprature, as well as the composition of quenching solutions, should be considered in order to optimize the assay for greater sensitivity.

Materials

1. Transfer buffer: 25mM Tris, 192 mM glycine, 20% methanol.
2. TBS (Tris buffered saline) 10mM Tris (pH 7.4): 150 mm NaCl.
3. Bovine serum albumin (BSA) or fetal calf serum (FCS).
4. An electrophoretic transfer apparatus.
5. An SDS-polyacrylamide slab gel.
6. Immobilizing matrix: nitrocellulose filter (NC).
7. Gloves.

Electrophoretic transfer

1. Prepare transfer buffer 24 h before blotting and precool. Volume should be enough to fill the apparatus and wet the NC.
2. Pour the cold transfer buffer into the transfer apparatus to wet the supportive Scotch-Brite pads.
3. Cut pieces of NC to the size of the gel(s) and wet by floating the NC on the surface of the transfer buffer so that trapped air is expelled from the NC.
4. Once the gel is taken out from between the glass plates, cut off the stacking gel.
5. The gel is then placed on a wet Whatmann 3 mm blotting paper and onto the pre-wet Scotch-Brite pad.
6. Rinse the surface of the gel with transfer buffer avoiding formation of bubbles and providing a wet surface for the NC to adhhere.
7. Apply a wet piece of the NC to the gel and take care not to trap air bubbles between the gel and the NC.
8. A second filter paper and a second Scotch-brite pad are then placed on the NC. This assembly should be well supported between plastic grids, held together and placed into the buffer-filled transfer apparatus. The NC should face the anode side of the transfer apparatus.
9. Transfer should continue for at least two h at 200 mA constant current.
10. At the end of the transfer remove the gel/NC composite and separate the two. The transfer dye front and any other signs providing easy identification can be marked on the NC with a pen or a pencil.
11. The wet membrane (NC) can be used immediately, stored dry between blotting paper, or kept in TBS.

Immunoblotting

All the following incubations and washes are performed while shaking or rocking the blots in the various solutions.

1. Incubate the blots in TBS containing 1-10% (w/v) BSA or FCS and 0.05% Tween 20 at room temperature (RT) for 1-12 h.
2. Wash NC with TBS/Tween for 30 sec with agitation.

3.   Incubate with antibodies for 1-2 h at RT or overnight at RT. Incubations should be done in sufficient volume so as to allow the blot to freely float in the solution mixture. Dilution should be done in protein containing solution as TBS/Tween/FCS. Determine concentration of the antibodies, *i.e.*. dilution, empirically.
4.   Wash the blots, 2 X TBS/T and 2 X TBS, for 10 min each.
5.   Incubate the blot in the labeled second antibody, *e.g.*, peroxidase labeled anti-human IgG, diluted in TBS/Tween/FCS (1:1000), for 1 h at RT with agitation.
6.   Wash as in 4.
7.   Detection of enzyme conjugate: prepare substrate solution just before use, and store in the dark: 50 mg of DAB (diaminobenzidine) in 100 ml of 10 mM phospate buffer pH 7.0, to which 50 µl of 30% H_2O_2 is added.
8.   Develop the blot at RT with agitation until the protein bands are suitably dark. A typical incubation would be 1-5 min. and the reaction is stopped by rinsing with water.

REFERENCES

Andersen, H., Birkelund, S., Christiansen, G. and Freundt E. A. 1987. Electrophoretic analysis of proteins from *Mycoplasma hominis* strains detected by SDS-PAGE, two-dimensional gel electrophoresis and immunoblotting. J. Gen. Microbiol. 133:181-191.

Baseman, J. B. The cytadhesins of *Mycoplasma pneumoniae* and *Mycoplasma genitalium*. In: "Subcellular Biochemistry: Mycoplasma Cell Membrane". (S. Rottem and I. Kahane, eds). Plenum Publishers Inc. 1993. (in press).

Boyer, M. J. and Wise, K. S. 1989. Lipid modified surface protein antigens expressing size variation within the species *Mycoplasma hyorhinis*. Infect. Immun. 57:245-254.

Cassell, G. H., Watson, H. L., Blalock, D. K., Horowitz, S. A. and Duffy, L. B. 1988. Protein antigens of genital mycoplasmas. Rev. Infect. Dis. 10:S391-S398.

Chandler, D. K. F., Olson, L. D., Kenimer, J. G., Probst, P. G., Rottem, S. Grabowski, M. W. and Barile, M. F. 1989. Biological activities of monoclonal antibodies to *M. pneumoniae* membrane glycolipids. Infect. Immun. 57:1131-1136.

Cole, B. C., Naot, Y., Stanbridge, E. J. and Wise, K. S. 1985. Interaction of *Mycoplasmas* and their products with lymphoid cells *in vitro*. p. 203-207. In: "The Mycoplasmas" (S. Razin and M. F. Barile, Eds.) Vol. 4, Academic Press, Inc., New York.

Davidson, M. K., Lindsey, J. R., Davis, J. K., Parker, R. F., Ross, S. E., Watson, H. L. and Cassell G. H. 1988. Alternative approach to identification of virulence mechanisms of *Mycoplasma pulmonis*. Zbl. Bakt. Suppl. 20:695-697.

Gois, M., Kuksa, J., Franz, J. and Taylor-Robinson, D. 1974. The antigenic differentiation of seven strains of *M. hyorhinis* by growth inhibition, metabolism inhibition, latex-agglutination and polyacrylamide-gel electrophoresis tests. J. Med. Microbiol. 7:105-115.

Grabowski, M. W. and Barile, M. F. 1989. Biological activities of monoclonal antibodies to *M. pneumoniae* membrane glycolipids. Infect. Immun. 57:1131-1136.

Horowitz, S. and Gal, H. 1991. Isolation and purification of viable *Ureaplasma urealyticum* cells free from medium components. J. Gen. Microbiol. 137:1087-1092.

Horowitz, S. A. and Gal, H. 1991. Isolation and purification of viable *Ureaplasma urealyticum* cells free from medium components. J. Gen. Microbiol. 137:1087-1092.

Horowitz, S. A., Garrett, B., Davis, J. K. and Cassell, G. H. 1987. Isolation of *M. pulmonis* membranes and identification of surface antigens. Infect. Immun. 55:1314-1320.

Horowitz, S. A., Duffy, L., Garrett, B., Stephens, J., Davis, J. K. and Cassell G. H. 1986. Can group- and serovar-specific proteins be detected in *Ureaplasma urealyticum*? Pediatr. Infect. Dis. 5:S325-S331.

Hu, P. C., Cole, R. M., Huang, Y. S, *et al.*, 1982. *Mycoplasma pneumoniae* infection: Role of surface protein in the attachment organelle. Science 216:313-315.

Lee, G. Y. and Kenny G. E. 1987. Humoral response to *Ureaplasma urealyticum* polypeptides. J. Clin. Microbiol. 25:1841-1844

Morrison-Plummer, J., Lazzell, A. and Baseman, J. B. 1987. Shared epitopes between *Mycoplasma pneumoniae* major adhesin protein P1 and a 140 kilodalton protein of *Mycoplasma genitalium*. Infect. Immun. 55:49-56.

Olsson, B., Bölske, G., Bergstrom, K., Johansson, K. E. 1990. Analysis of caprine mycoplasmas and mycoplasma infection in goats using two-dimensional electrophoresis and immunoblotting. Electrophoresis. 11:861-869.

Rosengarten, J. A. and Wise, K. S. 1990. Phenotypic Switching in *Mycoplasma*: Phase variation of Diverse Surface Lipoproteins. Science 247: 315-318.

Sasaki, T. 1991. Evidence that mycoplasmas, gram-negative bacteria and certain gram-positive bacteria share a similar protein antigen. J. Bacteriol. 173:2398-2400.

Schalla, W. O. and Harrison, H. R. 1987. Western blot analysis of the human response to *Mycoplasma hominis*. Isr. J. Med. Sci. 23:613-617.

Taylor-Robinson, Furr, F. M. and Tully, J. G. 1983. Serological cross-reaction between *Mycoplasma genitalium* and *M.pneumoniae*. Lancet 1:527

Towbin , H., Staehlin, T. and Gordon J. 1979. Electrophoretic transfer of proteins from polyacrylamide gels to nitrocellulose sheets: Procedure and some applications. Proc. Natl. Acad. Sci. USA 76:4350-4354.

Watson, H. L., Cox, N. R., Davidson, M. K., Blalock, D. K., Davis, J. K., Dybvig, K., Horowitz, S. A. and Cassell, G. H. 1987. *Mycoplasma pulmonis* proteins common to murine mycoplasmas. Isr. J. Med. Sci. 23:442-447.

Watson, H. L., McDaniel, L. S., Blalock, D. K., Fallon, M. T. and Cassell, G. H. 1988. Heterogeneity among satrains and a high rate of variation within strains of major surface antigen of *Mycoplasma pulmonis*. Infect. Immun. 56:1358-1363.

DETECTION OF HUMAN MYCOPLASMAS BY *IN VITRO* DNA AMPLIFICATION

Bertille de Barbeyrac, Cecile Bernet, Rémy Teyssou,
Francoise Poutiers, Christiane Bébéar

Laboratoire de Bactériologie, Université de Bordeaux II
146, rue Léo Saignat, 33076 Bordeaux, France

INTRODUCTION

Mycoplasmas are infectious agents of humans, animals, insects and plants. At least twelve different species have been isolated from humans. Most of them are simple commensals of respiratory and genital tracts. Three mycoplasma species are considered to be significant human pathogens. *Mycoplasma pneumoniae*, an important cause of respiratory infections, is also associated with non-respiratory symptoms. *M. hominis* and *Ureaplasma urealyticum* are responsible for various diseases of the urogenital tract, as well as other infections in immunosuppressed patients and newborn infants. The role of two other species, *M. genitalium* and *M. fermentans*, is still unknown. *M. genitalium*, originally isolated from the urethra of men with non-gonococcal urethritis, then suspected to be involved in pelvic inflammatory disease, has also been found in respiratory tract specimens associated with *M. pneumoniae*. Recently, *M. fermentans*, a mycoplasma rarely isolated from the genital tract of healthy people, was detected in various tissue samples of patients with AIDS (Lo *et al.*, 1989).

Several methods can be used for the microbiological diagnosis of mycoplasmal infections. Cultivation is well adapted to some species such as *M. hominis* and *U. urealyticum* which can be isolated easily and rapidly from clinical specimens. However, this procedure is not fully satisfactory for the detection of *M. pneumoniae*, *M. fermentans* and especially *M. genitalium*, which are fastidious microorganisms and may require several weeks for results. Serological techniques are the most widely used procedures for *M. pneumoniae*. However, this method allows only a retrospective confirmation of the etiology.

Several other procedures have been reported for the direct detection of mycoplasmas in clinical samples. Mycoplasma DNA staining is a rapid technique, currently used for the detection of cell culture contaminants, but is not well adapted to the diagnosis of mycoplasmal infections because of its lack of specificity. Enzyme immunoassays for the detection of *M. pneumoniae* antigens in clinical samples have been proposed (T. W. Kok *et al.*, 1988). Hybridization with DNA probes, a rapid and specific procedure, has been tested for the diagnosis of *M. pneumoniae* and *M. genitalium* infections (Hyman *et al.*, 1987). Unfortunately this procedure lacks sensitivity.

The polymerase chain reaction (PCR) was recently developed to amplify short segments of DNA. This technique, used for the diagnosis of genetic diseases, viral infections, is also an effective tool for bacteriological diagnosis. It has been recently applied to the diagnosis of mycoplasmal infection. This technique is simple, easy to perform, very sensitive, does not require the presence of viable organisms and seems to be particularly indicated for the detection of *M. pneumoniae* and *M. genitalium*. This chapter reports how PCR can be applied to the diagnosis of these two mycoplasmal infections. Furthermore, other possible applications of PCR to the detection of human mycoplasmal infections will be reviewed.

PCR DEVELOPMENT STEPS

Application of PCR to the detection of a microorganism requires several steps, briefly: (i) choice of the sequence to be amplified; (ii) treatment of the samples; (iii) optimization of the PCR parameters; (iv) detection and characterization of the amplified product; (v) determination of the sensitivity and control of the specificity of the detection; and (vi) validation of the technique.

The sequence to be amplified can be chosen in a published gene sequence or in a randomly cloned DNA fragment demonstrated to be specific for the organism to be detected. Using two different targets may be recommended, especially in the early steps of development of PCR.

DNA purified from microorganisms is generally used for developing PCR. Organisms in culture and clinical specimens have to be treated before amplification. Various treatments can be used, according to the organisms to be detected and the kind of specimens in which they occur. Since mycoplasmas do not possess any cell wall, boiling the sample is often sufficient to make the genetic material accessible. However, with certain specimens, DNA extraction is necessary. This has to be tested on the specimens. Since PCR is a very sensitive technique, many controls have to be used, including controls for the detection of PCR inhibitors in samples, negative and positive controls. These controls, essential for the interpretation of the results, allow the detection of false negative and false positive results due to a contamination.

The parameters of PCR to be optimized include the composition of the mix (dNTP, primers, Taq DNA polymerase, assay buffer), the volume to be used, and the amplification cycle (temperatures of the different steps, number of cycles).

The detection of the amplified product is usually performed by using either agarose or polyacrylamide gel electrophoresis, according to the size of the amplified fragment and staining by ethidium bromide. Identification of the amplified product is based upon its size, the detection of a specific restriction site, hybridization with an internal labelled probe after Southern transfer.

The sensitivity and the specificity of the detection have to be checked by testing dilutions of purified DNA or of grown organisms that may be diluted in clinical samples. Different results can be observed according to the sample tested. The sensitivity is generally extremely high for purified DNA but much lower in clinical samples. The specificity is controlled by testing other species as closely related as possible to the mycoplasma to be detected, and to other organisms that can be found in the same samples.

The last step of PCR development is the validation of the technique. This can be performed on experimental model or clinical samples by comparing the results obtained with PCR to those given by other techniques. However, since PCR is a more sensitive technique than culture, for instance, and since it is generally used for organisms difficult to grow, this step is often difficult to manage.

DETECTION OF *M. PNEUMONIAE* BY PCR

The PCR technique has been applied to the detection of *M. pneumoniae* by two groups (Bernet *et al.*, 1989; Skov-Jensen *et al.*, 1989). The fragments to be amplified were taken either in a randomly cloned small DNA sequence demonstrated to be specific for *M. pneumoniae* (Bernet *et al.*, 1989), or in the published sequence of the P1 adhesion protein of this organism (Skov-Jensen *et al.*, 1989), or in the variable region of the 16S rDNA (Skov-Jensen *et al.*, 1989). Details concerning the application of these different amplifications are indicated in Table 1. The estimated detection limits were comparable in the different studies: 40 Colour Forming Units or 10 Colour Changing Units (CCU) in artificially seeded bronchoalveolar lavages.

The validity of the assay was checked on an experimental model, hamsters inoculated intranasally by *M. pneumoniae* (Bernet *et al.*, 1989). Throat swab specimens were collected before and at various times after inoculation. PCR was found to be more sensitive and more reproducible than the culture method. Furthermore, PCR was completely unaffected by bacterial contamination that impaired mycoplasma culture. Next, PCR has to be validated by application to clinical samples. However, the low number of samples positive by culture makes this step difficult to achieve.

An example of amplification of *M. pneumoniae* DNA is shown in Figs. 1 and 2. The primers chosen in that experiment were taken in the sequence of the adhesin gene (MP-P11:5'TGCCATGAACCCGCGCTTAAC3', MP-P12: 'CCTTTGCAACTGCTCATAGTA3') and allowed the amplification of a 473 bp fragment. The samples examined were simulated positive specimens. They consisted of throat swab specimens collected from healthy persons in 2 ml

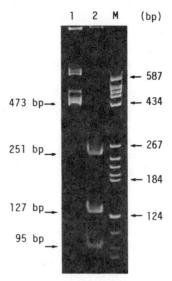

Figure 1. Electrophoretic analysis of the PCR products obtained with *M. pneumoniae* positive simulated throat swabs (10⁴ CCU) before (lane 1) and after cleavage with *Taq*I (lane 2). Lane M: molecular weight marker (pBR 322/ *Hae*III, Boehringer, Mannheim).

Table 1. *M. pneumoniae* detection by *in vitro* DNA amplification

Target	Size of the amplified fragment (bp)	Restriction site detected	No. of organisms detected in positive simulated samples	Reference
Randomly cloned DNA	144	DdeI	10 CCU*	Bernet[4]
P1 adhesin	473	TaqI	10 CCU	Bernet (unpub-lished data
	153	NA***	40 CFU**	Skov-Jensen[5]
16S rDNA	583	NA	NA	Skov-Jensen[5]

* CCU: colour changing unit
** CFU: colony forming unit
*** NA: not available

sucrose phosphate medium supplemented with 10% fetal calf serum and artificially seeded with known amounts of a *M. pneumoniae* culture. Samples were boiled for 10 min, then chilled on ice. Amplification of samples (10 µl) was performed in volumes of 50 µl. The reaction mixture consisted of 1 unit *Taq* DNA polymerase (Promega Corp., Madison, WI, USA); 200 µM each dNTP; 1 µM each primer MP-P11, MP-P12; 1 X assay buffer supplied with the enzyme by the manufacturer. Thirty- five cycles of amplification (hybridization of the primers on the target DNA 55°C 1 min, synthesis 72°C 1 min, denaturation 95°C 1 min) were performed. The amplified fragment was identified by hydrolysis with the restriction enzyme *Taq*I (Figure 1 lane 2) and by hybridization with an internal probe MP-I: 5'CAAACCGGGCAGATCACCTTT3' (data not shown). Figure 2 shows an example of the sensitivity and the specificity of the detection: 10 CCU of *M. pneumoniae* were detected (lane 4) while no amplification was obtained with 10^4 CCU of the other mycoplasma species examined, *M. salivarium M. orale, M. buccale* (lanes 8-10), *M. fermentans* PG18, K7, strain incognitus, and 6 different strains of *M. genitalium* (data not shown).

DETECTION OF *M. GENITALIUM* BY PCR

All the reports concerning the application of PCR to *M. genitalium* are based on the detection of nucleotide sequences of the adhesin gene. Table 2 shows the main characteristics of the amplification reaction, as described in different studies (Palmer *et al.*, 1991; Skov-Jensen *et al.*, 1991), as well as our own. All the *M. genitalium* strains tested could be amplified and the presence of an *Eco*RI site in the amplified fragment could be demonstrated. Next PCR was applied to clinical samples. In our study, specimens (throat swabs) from healthy patients , from patients presenting respiratory infections (throat samples and bronchoalveolar lavages) and from patients presenting genital infections (cervico-vaginal and urethral samples) were examined in parallel by PCR and culture in SP4 medium. All respiratory specimens were negative while 3 out of 50 genital samples tested were positive by PCR but not by culture. Similarly, 10 out of 150 genital samples tested by Skov-Jensen were found positive by PCR. In both studies, amplified fragments hybridized with internal probes, but none of them contained the *Eco*RI restriction site. The reason why the *Eco*RI site is absent is not resolved; it could be a point mutation or variability in that region of the adhesin gene as suggested by Skov-Jensen.

DETECTION OF OTHER MYCOPLASMA SPECIES BY PCR

PCR amplification applied to the detection of *M. pneumoniae* or *M. genitalium* is most useful for the diagnosis of respiratory or genital infections. However these amplifications are specific and not adapted to the detection of other known or unknown species.

The detection of genital mycoplasmas such as *U. urealyticum* or *M. hominis* does not currently require the use of hybridization methods since these organisms grow easily. However, PCR could be useful for their detection in samples where they are not viable. PCR primers allowing the amplification

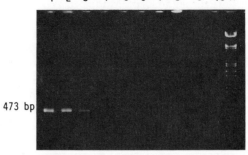

1 2 3 4 5 6 7 8 9 10 M

473 bp

Figure 2. Agarose gel showing sensitivity of PCR on *M. pneumoniae* positive simulated throat swabs (lane 1: 10^4 CCU; lane 2: 10^3 CCU; lane 3: 10^2 CC; lane 4: 10 CCU lane 5: 1 CCU) and specificity of PCR on heterologous mycoplasma positive simulated throat swabs (lane 8: 10^4 CCU; *M. salivarium*; lane 9: 10^4 CCU *M. orale*; lane 10: 10^4 CCU *M. buccale*), on negative throat swabs (lane 6) and on culture medium (lane 7). Lane M: molecular weight marker (λDNA/*Hind*III - *Eco*RI, Boehringer, Mannheim).

Table 2. *M. genitalium* detection by *in vitro* DNA amplification

	Size of the amplified fragment (bp)* detected	Restriction site	No. of organisms detected	Application
Skov Jensen[7]	281	*Eco*RI + 4 others	50 (EtBr) 4 (probe)	clinical samples
Palmer[6]	374	*Eco*RI	~10	mouse model
Bébéar (Unpublished data)	371	*Eco*RI	10 CCU	clinical samples

* Amplified fragments taken in the adhesin gene

of a sequence of the urease gene of *U. urealyticum* have been described recently (Blanchard, 1990; Willoughby *et al.*, 1991). A fragment of 460 bp was amplified specifically in all 14 human serotypes of *U. urealyticum*, but not in other mycoplasmas or urease positive bacteria (Willoughby *et al.*, 1991).

Other mycoplasma species may be responsible for human infections. PCR applied to the detection of *M. fermentans*, strain incognitus, has been reported recently (Lo *et al.*, 1989). Other unknown mycoplasma species should be detected by a universal PCR. Blanchard *et al.* (1991) reported a pair of PCR primers that allowed the detection of four human parasites *(M. genitalium, M.hominis, M. salivarium* and *M. orale)*. In a collaborative work with Bové and colleagues, by screening 16S rDNA sequences available in data banks, we have found a couple of primers (Molli-1, Molli-2a) able to promote the amplification of all *Mycoplasma, Ureaplasma* and *Spiroplasma* species tested, while a second couple (Molli-1, Molli-2b) allowed the amplification of *Acholeplasma* (Saillard *et al.*, 1990). These two sets of oligonucleotides should be useful to detect known, as well as unknown, mycoplasmas in various specimens.

PROSPECTIVE

As described here, PCR technology for the diagnosis of mycoplasma infection is still in the developing stage. Many problems will have to be solved before using PCR for current clinical diagnosis. The most important is actually the problem of DNA contamination, which is required to be avoided in order to take specific precautions. Other improvements, such as rapid sample preparation, elimination of PCR inhibitors, automation of the detection, are also requested. Furthermore, since this new technique is much more sensitive than previous methods, interpretative problems will arise and might make it necessary to define new diagnostic rules.

REFERENCES

Bernet, C., Garret, M., de Barbeyrac, B., Bébéar, C. and Bonnet, J. (1989). Detection of *Mycoplasma pneumoniae* by using the polymerase chain reaction, J. Clin. Microbiol. 27:2492-2496.

Blanchard, A. (1990). *Ureaplasma urealyticum* urease genes; use of a UGA tryptophan codon, Mol. Microbiol. 4:669-676.

Blanchard, A., Gautier, M. and Mayau, V. (1991). Detection and identification of mycoplasmas by amplification of rDNA, FEMS Microbiol. Lett. 81:37-42.

Hyman, H. C., Yogev, D. and Razin, S. (1987) DNA probes for detection and identification of *Mycoplasma pneumoniae* and *Mycoplasma genitalium*. J. Clin. Microbiol. 25:726-728.

Kok, T. W., Varkanis, G. and Marmion, B. P.. (1988). Laboratory diagnosis of *Mycoplasma pneumoniae* infection. 1 - Direct detection of antigen in respiratory exudates by enzyme immunoassay, Epidem. Inf. 101:669-684.

Lo, S .C., Shih, J. W. K., Yang, N. Y., Ou, C. Y. and Wang, R. Y. H. (1989) A novel virus-like infectious agent in patients with AIDS. Am. J. Trop. Med. Hyg. 40:213-225.

Palmer, H. M., Gilroy, C. B., Furr, P. M. and Taylor-Robinson, D. (1991). Development and evaluation of the polymerase chain reaction to detect *Mycoplasma genitalium.*. FEMS Microbiol. Letts. 77:199-204.

Saillard, C., Teyssou, R., Grau, O., Poutiers, F. Laigret, F., Bové, J. M. and C. Bébéar. Toward the amplification by PCR of all mollicutes species. 8th Intl. Cong. IOM, Istanbul, July 8-12, 1990, IOM Lett. Vol. 1, p. 446-447.

Skov-Jensen, J., Sondegard-Andersen, J., Uldum, S. A. and Lind, L. (1989). Detection of *Mycoplasma pneumoniae* in simulated clinical samples by polymerase chain reaction, APMIS. 97:1046-1048.

Skov-Jensen, J., Uldum, S. A., Sondegard-Andersen, J., Vuust, J. and Lind, K. (1991). Polymerase chain reaction for detection of *Mycoplasma genitalium* in clinical samples. J. Clin. Microbiol. 29:46-50.

Willoughby, J. J., Russell, W. C., Thirkel, D. and Burdon, M. G. (1991). Isolation and detection of urease genes in *U. urealyticum*, Infect. Immun. 59:2463-2469.

SENSITIVE DETECTION OF MYCOPLASMAS IN CELL CULTURES BY USING TWO-STEP POLYMERASE CHAIN REACTION

Ryô Harasawa[1], Takashi Uemori[2],
Kiyozo Asada[2] and Ikunoshin Kato[2]

[1] Animal Center for Biomedical Research, Faculty of Medicine
The University of Tokyo, Bunkyo-ku, Tokyo 113, Japan
and [2]Biotechnology Research Laboratories, Takara
Shuzo Co., Ltd., Otsu-shi, Shiga 520-21, Japan

INTRODUCTION

Mycoplasma contamination of cell cultures has been a serious problem in biomedical research. The incidence of mycoplasma contamination is higher than might be expected, and it is difficult to eliminate mycoplasmas from contaminated cell cultures (Barile *et al.*, 1978; McGarrity and Kotani, 1985). Several techniques for the detection of mycoplasma contamination of cell cultures have been described (Barile and McGarrity, 1983). They are the direct culture procedure (Ogata and Koshimizu, 1967), enzyme activity tests (Barile and Schimke, 1963; Levine, 1972; Uitendall *et al.*, 1979), fluorescent staining by DNA-binding dyes (Chen, 1977). The direct culture technique takes time and sometimes fails to detect fastidious mycoplasmas such as *Mycoplasma hyorhinis* (Hopps *et al.*, 1973), and the enzyme activity test frequently leads to false results. Immunoenzyme techniques (Chasey and Woods, 1984; Kotani and McGarrity, 1985), and DNA-DNA hybridization by Southern blotting

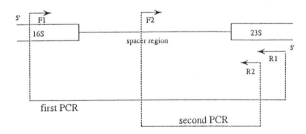

Figure 1. Diagram of the mycoplasmal 16S/23S rRNA intergenic region with locations and orientations of the primers.

Rapid Diagnosis of Mycoplasmas, Edited by I. Kahane
and A. Adoni, Plenum Press, New York, 1993

Table 1.   Spacing between Each Pair of the Primers

Mycoplasma Species	F1 and R1	F2 and R2 (bp)
M. fermentans	491	195
M. hyorhinis	448	211
M. orale	423	179
M. salivarium	403	151
M. hominis	369, 370[a]	147, 148
M. arginini	369	145

[a]M. *hominis* has two 16S/23S rRNA intergenic spacers in different size.

(Razin *et al.*, 1984) or by using hydroxyapatite columns (Harasawa *et al.*, 1986) have been reported as alternative and useful methods.

A novel *in vitro* DNA amplification through the polymerase chain reaction (PCR) was recently devised (Saiki *et al.*, 1988), and this provides an important advance in the diagnostic research (Schochetman *et al.*, 1988). The PCR technique has been applied to detect a variety of viruses and bacteria. We examined the use of PCR to detect mycoplasmas contaminating in cell cultures.

This paper describes a two step PCR which is able to detect light contamination (13 CFU/ml) of mycoplasmas in cell cultures.

Universal primers used for the PCR

We have previously sequenced the spacer regions between the 16S and 23S rRNA genes of the major *Mycoplasma* species contaminating in cell cultures and deposited their sequences to the EMBL Data Library under the accession numbers given in brackets (Uemori *et al.*, 1991): M. *fermentans* PG18 [X58553], M. *hyorhinis* BTS-7 [X58555], M. *orale* CH 19299 [X58556], M. *salivarium* PG20 [X58558], M. *hominis* PG21 [X58559] and M. *arginini* G230 [X58560]. We selected the following four universal primer sequences from the conserved regions between the 16S/23S intergenic spacers of these *Mycoplasma* species:

```
Primer F1   5'-ACACCATGGGAGCTGGTAAT-3'
Primer R1   5'-CTTCATCGACTTTCAGACCCAAGGCAT-3'
Primer F2   5'-GTTCTTTGAAAACTGAAT-3'
Primer R2   5'-GCATCCACCAAAAACTCT-3'
```

These universal primers were synthesized in an Applied Biosystem DNA synthesizer (Foster City, CA). The spacing length between each pair of the primers is given in Table 1.

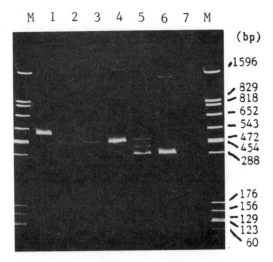

Figure 2. Sodium dodecyl sulfate-polyacrylamide gel electrophoretic paterns of the first PCR products. Lane 1, *M. fermentans* PG18; lane 2, *M. hyorhinis* DBS 1050 (=ATCC29052); lane 3, *M. orale* ATCC 15539; lane 4, *M. salivarium* PG20; lane 5, *M. hominis* PG21; lane 6, *M. arginini* G230; lane 7, *A. laidlawii* PG8. Lane N indicates molecular mass obtained by cleaving the phage M13 replicative form DNA with restriction endonuclease *Hap*II.

Conditions for the two-step PCR

The PCR was performed in a Perkin-Elmer Cetus DNA Thermal Cycler (Norwalk, CT) by using a GeneAmp kit (Perkin-Elmer Cetus). Reaction mixture contained 1 µl of 10X reaction buffer, 20 nmol of each deoxynucleotide, samples as templates and water to a volume of 95 µl, and was overlaid with 50 µl of mineral oil. After incubation at 94°C for 5 minutes, 0.5 U (5 µl) of *Taq* polymerase was added, and amplification was achieved with 30 cycles of denaturation at 94°C for 30 sec, renaturation at 55°C for 2 min, and elongation at 72°C for 2 min. A 10-µl amount of each amplified product was mixed with 2 µl of 6X dye solution consisting of 0.25% xylene cyanol, 0.25% bromophenol blue and 40% sucrose in water, and resolved by 10 to 20% gradient sodium dodecyl sulfate-polyacrylamide or 1.4% agarose gel electrophoresis. After electrophoresis, gels were stained for 30 min in aqueous ethidium bromide (0.4µg/ ml) and visualized with shortwave ultraviolet light on a Chromato-Vue transilluminator model C-61 (Ultra-Violet Products, San Gabriel, CA). Photographs were taken with Polaroid type 55 films, using a Polaroid MP-4 land camera with a Kodak 23A Wratten gelatin filter.

The first PCR was performed in a 100-µl volume containing the primers F1 and R1 and 10 µl of cell culture fluid. The supernatant fluid of Vero cell cultures contaminated with known *Mollicutes* species was directly subjected to the PCR without extraction of DNA. Test organisms include *M. fermentans,*

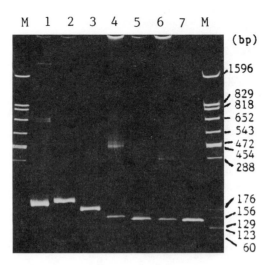

Figure 3. Sodium dodecyl sulfate-polyacrylamide gel electrophoretic patterns of the second PCR products. Lane designations are the same as Figure 2.

M. *hyorhinis, M. orale, M. salivarium, M. hominis, M. arginini* and *Acholeplasma laidlawii.* As shown in Fig. 2, although the six *Mycoplasma* species titers of which were between 10^4 and 10^6 CFU/ml in cell cultures were detected by the first PCR, no bands were apparent in the *A. laidlawii* lane because of low titer (10^3 CFU/ml). Size of the first PCR products from the six*Mycoplasma* species was the same as expected from the nucleotide sequence data.

The second PCR was performed in a 100-µl volume containing the inner primers F2 and R2 and 1 µl of the first PCR product. The size of the second PCR products was the same as expected from the nucleotide sequences (Fig. 3). The second PCR using the inner primers substitutes the blot hybridization with an inner probe, and confirms the specificity of the first PCR. The first PCR may amplify the DNA of *Escherichia coli* and *Bacillus subtilis* under low stringent conditions of renaturation, but the second PCR does not. The second PCR increased sensitivity of detection and was able to detect light contamination (10^3 CFU/ml) with *A. laidlawii.*

Sensitivity of the two-step PCR

Detection limits of the first and second PCR were compared by sodium dodecyl sulfate-polyacrylamide gel electrophoresis (data not shown). The two-step PCR was 100 times more sensitive than the first PCR alone. The two-step PCR was able to detect at least 10 mycoplasmal cells in 10 µl of cell culture fluid after all. We have collected several mammalian cell lines from different laboratories and examined them by using the two-step PCR. As shown in Fig. 4, the second PCR was able to detect mycoplasma contaminations which were not detected by the gel electrophoresis of the first PCR alone. Therefore, it is always necessary to perform both the first and second PCR to detect a small number of mycoplasma cells in cell cultures.

During the course of examination of mycoplasma contamination in animal cell cultures, we found dimethyl sulfoxide in frozen cell cultures is inhibitory to the PCR, and conventional broth media for mycoplasmas contain inhibitory factors against the PCR. Therefore, it is important to check the sample to be amplified by the PCR being free from these inhibitors.

Size of the PCR products was distinct to each *Mycoplasma* species, and may be used for species identification. Different restriction sites in the PCR products may also provide useful markers for species identification (Uemori *et al.*, 1992).

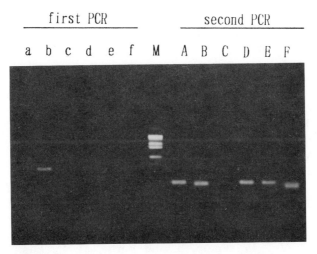

Figure 4. Agarose gel electrophoretic patterns under examination of mycoplasma contamination in six mammalian cell cultures by the two-step PCR. Lanes a through f, the first PCR products; lane M, molecular mass marker; lanes A through F indicate the second PCR products amplified from the first PCR products of lanes a through f, respectively.

CONCLUSIONS

The two-step PCR had proven very sensitive for detection of mycoplasma contamination in cell cultures. The universal primers used in this study can be used for amplification of the 16S/23S rRNA intergenic spacers of the other *Mollicutes* species. Different size and restriction sites of the PCR products may provide useful markers for species identification. We believe the two- step PCR described here is also applicable to detection of mycoplasma contamination in foods and biologics such as virus vaccines, sera and medicine prepared by using animal cell cultures.

REFERENCES

Barile, M. F., Hopps, H. E. and Grabowski, M. (1978) Incidence and source of mycoplasma contamination: a brief review, In: "Mycoplasma Infection of Cell Cultures" (McGarrity, G.J., Murphy, D.G., and Nichols, W.W., Eds.), pp. 35-46. Plenum Press, New York.

Barile, M. F. and McGarrity, G. J. (1983) Special techniques for isolation and identification of mycoplasmas from cell cultures, In: "Methods in Mycoplasmology, Vol. II (Tully, J. G. and Razin, S., Eds.), pp. 154-208. Academic Press, New York.

Barile, M. F. and Schimke, R. T. (1963) A rapid chemical method for detecting PPLO contamination of tissue cell cultures. Proc. Soc. Exp. Biol. Med. 114:676-679.

Chasey, D. and Woods, S. B. (1984) Detection of immunoperoxidase labeled mycoplasmas in cell cultures by light microscopy and electron microscopy. J. Med. Microbiol. 17:23-30.

Chen, T. R. (1977) *In situ* demonstration of mycoplasma contamination in cell cultures of fluorescent Hoechst 33258 stain. Exp. Cell Res. 104:255-262.

Harasawa, R., Mizusawa, H. and Koshimizu, K. (1986) A reliable and sensitive method for detecting mycoplasmas cell cultures. Microbiol. Immunol. 30:919-921.

Hopps, H. E., Meyer, B . C., Barile, M. F. and DelGiudice, R. A. (1973) Problems concerning "non-cultivable" mycoplasma contamination in tissue cultures. Ann. N.Y. Acad. Sci. 225:265-276.

Kotani, H. and McGarrity, G. J. (1985) Rapid and simple identification of mycoplasmas by immunobinding. J. Immunol. Methods 85:257-267.

Levine, E. M. (1972) Mycoplasma contamination of animal cell cultures: a simple, rapid detection method. Exp. Cell Res. 74:99-109.

McGarrity, G. J. and Kotani, H. (1985) Cell culture mycoplasmas In: "The Mycoplasmas", Vol. IV (Razin, S. and Barile, M. F., Eds.), pp. 353-390. Academic Press, New York.

Ogata, M. and Koshimizu, K. (1967) Isolation of mycoplasmas from tissue cell lines and transplantable tumor cells. Jpn. J. Microbiol. 11:289-303.

Razin, S., Gross, M., Wormser, M., Pollack, Y. and Glaser, G. (1984) Detection of mycoplasmas infecting cell cultures by DNA hybridization. In Vitro 20:404-408.

Saiki, R. K., Gelfand, D. H., Stoffel, S., Scharf, S. J., Higuchi, R. G., Horn, G. T., Mullis, K. B. and Erlich, H.A. (1988) Primer directed enzymatic amplification of DNA with a thermostable DNA polymerase. Science 239:487-491.

Schochtetman, G., Ou, C.-Y. and Jones, W. K. (1988) Polymerase chain reaction. J. Infect. Dis. 158:1154-1157.

Uemori, T., Asada, K., Kato, I. and Harasawa, R. (1992) Amplification of the 16S-23S spacer region in rRNA operons of mycoplasmas by the polymerase chain reaction. Syst. Appl. Microbiol. 15:181-186.

Uitendall, M. P., DeBruyn, D. H. M. M., Hatanaka, M. and Hosli, P. (1979) An ultramicrochemical test for mycoplasmal contamination of cultured cells. In Vitro 15:103-108.

RAPID DETECTION OF MYCOPLASMAS: GOALS FOR THE FUTURE

I. Kahane[1] and A. Adoni[2]

[1]The Hebrew University-Hadassah Medical School
and [2]The Department of Obstetrics and Gynecology
Hadassah University Hospital, Mt. Scopus
Jerusalem, Israel

The presentations and discussions in this workshop illuminated the great need for methods for rapid detection of mycoplasmas, as well as some directions and achievements.

Of the various methods discussed, it seems that the ELISA, the DNA hybridization and the *in vitro* DNA amplification, *e.g.*, PCR, have the largest potential in the rapid detection of mycoplasmas.

The ELISA can be employed for the detection of mycoplasma antigen or antibodies raised against mycoplasma. The major advantages of the ELISA is its use for screening of large numbers of samples. In the development of the methods for detection of the mycoplasma antigen, we should seek the most specific antigen. An example of that was presented by Dr. E. Jacobs group (1992) for the detection of *M. pneumoniae*. The screening of antibodies for *M. pneumoniae* using the ELISA can be easily done since commercial kits are already available. The data about the possible role of *U. urealyticum* in pathogenesis and the accumulating data on *M. fermentans* pathogenicity indicate the need for ELISA tests for these organisms.

The use of DNA probes for rapid detection of mycoplasmas was discussed in detail by Bové (1992) and by Johansson (1992). This approach was also developed into several commercial kits. However, more are needed to cover the entire range of mycoplasmas. In developing DNA probes, efforts should be made to employ nonradioactive methods for the detection of the probes. This is feasible and was actually successfully done, even with one of the commercial kits (Orgenics, Ltd., Israel). In this way, the probe not being labeled by the short-lived radioisotope has a longer shelf life and the use is not limited to laboratories that are licensed for radioactive protocols.

The *in vitro* DNA amplification, *e.g.*, PCR, seems, as in many other fields of microbiology and virology, the most promising procedure for rapid detection having a very high sensitivity. Obviously, this procedure also has its flaws. The protocols for the detection of mycoplasmas by PCR were discussed by Bébéar *et al.* (1992) and a two-stage procedure was discussed by Harasawa (1992). The great potential of this method may increase, especially if future studies of mycoplasmas' genome reveal common sequences that will be used for detection of several groups of mycoplasmas.

We would like to stress that other approaches should be searched for rapid detection of the mycoplasmas which will allow the rapid diagnosis and prevention of their disease. This is especially important since it has been reported that at least some mycoplasmas can be life threatening.

REFERENCES

Gerstenecker, B. and Jacobs, E. 1993. Development of a capture-ELISA for the specific detection of *Mycoplasma pneumoniae* in patients'material. In:"Rapid Diagnosis of Mycoplasma" (I. Kahane and A. Adoni, Eds.) Plenum Press, New York and London.

Bové, J. M. 1993. Biology of mollicutes. In: "Rapid Diagnosis of Mycoplasma" (I. Kahane and A. Adoni, Eds.) Plenum Press, New York and London.

Johansson, K.-E. 1993. Detection and identification of mycoplasmas by diagnostic DNA probes complementary to ribosomal RNA. In: "Rapid Diagnosis of Mycoplasma" (I. Kahane and A. Adoni, Eds.) Plenum Press, New York and London.

de Barbeyrac, B., Bernet, C., Teyssou, R., Poutiers, F. and Bébéar, C. 1993. Detection of human mycoplasmas by *in vitro* DNA amplification. In: "Rapid Diagnosis of Mycoplasma" (I. Kahane and A. Adoni, Eds.) Plenum Press, New York and London.

Harasawa, R., Uemori, T., Asada, K. and Kato, I. 1993. Sensitive detection of mycoplasmas in cell cultures by using two-step polymerase chain reaction. In: "Rapid Diagnosis of Mycoplasma" (I. Kahane and A. Adoni, Eds.) Plenum Press, New York and London.

Case 5-1992: Presentation of a case. 1992. New England J. Med. 326; 324-336.

Lo, S.-C., Dawson, G., Wong, D. M.,Newton III, P. B., Sonoda, M. A., Engler, W. F., Wang, R. Y.-H. Shih, J. W.-K., Alter, H. J. and Wear, D . J. 1989. Identification of *Mycoplasma incognitus* infection in patients with AIDS: an immunohistochemical, in situ hybridization and ultrastructural study. Am. J. Trop. Med. Hyg. 41:601.c

INDEX